"It's hard to imagine a more needed book today than this searching exploration of the vicissitudes of our moral sense. Freud said that the 'normal' person was both more immoral and moral than s/he knew. Paul Marcus combines studies and thought from psychoanalysis and social psychology to illuminate eddies, corners and creative streams of the meaning of morality and links with wisdom. The work opens vistas that combine everyday dilemmas with our deepest hopes and touches what it means to be alive and a human being."

Michael Eigen, *The Challenge of Being Human* and *Dialogues with Michael Eigen: Psyche Singing*

"Having taught these 'mind-blowing' classic social psychological studies for over thirty years in my sociology courses, I believed just about everything worth saying about them has been said –until I read Paul Marcus's splendid book. His psychoanalytically glossed interpretation of the classics, his finding common ground between experimental social psychology and psychoanalysis, and most importantly, his illumination of the significance of these classics for living a moral life, provide much 'food for thought' and, I hope, productive conversation between the disciplines and beyond."

William B. Helmreich, Professor of Sociology and author of *The Things They Say Behind Your Back: Stereotypes and the Myths Behind Them*

"Is our behavior shaped by our unconscious internal drives, or demands of the external environment? Or both? Sadly, psychoanalysis and social psychology science (SPS) have remained totally separate paths to understanding human behavior, due to their 180-degree differences in concepts, methods, and outlook. Happily, this new volume by Paul Marcus offers us a long-overdue 'conversation,' applying psychoanalytic concepts to nine classic SPS experiments. Dr. Marcus is a distinguished, articulate, and erudite psychoanalyst who invites us to see more than 'half the picture,' by offering this book as a valuable opportunity to more fully understand behavior – reconciling the insights of social psychology and psychoanalysis."

Harold Takooshian, PhD, past-President of the American Psychological Association's divisions of International Psychology and General Psychology

PSYCHOANALYSIS, CLASSIC SOCIAL PSYCHOLOGY AND MORAL LIVING

In *Psychoanalysis, Classic Social Psychology and Moral Living: Let the Conversation Begin*, Paul Marcus uniquely draws on psychoanalysis and social psychology to examine what affects the ethical decisions people make in their everyday life.

Psychoanalysis traditionally looks at early experiences, concepts and drives which shape how we choose to behave in later life. In contrast, classic social psychology experiments have illustrated how specific situational forces can shape our moral behavior. In this ground-breaking fusion of psychoanalysis and social psychology, Marcus gives a fresh new perspective to this and demonstrates how, in significant instances, these experimental findings contradict many presumed psychoanalytic ideas and explanations surrounding psychoanalytic moral psychology. Examining classic social psychology experiments, such as Asch's line judgement studies, Latané and Darley's bystander studies, Milgram's obedience studies, Mischel's Marshmallow Experiment and Zimbardo's Stanford Prison Experiment, Marcus pulls together insights and understanding from both disciplines, as well as ethics, to begin a conversation and set out a new understanding of how internal and external factors interact to shape our moral decisions and behaviors.

Marcus has an international reputation for pushing boundaries of psychoanalytic thinking and, with ethics being an increasingly relevant topic in psychoanalysis and our world, this pioneering work is essential reading for psychoanalysts, psychoanalytic psychotherapists, moral philosophy scholars and social psychologists.

Paul Marcus is a training and supervisory analyst at the National Psychological Association for Psychoanalysis in New York City and the author/editor of twenty books, including *The Psychoanalysis of Overcoming Suffering: Flourishing Despite Pain* (Routledge, 2019).

Recently published titles by Paul Marcus

The Psychoanalysis of Overcoming Suffering: Flourishing Despite Pain (Routledge 2018)

The Psychoanalysis of Career Choice, Job Performance, and Satisfaction: How to Flourish in the Workplace (Routledge, 2017)

Creating Heaven on Earth: The Psychology of Experiencing Immortality in Everyday Life (Karnac, 2015)

How to Laugh Your Way Through Life: A Psychoanalyst's Advice (Karnac, 2013)

In Search of the Spiritual: Gabriel Marcel, Psychoanalysis and the Sacred (Karnac, 2013)

In Search of the Good Life: Emmanuel Levinas, Psychoanalysis and the Art of Living (Karnac, 2010)

PSYCHOANALYSIS, CLASSIC SOCIAL PSYCHOLOGY AND MORAL LIVING

Let the Conversation Begin

Paul Marcus

Routledge
Taylor & Francis Group
LONDON AND NEW YORK

First published 2020
by Routledge
2 Park Square, Milton Park, Abingdon, Oxon OX14 4RN

and by Routledge
52 Vanderbilt Avenue, New York, NY 10017

Routledge is an imprint of the Taylor & Francis Group, an informa business

British Library Cataloguing-in-Publication Data
A catalogue record for this book is available from the British Library

Library of Congress Cataloging-in-Publication Data
A catalog record has been requested for this book

ISBN: 978-0-367-41559-4 (hbk)
ISBN: 978-0-367-41560-0 (pbk)
ISBN: 978-0-367-81523-3 (ebk)

Typeset in Bembo
by Taylor & Francis Books

In gratitude to Ronna.

CONTENTS

ACKNOWLEDGMENTS

I wish to thank my three thoughtful readers who critically commented on every chapter of my book, though I, of course, take full responsibility for its contents: my wife, Irene Wineman-Marcus, a child and adult psychoanalyst; Ronna Kabatznick, a social psychologist/psychotherapist; and Distinguished Professor of Sociology, William B. Helmreich. Without their helpful criticisms and suggestions, I doubt my book would be as good as it can be. I also would like to thank my editor, Stefanie Bendik, who has made my occasionally turgid prose easily accessible. Finally, I would like to express my gratitude to Kate Hawes of Routledge for her continuing support of my work, as well as her superb staff that has brought this book to publication.

1

INTRODUCTION

Psychoanalysis and social psychology: Let the conversation begin

"Normal man is not only far more immoral than he believes," said Freud, "but also far more moral than he knows" (1974, p. 52). Indeed, he noted that the psychoanalysts' "art consists in making it possible for people to be moral and to deal with their wishes philosophically" (Hale, 1971, p. 121); that is, more kind, humane, reasonable and rational. Psychoanalysis has often prided itself on being the most comprehensive psychology of human behavior, a claim that includes understanding and promoting the moral life, by which I mean "a commitment to a rigorous and truthful account of the psyche that is itself trying to promote what it finds to be good about human being" in the world (Lear, 2017, p. 191). In psychoanalysis, a moral life is typically instantiated by a person's capacity for deep and wide love and creative and productive work, a life that is guided by reason and ethics and is aesthetically pleasing (a judgment that the analysand makes, usually in consultation with the analyst).

While the overused term, moral psychology, is at the interface of ethics, psychology and philosophy, I wish to mainly address the issue of moral behavior, the way in which one acts or conducts oneself, especially toward others in morally challenging circumstances. I focus on behavior that is lodged in moral emotions such as the four "social," "higher-order" or "self-conscious" emotions of guilt, shame, embarrassment and pride (Simons, 2009).[1] These are judged by the person and by the consensus of others to be life-affirming and life-promoting. The moral life, "ethics," is "consciousness of a responsibility towards others" (Levinas, 1996, p. 76). In this view, says the eminent sociologist Zygmunt Bauman, the "I being *for* the Other, I bearing *responsibility* for the Other," is what matters most (1992, p. 42).[2] Indeed, such a view resonates with the wisdom of the great religious/spiritual traditions that affirm that man is never closer to God, never more animated by the spirit of the Divine, than when he behaves compassionately (Marcus, 2003). Moreover, such behavior, and the virtue-based outlook it is typically associated with, can be designated as reflecting a well-lived life, what has been aptly called a "flourishing" or "good" life by the great Greek philosophers (i.e., *eudaimonia*).[3]

Psychoanalysis has been masterful in describing the wide range of alleged reasons and ways that individuals act immorally, focusing on their warped and corrupted internal life (e.g., irrationality and deviant wishes), the so-called dispositional perspective (roughly, the concepts and drives of personality and what makes individuals respond in certain manners). What both devotees and critics of psychoanalysis have criticized about the theory and practice is that it has not developed an adequate social psychology. This especially includes a social psychology that gives a prominent role to the external environment, the circumstances and perceived "reality" considerations that are pertinent to understanding and explaining important moral conflicts and the resultant behavior. It also centrally focuses on group dynamics and situational forces rather than mainly intra-psychic ones to account for moral and immoral behavior. It is these conscious and non-conscious group dynamics that powerfully influence the moral and immoral behaviors of individuals in striking and unanticipated ways. The nine groundbreaking studies discussed in this book create significant moral dilemmas and the requirement is to examine the situational forces that influence and create individual responses. While the general assumption is that the individual is in control of decisions and actions from within, these studies show that there are dramatic and often invisible forces at work that influence behavior in surprising and unpredictable ways that are relevant to psychoanalytic theory and clinical work (like helping analysands to enhance their social intelligence and sharpen their social cognition).[4] Such situational forces within the everyday realms of love, work, consumerism, political action and helping or harming others can have the power to shift behavior in important ways.

With regards to the social environment, Bruno Bettelheim, a former Nazi concentration camp prisoner, noted that during his imprisonment, "The impact of the concentration camp … within a few weeks, did for me what years of useful and quite successful analysis had not done" (1960, p. 12). It significantly reduced his sense of autonomy, integration and humanity. Moreover, he said,

> I only wish to suggest that the psychoanalytic theory of personality [i.e., classical theory] is deficient in suggesting what makes for a 'desirable' well integrated personality; and this because it over stresses the importance of the inner life to the neglect of the total man as he deals with human and social environment.
>
> *(ibid., p. 21)*[5]

In light of the fact that the "extreme" environment of the concentration camp so swiftly and invasively shaped the person for better or worse, Bettelheim concluded, "What psychoanalysis has achieved for the personality within a stable social context must now be done for personality and social context in their interaction, when both of them are changing" (ibid., p. 57). Bettelheim thus recognized some of the deficiencies in psychoanalytic personality theory which, as he intimates, forced him to modify his psychoanalytic perspective with insight from the field of social psychology and sociology[6] (i.e., the role of the social environment in changing personality). Social psychology questions the assumption of "personality" as a disposition, since the "classic" experiments described in this book point to the fluidity of personality—that it is not fixed but dependent on situational forces, usually unacknowledged.

This being said, Martin Bergmann, a prominent psychoanalyst, noted that "we have a very rudimentary social psychology as psychoanalysts" (Luel & Marcus, 1984, p. 216), while the former President of the American Psychoanalytic Association, Robert Wallerstein, wrote that "the psychoanalytic study of reality" has been "relatively neglected or taken for granted in usual psychoanalytic discourse" (Wallerstein, 1973, p. 5). He believes that this neglect is implicit in the long-standing belief in a fixed world "out there," of an unvarying "average expectable environment" (ibid., p. 7). More recently, psychodynamic psychologist Tamara McClintock Greenberg noted, "within mainstream psychoanalysis, there has been relatively little emphasis on 'real events,' including the effects of adult-onset trauma," such as illness in old age (2016, p. 43). Indeed, a recent definition of reality reinforces my claim that not much has changed in how psychoanalysis reckons with the notion of reality since Wallerstein made his observation: "By 'reality,' psychoanalysis means what is *actually out there*, can be objectively perceived and consensually agreed upon" (Akhtar, 2009, p. 240, italics added). For example, Freud described a particular kind of psychosis called "hallucinatory confusion" wherein the "ego breaks away from the incompatible idea" (an idea that is overpoweringly painful or distressing) so that it has "detached itself wholly or in part from reality" (1962, p. 59). Social psychology questions this foundational assumption by suggesting that reality is perception, not fixed. Kurt Lewin, "the founding father of experimental social psychology" (Aronson et al., 2014, p. 16), emphasized this point when he wrote,

> If an individual sits in a room trusting that the ceiling will not come down, should only the 'subjective probability' be taken into account for predicting behavior or should we also consider the 'objective probability' of the ceiling's coming down as determined by engineers? To my mind, only the first has to be taken into account.
> *(ibid., p. 18)*

The counter-intuitive claim of my book is that experimental/scientific social psychology (henceforth, social psychology), especially the classic experiments like Asch's line judgment studies (highlighting the moral conflict of "conformity versus independence"), Latané and Darley's bystander studies (highlighting the moral conflict of "helping versus indifference"), and Milgram's obedience studies (highlighting the moral conflict of "obedience versus resistance"), have experimentally demonstrated that what is "actually out there," how it "hangs" together, what we expect of it and how we behave, is not entirely obvious. As John Lennon allegedly said, "Reality takes a lot of imagination" (Frank, 2013, p. 79). Indeed, in significant instances these experimental findings challenge many presumed psychoanalytic ideas and explanations regarding issues pertinent to psychoanalytic moral psychology and the analysand's efforts to help fashion a moral life (what might be called clinical ethics). Even more importantly, these experiments suggest what is psychologically necessary for people to develop to resist these potentially dangerous social dynamics: by acting in ways that are humane, life-affirming and life-promoting. Other examples of classic experiments include: Zimbardo's Stanford Prison Experiment, which highlights the way social influences, like assigned roles, can contribute to "normal" people engaging in brutal tyranny while other assigned roles can contribute to "normal" people engaging in behaviors associated with extreme victimization (Haney et al., 1973); Festinger's cognitive dissonance studies, in which individuals aim for consistency between attitudes and behaviors, and may not use rational or moral methods to achieve it (Festinger et al., 1956); and the Rosenhan experiment, which highlights the lack of validity and reliability of psychiatric diagnosis about what is "normal" versus "abnormal," and the disempowering and demeaning nature of patient care experienced by the study participants (Rosenhan, 1973). This path-breaking experiment is particularly pertinent to psychoanalysis because it raises intriguing questions, such as whether madness is the inability to fake sanity, or as sociologist Erving Goffman implied, whether society is an insane asylum run by the inmates. In other words, I will consider how these divisions of sane and insane operate, often negatively, for the clinician and analysand, patient or client.

This book can be described as a social psychology of "witness" in that it has an overarching goal of increasing the individual's capacity to act in an autonomous, integrated and humane manner amidst the moral challenges one faces in the attempt to fashion a flourishing moral life that includes an understanding of the visible and invisible external social forces that influence behavior. As Foucault noted, the role of philosophy, and I would add the role of social psychology and psychoanalysis, is not so much "to discover what is hidden, but to render visible what precisely is visible, which is to say, to make appear what is so close, so immediate, so intimately linked to ourselves that, as a consequence, we do not perceive it" (Cavell, 2004, p. 33). In this way one can "think differently" about one's situation: "Thought is freedom in relation to what one does, the motion by which one detaches oneself from it, establishes it as an object, and reflects on it as a problem" (Foucault, 1984a, p. 388). For instance, there were individuals in Asch's line drawing studies (1951) who did not cave in to group pressure and told the truth as they perceived it, there were people in Latané and Darley's bystander study (1968) who intervened in an emergency situation, and there were individuals who refused to shock an innocent victim in Milgram's study (1974). In this book, I use these classic social psychology studies, which together can be called the "sacred cannon," as analogous to compelling, modern "morality plays": to delineate the important insights about the conditions of possibility for potentiating the "worst" and "best" about human behavior, what psychoanalysis needs to integrate into its understanding of the human condition,[7] and how these social-psychological findings can be pragmatically integrated into clinical practice. For example, helping the analysand develop better "situational awareness," defined as increased awareness of one's surroundings (e.g., of time and space) and identifying potential threats and dangerous situations, is a mind-set and an ego-strength that has enormous benefit in helping an analysand maintain personal and collective security. This increased awareness goes against denial and complacency in a world that feels—and often is—menacing. Such skillful situational awareness is in sync with how sociologist Anthony Giddens describes the modern self: "as a reflexive project, for which the individual is responsible" (1991, p. 75). Rather than taking for granted or passively inheriting who we are, as in traditional culture, we actively shape, reflect on and monitor our selves, fashioning our biographical narratives as we move through life. We view our identities as a project, something that we actively construct and are alone responsible for. Any psychoanalytic social psychology worth its salt includes responsibility as a core valuative attachment of its intellectual and practical activities.[8] Indeed, throughout this book, in part drawing from social psychologist Milton Rokeach, I suggest that the person who fashions a self-identity that includes strongly felt, flexibly and creatively applied, transcendent-pointing moral beliefs and values that are primarily other-directed, other-regarding and other-serving, tends to behave in morally praiseworthy, life-affirming and life-promoting ways.

Many eminent psychoanalytic personality and social theorists have investigated the role of culture on the individual, such as the way that one socially constructs a self within the context of family and the broadly conceived environment (e.g., the role of gender, patriarchy, race, economics, etc.). While these theorists have tried to delineate the ways that individuals are shaped by social circumstances, including acknowledging social context as being a primary determinant of behavior, intra-psychic properties (e.g., desire and fantasy) tend to dominate the analysis of why people behave the way they do. For example, one psychoanalytically influenced sociologist, Anthony Elliott, points out that the analyst and analysand attempt to understand how social and cultural forms are given shape internally, involving critically reflecting on how the self is constituted culturally as a manifestation of "internal depth": "[T]he self is a work of active construction and reconstruction, built on inner workings of fantasy and its unconscious contortions—anxieties about difference, about otherness and strangeness, about intimacy and proximity—in the wider frame of culture, society and politics" (2015, p. 187). Elliott further emphasizes the importance of psychoanalytic reflections on modern culture and what the individual represses: Freud viewed modern culture in terms of the self and society structured and organized via ambivalence, such that culture was reproduced through unconscious repression; Erich Fromm viewed modern society in terms of how it distorted human needs, desires and interpersonal relationships; Herbert Marcuse claimed modern societies reproduced through surplus repression, those forces that are socially dominating of individual instinctual life and sense of reality; Frantz Fanon and Homi Bhabha viewed modern culture in terms of colonialism and decolonization analyzed as cross-cutting forms of ambivalence and cultures of resistance; Joel Kovel, an eco-socialist, claimed that narcissistic pathology was a function of the worst aspects of self-serving capitalism and globalization; and Christopher Lasch argued that Western society's inordinate narcissism was linked to overall social conditions of modernity, such as the inward turn related to the impact of World War II and consumer culture (Elliott, 2015, p. 62). All of these thinkers have drawn mainly from sociology, the investigation of human social relationships and institutions, specifically comprehending how human action and consciousness both form and are formed by encircling cultural and social structures.

While sociology tends to have a macro-focus on the broad social, economic, political and historical forces at play, social psychology tends to be micro-focused on the psychology of the individual in the service of identifying "universal properties of human nature that make everyone, regardless of social class or culture, susceptible to social influence" (Aronson et al., 2014, p. 10).

What Elliott is saying is surely good, but, I believe, incomplete. What psychoanalysis has not done, which I believe is a huge deficit in psychoanalytic theory and practice, is to develop a sophisticated psychology of everyday "situational" behavior that gives robust consideration to specific contextual factors in determining behavior on vitally important moral issues. Put differently, the most important feature of the classic social psychology studies is that they focused on "fundamental questions about human sociality such as, 'Why do we conform and obey? Why do we oppress? Why do we help and support?'" (Haslam & Smith, 2017, p. 2). It does this by providing a scientific analysis of the relationship between "mind and society" (ibid., p. 1) that challenges mainstream psychoanalytic thinking. That is, social psychology concentrates on scientifically explaining and understanding people engaging in "real" behavior in "real" situations. William James called himself a "childish idiot" in a letter to a colleague regarding his own arrogant and ignorant desire to formulate truths as an expression of personal ambition, writing, "… as if formulas about the Universe could ruffle its majesty and as if the commonsense world and its duties were not eternally the really real" (1987, p. 1344). This real-life experimental/scientific methodology is in sync with those who have argued for an "evidence-based" psychoanalysis that focuses on the "here-and-now" and therapeutic immediacy between analyst and analysand (Luyten et al., 2015).

There have been numerous related experimental/scientific investigations into the effects of social circumstances on the individual since the original studies, some of which challenge the earlier studies. Like in psychoanalysis, social psychology has shown great "internal diversification and substantive sprawl" in its contemporary developments (Smelser, 2014, p. 107). These investigations and the canon in which they are lodged are extremely pertinent to mainstream psychoanalytic theory and technique, and, as I will argue, to the development of a scientifically grounded psychoanalytic social psychology. These studies have dramatically demonstrated that particular characteristics of situations at a given moment can sharply alter behavior and be more useful in predicting behavior than knowledge of personality characteristics, as mainstream analysts usually prioritize. Nevertheless, the psychoanalytic community has been slow and resistant to absorb the implications of these compelling findings and the ways in which they influence the judged "pathology" and "health" of their analysands. In fact, all of the major contemporary psychoanalytic textbooks, handbooks and dictionaries I consulted do not even have an entry for social psychology, let alone experimental/scientific social psychology, nor are there any references to any of the classic experiments or researchers in their table of contents or indices. A search indicated there was no book on the interface of social psychology and psychoanalysis, and only one psychoanalytic text that had the words social psychology in it (Curtis, 1991), which mainly deals with relational therapy. It is my belief that psychoanalysts will strengthen their theoretical viewpoint and interpretive powers, as well as their therapeutic efficacy, as they integrate these classic social psychology findings into the existing psychoanalytic frameworks, on the way to developing a sound psychoanalytic social psychology.

A "match made in heaven"?

In order to better contextualize the main terms of this book, psychoanalysis and social psychology, I will define them in more detail as they are used throughout the following nine chapters. I will then briefly compare and contrast some of the assumptions that animate psychoanalysis and social psychology and have caused these two psychological disciplines to avoid having any sustained cross-fertilization despite them being beautifully complementary, "a match made in heaven." Psychoanalysis can greatly benefit from the social-psychological analysis of specific context and setting, while social psychology can benefit from a psychoanalytic understanding of character/personality structure on the psychological level. In this way, each approach can expand their theoretical grounds and enhance their practical effectiveness, whether in the psychoanalyst or psychotherapist's office, the school, workplace or other organizational setting. While this book does not attempt to develop a comprehensive psychoanalytically based scientific social psychology, it does suggest that it is worthwhile to attempt to begin to build a modulating bridge between these two intellectual approaches, especially as they work slowly to improve specific morally compelling individual "problems in living" and social toxicity.

What is Psychoanalysis?

Psychoanalysis as I conceive it is a form of life, a meaning-giving, affect-integrating and action-guiding resource for individuals who can appropriate the life- and identity-defining narrative of psychoanalysis when they seek to understand, endure and possibly gain some self-mastery over the problems that affect, if not assault, their lives, such as despair, loss, tragedy, anxiety and conflict. Psychoanalysis can be viewed as what Michel Foucault called a "technology of the self": "an exercise of the self, by which one attempts to develop and transform oneself, and to attain a certain mode of being" (1989, p. 433). As philosopher Pierre Hadot noted about ancient Greek philosophy, psychoanalysis can be understood as a "spiritual exercise," a tool for living life skillfully, fully and wisely (1997, p. 83). Erik Erikson may have had this in mind when he wrote that "free association" was a "western form of meditation" (Hoare, 2001, p. 88), while Symington explicitly states "that psychoanalysis has a spiritual function," such that "purifying motivation" becomes "the organizing center of his activities" (1993, p. 47). The aim of a spiritual exercise is to foster a deep modification of an individual's way of "seeing and being," a decisive change in how one lives one's practical, everyday life. Most importantly, the objective of a spiritual exercise is "a total transformation of one's vision, life-style, and behavior" in the service of increased personal freedom and peace of mind

(Hadot, 1997, pp. 83, 103, 14), to which I would add, a less self-centric outlook and behavior (this being one of the important ports of entry into moral living). According to this view, as Levinas described "Jewish Humanism" at its best, psychoanalysis is "a difficult wisdom concerned with truths that correlate to virtues" (1989, p. 275). Psychoanalysis is a painful, deconstructive, demythologizing and defamiliarizing process for acquiring greater self-awareness and self-understanding, especially of one's destructive unconscious emotional activity, and one that transforms moral consciousness by expanding and deepening one's capacity to love. As the great Axial period[9] sages viewed it, self-understanding leads to self-mastery, which leads to self-transcendence. In fact, Freud described psychoanalytic treatment as the "scientific cure by love" (McGuire, 1974, pp. 12–13). In this sense, psychoanalysis is animated by both the "love of wisdom" and the "wisdom of love" by Greek and Hebrew values, and is a powerful tool for the art of living a flourishing or good life, as one construes and fashions it.

What is social psychology?

Social psychology has been defined as "a scientific analysis of the relationship between 'mind and society'" (Haslam & Smith, 2017, p. 1). More specifically, it is "the scientific study of the effects of social and cognitive processes on the way individuals perceive, influence, and relate to others" (Smith et al., 2015, p. 3). It should be emphasized that for social psychologists, underlying "emotion and motivation," the bailiwick of psychoanalysis, "are intrinsic parts of every cognitive process" and its "central concern is how people understand and interact with others" (ibid., p. 4).

As Smith et al. unpack their definition, "the scientific study" refers to the method that social psychologists use to comprehend, predict and influence people's thoughts, feelings and perhaps most importantly in terms of moral psychology, overt social behavior. It is precisely this methodological feature, the systematic method of collecting data and the mindfulness of the possibility of error, that has allowed social psychology to generate findings that go against "common sense knowledge" (ibid., p. 3). Indeed, all of the classic studies in this book have generated radically counter-intuitive findings about moral process and behavior.

The phrase "of the effects of social and cognitive processes" refers to the fact that it is the attendance of other people, the knowledge and opinions they transmit to us and the feelings regarding the groups that we belong to, that profoundly influence us via social processes, regardless of whether we are in the company of others or alone. Social processes "are the way in which input from the people and groups around us affect our thoughts, feelings and actions" (ibid., p. 4). Moreover, our emotions, motivation, perceptions and memories exercise an all-encompassing influence on us via cognitive processes. Cognitive processes, are "the ways in which our memories, perceptions, thoughts, emotions and motives influence our understanding of the world and guide our actions" (ibid.). The impacts of these social and cognitive processes are never discrete; rather, they are interdependent, interrelated and interactive.

Lastly, the phrase "on the way individuals perceive, influence, and relate to others" refers to the fact that it is grasping the effect of the aforementioned social and cognitive processes on the way individuals perceive, influence and relate to others that matters most (i.e., social behavior), in terms of explaining why people behave the way they do. These insights can aid in solving (or improving) important social problems that have serious moral import and ramifications. As Lewin noted, while theory is important, theories needed to have practical applications that make things better.

Thus, on the face of it, there are many common thematics between psychoanalysis and social psychology, such as their devotion to systematic empirical inquiry (clinically for psychoanalysis and experimentally for social psychology), their respective interest in understanding the relationship between mind and society, and helping people to feel, think and act better in the moral realm. And yet, this is a "marriage" between two intellectual disciplines that never happened; in fact, they have hardly spoken to each other.

The divergent optics of psychoanalysis and social psychology

It will be helpful to the reader of this book to appreciate some of the differences between how psychoanalysis and social psychology tend to view their subject matter, human behavior and its improvement, that have led to the aforementioned missed opportunity. This comparison is in no way comprehensive. It is meant to give the reader a sense of the divergent ways that these two perspectives approach understanding human experience and its enhancement, including in the realm of moral psychology. I will list four points as simplified generalizations as there are always exceptions and the matter is much more complicated.

1 Psychoanalysis tends to focus on the "internal world," the depth of feeling, wish, fantasy and memory of the individual, while social psychology tends to focus on the "external world," in particular the specific context and setting in which behavior occurs. While psychoanalysis is immensely interested in social relations, in particular family relations (the external world), social psychology tends to focus on specific situational forces that impact behavior in "real" time (though it, too, is interested in the internal world, like cognition, emotion and motivation). In a certain sense, internal and external are arbitrary human categories, as human existence is "being-in-the-world" as Heidegger noted. That is, while these broad distinctions are heuristically helpful in constructing intelligible differences, one must be mindful that human being-in-the-world is best conceptualized as an individual unity of thought, feeling/kinesthetic and action engaged in the lived actuality of his everyday life. Thus, psychoanalysis is at its "best" when it focuses on the personal levels of human experience while social psychology is at its "best" when focusing on the experimentally verifiable social level of experience.

2 Psychoanalysis tends to focus on individuals in all of their uniqueness and it usually builds its arguments working from the individual to the group, from individual motivation to social behavior and collective action. Individual causality is its emphasis. Social psychology tends to work in the opposite direction—it begins with social behavior and collective action and relates this

to individual motivation and explanation. Social causality is its emphasis. Both approaches are prone to individual and social reductionism, respectively. Indeed, psychoanalysis tends to view social psychology as providing a "superficial snapshot of social process which in real life occur over time and a social context" (Hayes, 1995, p. 65), while social psychologists believe that explaining behavior with reference to personality psychology is "superficial" because it leaves out or underplays the powerful role of social influence (Aronson et al., 2014, p. 11). Thus, while psychoanalysis tends to underestimate the influence of situational factors and has difficulties in making verifiable normative generalizations about behavior, social psychology underestimates individual differences in behavior such that it does not adequately explain why some people depart from the expected norm in any given social situation. That is, the individual is always in the social and the social is always in the individual, hence a multi-dimensional approach is the most prudent way to think about mind and society (Chancer & Andrews, 2014, p. xvii).

3 Psychoanalysis does not have one notion of "human nature," but rather, "Psychoanalytic models rest upon … irreconcilable claims concerning the human condition" (Greenberg & Mitchell, 1983, p. 404). While there are common thematics in all versions of psychoanalysis, such as the importance of the unconscious, sexuality, repression, childhood experiences and trauma, it would be false to claim that contemporary psychoanalysis has a single, explicit manner of conceptualizing "human nature." Indeed, Freud, like Homer, Aristotle, the Church Fathers, Galileo and Marx, was one of the "founders of discursivity," in that he was not just an author of his own work. He has "produced the possibilities and the rules for the formation of other texts … an endless possibility of discourse" (Foucault, 1984b, p. 114). Freud is the author of a theory, tradition and discipline in which all subsequent analysts must situate themselves one way or another. Analysts have very different narratives, carved out of the "master narratives," about the self: the self fashioned by its defenses against instincts (Freud), the self formed by its inner objects (Klein), the self shaped by its internalized relationships (Kohut) (Jones, 1991, p. 135) and "the self as a narcissistic misrecognition, represented through the symbolic order of language" (Lacan) (Elliott, 2015, p. 123). Moreover, depending on which master narrative one is lodged in, the goals of psychoanalytic treatment tend to be conceptualized differently: We have "the taming of the beast within" through reason and love (Freud), the "mad person within raging about" who becomes transformed through compensatory reparative activities (Klein), the "discovery of the self within" and the development of compensatory self-structures (Kohut), and "to speak what [had] heretofore been unspeakable," to reclaim the voice of one's desires (Lacan) (Roth, 1998, p. 327). Moreover, social behavior is understood through the frame and filter of the view of the human condition or human nature that is in play.

Somewhat in contrast, most social psychologists share in an experimental/scientific outlook with positivistic gloss (similar to versions of psychoanalysis that are associated with the medical model). Such a perspective assumes that whatever exists can be verified via experiments, observation and mathematical/logical proof, a manifestation of a belief in realism. For the social psychologist, the "core values" are "accuracy," that is, gathering information about social behavior in as careful, exacting and error-free way as possible; "objectivity," that is, gathering information without human bias; "skepticism," that is, embracing evidence only to the extent that it has been verified by replication; and "open-mindedness," that is, being willing and able to revise one's views in the face of contradictory evidence (Baron & Byrne, 2003, p. 6). Moreover, positivists often maintain that scientific progress will significantly reduce social problems. This being said, there are many social-psychological communities that only partially overlap and they have different ideal characterizations of methodological practice, including credible exceptions to any generalizations (Cook & Groom, 2004). However, all social psychologists pride themselves on their scientific methodology in understanding the person in a social context and setting, the mind and society in dynamic, reciprocal interaction.[10] Indeed, while not usually viewed as one of the founders of discursivity, Kurt Lewin, influenced by Gestalt psychology, brilliantly argued that human behavior should be viewed, and scientifically studied, as a constituent part of a continuum with individual variations that depart from the norm, which can be seen as a consequence of tensions between perceptions of the self and of the environment. To adequately comprehend and predict human behavior, Lewin believed that the entire psychological field, or "lifespace," within which the person was lodged and acted had to be viewed, such that the totality of events in this lifespace determined behavior at any one instant.[11] Thus, Lewin's theory stressed the importance of individual personalities, interpersonal conflict, and situational forces, with it probably being the first theoretical depiction of the "imagery of human nature" (Smelser, 2014, p. 108) that was appropriated to some extent by all subsequent social psychologists. In all of the classics discussed in this book, and indeed, in most of mainstream social psychology, not one of the authors has seriously, let alone systematically, raised the issue that maybe the very mode of intelligibility and praxis (positivistic science), that is, the sense-making structure inside which phenomena are found, might be limited if not questionable, and can be usefully augmented by psychoanalysis, phenomenology or other fields of intelligibility.[12]

4 Psychoanalysis occurs mainly in the psychotherapist's office while social psychology is laboratory-based, which includes systematic field studies and research in naturalistic settings that have robust ecological credibility. While the "softer" clinical studies can resonate with aspects of these less controlled field studies, most often psychoanalysis relies on the single case study approach while social psychology strives to aggregate data on many people in order to make reasonable generalizations. Likewise, psychoanalytic argumentation draws on constructs that are not easily experimentally/scientifically studied, like the analysand's unconscious, infantile sexuality, early object relationships, ambivalence and the like, while social psychology prides itself on its ability to replicate its findings and tends

to focus on the actor being largely motivated by the perceived aspects of the immediacy of the situation.

Psychoanalysis and social psychology "need" each other now

It is worth noting that contemporary psychoanalysis and social psychology may need each other, or would at least benefit from a lively conversation, since both approaches have been described by sympathetic scholars in their communities as in crisis. As Marshall Edelson reflects, psychoanalysis is a "theory in crisis" characterized by "profound malaise" (1988, p. xiv) while Nathan G. Hale describes the psychoanalytic crisis as "a crisis of clashing theories, competing modes of therapy, and uncertainties of professional identity" (1995, p. 360). Not only does psychoanalysis lack what Thomas Kuhn called disciplinary matrix for its activities as a science (however conceived), and it "is too fragmented to be constituted as a unitary discipline" (Weinstein, 1990, p. 26),[13] but it has not been hospitable to heretical and dissident thinkers, thus "sucking the life" out of the psychoanalytic institute training experience. Otto Kernberg, the great psychoanalytic theorizer of narcissism and borderline conditions, recently noted in an interview that U.S. psychotherapy training is on the decline.[14] Psychoanalysis is hardly represented in the university training programs of psychiatrists and doctoral level clinical psychology psychologists but has instead been marginalized to institutes.[15]

There is also "a crisis of confidence" on "replicability in psychological science" (Pashler & Wagenmakers, 2012, p. 528), which was affirmed by two prominent social psychologists (Haslam & Smith, 2017, p. 6). The crisis involves improper research methods (e.g., playing fast and loose with statistics, reporting only positive findings), fake research (e.g., fabricating findings) and difficulties in replication, the hallmark of positivistic science. This crisis of confidence calls to mind what Freud said, "That psychoanalysis has not made the analysts themselves better, nobler, or of stronger character remains a disappointment for me. Perhaps, I was wrong to expect it" (Hale, 1971, pp. 163–164). More recently, Jane Brody noted in the *New York Times* (2018) that three of the studies discussed in this book, the Stanford Prison Experiment, the Marshmallow Experiment, and the research on "ego depletion," have not been adequately replicated (though there is debate about whether the methodological criticisms and alleged statistical bias are valid). Brian Nosek, one of the social psychologists who has researched the replication crisis, noted that about 60% of well-known psychology studies were not reproducible: "this is a phase of cleaning house, and we're finding that many things are not as robust as we thought….This is a reformation moment—to say let's self-correct, and build on knowledge that we know is solid" (Brody, 2018).[16]

Given the fact that psychoanalysis and social psychology are in crisis—one lacks a disciplinary matrix as a science, the other finds itself questioning it foundational texts and scientific methods—and that they share many conceptual and practical concerns, there may be potential if they "joined forces." Psychoanalysis, with its robust emphasis on the psychic, and social psychology, with its robust emphasis on the social, both embrace scientific methodologies. They could benefit from seeing themselves as "two sides of the same coin," as "complementary articulation[s]" (Smelser, 2014, p. 112) that are geared to understanding human behavior and making things better. This early stage of trying to integrate these two marvelously insightful intellectual traditions means tackling one individual problem in living and one social problem at a time, at least until the conditions of possibility are right such that a more comprehensive psychoanalytically inspired scientific social psychology can be fashioned.

Book layout

Seven of the nine studies discussed in this book were considered classics by Smith and Haslam (2017) in their wonderful volume that revisits the classic social psychology studies. Only Walter Mischel's Marshmallow Experiment (Mischel & Ebbesen, 1970) and David Rosenhan's study of diagnosis in psychiatric hospitals (1973) were not included by Smith and Haslam. I have also followed Smith and Haslam's lead in organizing each chapter chronologically with the exception of the Rosenhan study of being sane in insane places, which, because of its pertinence to the practice of psychoanalysis, is the last chapter. Each chapter is generally structured as follows: (1) an introduction that contextualizes the moral and practical problem; (2) a summary of the classic study and its implications; (3) social-psychological interpretations of the study, including criticisms and replication considerations; (4) psychoanalytic interpretations of the study, including conceptual and practical "contact points" between psychoanalysis and social psychology; and (5) therapeutic/practical implications for living a moral life that emanate from the aforementioned studies.

My hope is to begin a "conversation" between the two inspired and inspiring disciplines, psychoanalysis and social psychology, in the service of developing the rudiments of a scientifically rigorous, theoretically credible, psychoanalytic social psychology.

Notes

1 The moral emotions, some scholars believe, are felt only by organisms that have a well-developed capacity for self-reflection and self-criticality. It requires "position-taking," that is comprehending how one's behavior would impact and be judged by others, and how that behavior reflects back on self-appraisal, self-judged character (Simons, 2009). In social psychology, in general, there are three classes of moral emotions: emotions that inspire people to care about the suffering of others (e.g., sympathy, empathy, compassion), emotions that drive people to punish others (e.g., anger and disgust) and emotions that are self-punitive for breaching one's moral code (e.g., guilt and shame). Some researchers also include a class of emotions that are evoked when one views the positive moral acts of others, such as praise and a type of moral awe termed elevation (https://psychology.iresearchnet.com/social-psychology/emotions/moral-emotions/, retrieved 5/3/19).

2 I am aware that what constitutes alleged moral behavior and emotions is a judgment call and will vary depending on who is making the judgment. As the popular saying goes, "One man's terrorist is another man's freedom fighter." This being said, by moral behavior and emotion I have in mind a Levinasian sensibility, one in which "ethics is an 'optics'" (Levinas, 1969, p. 29). In this view, "ethics is no longer a simple moralism of rules which decree what is virtuous. It is the original awakening of an I responsible for the other; the accession of my person to the uniqueness of the I called and elected to responsibility for the other" (Levinas, 2001, p. 182). Levinas is one of my intellectual touchstones that I frequently draw from in this book.

3 What constitutes a flourishing or good life is also a judgment call. In positive psychology, a flourishing life has been defined as living "with an optimal range of human functioning, one that connotes goodness, generativity, growth and resilience" (Fredrickson & Losada, 2005, p. 678). Needless to say, this definition is heavily value-laden and boils down to the decision-making of the analysand and the clinician.

4 Briefly, social intelligence is an individual's competency at social skills and behaviors (i.e., roughly "street smarts" and "common sense"), while social cognition is the ability to collect information about and understand the rules and concepts that influence if not control their social interactions, the ways in which we comprehend social rules of etiquette, proximity, gestures, inferences, etc.

5 Self-psychologists and Holocaust survivors Paul and Anna Ornstein told me that, in their view, Bettelheim's statements are also true for self-psychology and other versions of psychoanalysis. My study of survival in the Nazi concentration camps supports this conclusion (Marcus, 1999). From time to time, I draw from the Holocaust literature, in particular the inmate's ordeal of suffering, as such an extreme is a "limit case, or the farthest borderland of human existence" (Sass, 1992, p. 15), and as such puts into sharp focus aspects of human behavior that may not be easily illuminated.

6 A recent anthology with a telling title, *The Unhappy Divorce of Sociology and Psychoanalysis: Diverse Perspectives on the Psychosocial*, suggests that the discipline of sociology (especially its empirical tradition) and psychoanalysis have not had much influence on each other (Chancer & Andrews, 2014).

7 "The human condition" is one of those phrases that implies there is a natural, essential, ahistorical and universal subject, a view I don't subscribe to. Indeed, what constitutes "the human condition" depends on the theory-animated model of "human nature" one assumes; hence, what constitutes the human condition and human nature is perspectival and historically situated. In psychoanalysis, for example, there are many incompatible versions of the human condition, much less so in social psychology where human nature as an objective thing is assumed (Marcus & Rosenberg, 1998).

8 www.routledgesoc.com/category/profile-tags/reflexivity, retrieved 6/22/18. Goffman has a similar view: "the self … is not an organic thing that has a specific location, whose fundamental fate is to be born, to mature, to die; it is a dramatic effect arising diffusely from a scene that is presented" (1959, p. 252). Some psychoanalysts influenced by postmodernism hold views about "the self" that resonate with Giddens and Goffman's formulations (see Elliott, 2015).

9 The Axial period as described by Karl Jaspers was between 800 and 200 B.C.E., when the great philosophers, religious leaders and teachers emerged throughout the world, such as Confucius, Lao Tzu, Zarathustra, Plato and Jeremiah. These creative geniuses shaped civilization as we know it (Marcus, 2019).

10 It should be mentioned that many of the classics used methodologies that may not be "up to snuff" by today's standards. Moreover, there are ethical issues that may trouble some scholars and researchers that were not problematic to the classic experimenters. This being said, all of these studies focused on "big questions" (Haslam & Smith, 2017, p. 2), the moral conundrums that are still pertinent to everyday individual and social existence and flourishing.

11 www.britannica.com/biography/Kurt-Lewin, retrieved 5/10/19. It is worth mentioning that there are psychoanalytic "field theories" that have drawn from Lewin's dynamic field concept as important to their psychoanalytic theory of the analyst/analysand interaction (e.g., the analytic dyad is bi-personal, ensconced in an interpersonal field, or a session is like an unmetabolized dreamscape). See Charles (2018) for a good overview of these different theories.

12 As is well known, all human comprehension is already lodged in a hermeneutical circle, in the experimenter's experiences, pre-suppositions, values and expectations.

13 While I can appreciate that there is something positive about diversity and difference in a discipline, that there can be a unity in multiplicity, this can reach a perilous threshold where it becomes a "veritable Babel of theories" (Kurzweil, 1989, p. 256). Whether this psychoanalytic landscape has improved or worsened is entirely perspectival.

14 www.psychotherapy.net/interview/otto-kernberg, retrieved 5/12/19.
15 Psychoanalysis has been marginalized by the biological revolution in psychiatry as well as the upsurge of cognitive behavioral therapy (including Dialectical Behavioral Therapy) and related forms of efficacy-based psychotherapies (Harrington, 2019).
16 Haslam and Smith (2017) believe, and I agree, that "the core findings" from the majority of the classic experiments have been replicated numerous times, drawing from a diverse range of subjects, from dissimilar cultural backgrounds and over varying time periods (p. 6).

References

Akhtar, S. (2009). *Comprehensive dictionary of psychoanalysis*. London: Karnac.

Aronson, E., Wilson, T. D. & Akert, R. M. (2014). *Social psychology* (4th ed.). Upper Saddle, NJ: Pearson.

Baron, R. A. & Byrne, D. (Eds.) (2003). *Social psychology* (10th ed.). Boston: Pearson Education.

Bauman, Z. (1992). *Mortality, immortality, and other life strategies*. Stanford, CA: Stanford University Press.

Bettelheim, B. (1960). *The informed heart: Autonomy in a mass age*. Glencoe, IL: The Free Press.

Brody, J. E. (2018). Psychology is having a 'reformation moment.' *New York Times*, 7/17/18, Science Times, D5.

Cavell, S. (2004). *Cities of words: Pedagogical letters on a register of the moral life*. Cambridge: Cambridge University Press.

Chancer, L. & Andrews, J. (2014). *The unhappy divorce of sociology and psychoanalysis: Diverse perspectives on the psychosocial*. Houndmills, UK: Palgrave Macmillan.

Charles, M. (Ed.) (2018). *Introduction to contemporary psychoanalysis: Defining terms and building bridges*. London: Routledge.

Cook, T. D. & Groom, C. (2004). The methodological assumptions of social psychology: The mutual dependence of substantive theory and method choice. In C. Sansone, C. C. Morf & A. T. Panter (Eds.), The Sage handbook of methods in social psychology (pp. 19–44). Thousand Oaks, CA: Sage Publications.

Curtis, R. C. (1991). *The relational self: Theoretical congruence in psychoanalysis and social psychology*. New York: Guilford.

Edelson, M. (1988). *Psychoanalysis: A theory in crisis*. Chicago: University of Chicago Press.

Elliott, A. (2015). *Psychoanalytic theory* (3rd ed.). London: Palgrave Macmillan.

Festinger, L., Riecken, H. W. & Schachter, S. (1956). *When prophecy fails*. Minneapolis, MN: University of Minnesota Press.

Foucault, M. (1984a). Polemics, politics, and problemizations. In P. Rabinow (Ed.), *Foucault reader* (pp. 381–390). New York: Pantheon.

Foucault, M. (1984b). What is an author? In P. Rabinow (Ed.), *Foucault reader* (pp. 101–123). New York: Pantheon.

Foucault, M. (1989). The ethics of the concern for self as a practice of freedom. In S. Lotringer (Ed.), *Foucault live: Collected interviews, 1961–1984* (pp. 432–449). New York: Semiotexte.

Frank, A.W. (2013). *The wounded storyteller: Body, illness & ethics* (2nd ed.). Chicago, IL: University of Chicago Press.

Fredrickson, B. L. & Losada, M. F. (2005). Positive affect and complex dynamics of human flourishing. *American Psychologist*, 60, 678–686.

Freud, S. (1962). The neuro-psychoses of defence. In J. Strachey (Ed. & Trans.), *Standard edition of the complete psychological works of Sigmund Freud* (Vol. 3, pp. 41–68). London: Hogarth Press. (Original work published 1894).

Freud, S. (1974). The Ego and the Id. In J. Strachey (Ed. & Trans.), *Standard edition of the complete psychological works of Sigmund Freud* (Vol. 19, pp. 3–66). London: Hogarth Press. (Original work published 1923).
Giddens, A. (1991). *Self and society in the late modern age*. Cambridge, MA: Polity Press.
Goffman, E. (1959). *The presentation of self in everyday life*. Garden City, NY: Doubleday Anchor.
Greenberg, J. R. & Mitchell, S. A. (1983). *Object relations in psychoanalytic theory*. Cambridge: Harvard University Press.
Greenberg, T. M. (2016). *Psychodynamic perspectives on aging and illness* (2nd ed.). Heidelberg, HR: Springer.
Hadot, P. (1997). *Philosophy as a way of life*. Oxford, UK: Blackwell.
Hale, N. (Ed.) (1971). *James Jackson Putnam and psychoanalysis*. J. B. Heller (Trans.). Cambridge: Cambridge University Press.
Hale, N.G. (1995). *The rise and crisis of psychoanalysis in the United States*. Oxford: Oxford University Press.
Haney, C., Banks, C. & Zimbardo, P. (1973). A study of prisoners and guards in a simulated prison. *Naval Research Reviews*, September, 1–17. Washington, DC: Office of Naval Research.
Harrington, A. (2019). *Mind fixers: Psychiatry's troubled search for the biology of mental illness*. New York: W.W. Norton & Company.
Haslam, S. A. & Smith, J. R. (2017). An introduction to classic studies in social psychology. In J.R. Smith & S.A. Haslam (Eds.), *Social psychology: Revisiting the classic studies* (2nd ed., pp. 1–10). Los Angeles: Sage.
Hayes, N. (1995). *Psychology in perspective*. New York: Macmillan.
Hoare, C. H. (2001). *Erikson on development in adulthood: New insights from the unpublished papers*. Oxford, UK: Oxford University Press.
James, W. (1987). *Writings: 1902–1910*. New York: Library of America.
Jones, J. (1991). *Contemporary psychoanalysis: Religion, transference and transcendence*. New Haven, CT: Yale University Press.
Kurzweil, E. (1989). *The Freudians: A comparative perspective*. New Haven: Yale University Press.
Latané, B., & Darley, J. M. (1968). *Group inhibition of bystander intervention in emergencies. Journal of Personality and Social Psychology*, 10, 215–221.
Lear, J. (2017). *Wisdom won from illness: Essays in philosophy and psychoanalysis*. Cambridge, MA: Harvard University Press.
Levinas, E. (1969). *Totality and infinity: An essay on exteriority*. A. Lingis (Trans.). Pittsburgh, PA: Duquesne University Press.
Levinas, E. (1989). *Difficult freedom: Essays on Judaism*. S. Hand (Ed.). Baltimore, MD: Johns Hopkins.
Levinas, E. (1996). *Proper names*. M.B. Smith (Trans.). Stanford, CA: Stanford University Press.
Levinas, E. (2001). *Is it righteous to be? Interviews with Emmanuel Levinas*. J. Robbins (Ed.). Stanford, CA: Stanford University Press.
Luel, S. A. & Marcus, P. (Eds.) (1984). *Psychoanalytic reflections on the Holocaust: Selected essays*. New York: University of Denver and KTAV Publishing House.
Luyten, P., Mayes, L. C., Fonagy, P., Target, M. & Blatt, S. J. (Eds.) (2015). *Handbook of psychodynamic approaches to psychopathology*. New York: Guilford.
McGuire, W. (Ed.) (1974). *The Freud/Jung letters*. Princeton: Princeton University Press.
Marcus, P. (1999). *Autonomy in the extreme situation: Bruno Bettelheim, the Nazi Concentration Camps and the mass society*. Westport, CT: Praeger.
Marcus, P. (2003). *Ancient religious wisdom, spirituality, and psychoanalysis*. Westport, CT: Prager.

Marcus, P. (2019). *The psychoanalysis of overcoming suffering: Flourishing despite pain.* London: Routledge.
Marcus, P. & Rosenberg, A. (Eds.) (1998). *Psychoanalytic versions of the human condition: Philosophies of life and their impact on practice.* New York: New York University Press.
Milgram, S. (1974). *Obedience to authority: An experimental view.* New York: Harper & Row.
Mischel, W. & Ebbesen, E. B. (1970). Attention in delay of gratification. *Journal of Personality and Social Psychology*, 16(2), 329–337. doi:10.1037/h0029815.
Pashler, H. & Wagenmakers, E.-J. (2012). Editor's introduction to the special section on replicability in psychological science: A crisis of confidence? *Perspectives on Psychological Science*, 7(6), 528–530.
Rosenhan, D. (1973). On being sane in insane places. *Science*, 179(4070), 250–258.
Roth, P.A. (1998). The cure of stories, self-deception, danger situations, and the clinical role of narratives in Roy Schaefer's psychoanalytic theory. In P. Marcus & A. Rosenberg (Eds.), *Psychoanalytic versions of the human condition: Philosophies of life and their impact on practice* (pp. 306–331). New York: New York University Press.
Sass, L. A. (1992). *Madness and modernism: Insanity in the light of modern art, literature and thought.* Cambridge: Harvard University Press.
Simons, I. (2009). The four moral emotions: Guilt, shame, embarrassment, and pride make societies work. *Psychology Today*. Retrieved from www.psychologytoday.com/us/blog/the-literary-mind/200911/the-four-moral-emotions.
Smelser, N. J. (2014). Sustaining an unlikely marriage: Biographical, theoretical, and intellectual notes. In L. Chancer & J. Andrews (Eds.), *The unhappy divorce of sociology and psychoanalysis: Diverse perspectives on the psychosocial* (pp. 101–121). Houndmills, UK: Palgrave Macmillan.
Smith, J. R. & Haslam, S. A. (Eds.) (2017). *Social psychology: Revisiting classic studies.* Los Angeles: Sage.
Smith, R., Mackie, D. M. & Claypool, H. M. (Eds.) (2015). *Social psychology* (4th ed.). New York: Psychology Press.
Symington, N. (1993). *Emotion and spirit: Questioning the claims of psychoanalysis and religion.* New York: St. Martin's Press.
Wallerstein, R. S. (1973). Psychoanalytic perspectives on the problem of reality. *Journal of the American Psychoanalytic Association*, 21, 5–33.
Weinstein, B. (1990). *History and theory after the fall.* Chicago: University of Chicago Press.

Internet sources

https://psychology.iresearchnet.com/social-psychology/emotions/moral-emotions/, retrieved 5/3/19.
www.britannica.com/biography/Kurt-Lewin, retrieved 5/10/19.
www.psychotherapy.net/interview/otto-kernberg, retrieved 5/12/19.
routledgesoc.com/category/profile-tags/reflexivity, retrieved 6/22/18.

2

CONFORMITY VERSUS INDEPENDENCE

Asch's line judgement studies (1951)

"In individuals, insanity is rare," said Nietzsche in *Beyond Good and Evil*, "but in groups, parties, nations, and epochs, it is the rule" (Christian, 2012, p. 494). Indeed, the Asch studies are a dramatic demonstration of "groupthink"—when ordinary people go along blindly with a group. When the individual acts in this way, "he turns his back on reality and truth" (Moscovici, 1985, p. 349). If, as Freud suggested, insanity has everything to do with repudiating reality and truth, then the participants in these iconic studies were possibly insane. But were they? Research has shown that the need to conform can lead ordinary people to change their perceptions of a situation so that conformity with the group appears entirely justified. As the iconoclastic economist John Kenneth Galbraith quipped, "Faced with the choice between changing one's mind and proving that there is no need to do so, almost everyone gets busy on the proof" (1971, p. 50). One of the key animating questions of this chapter is, why are ordinary people in a small group context willing and able to say and do things that they know don't correlate with objective reality? Or put differently, why do people go along with their peers who have no determinative authority over them, except the influence they permit?

The Asch experiments

As is often the case with great thinkers, there are childhood-based conscious and unconscious motivations that contribute to the thematics of their creative output. As Nietzsche noted, every great philosophy (or "classic" research) is "a kind of involuntary and unconscious memoir" (Solomon, 1996, p. 216). Moreover, to paraphrase Sartre, every book is an attempt to improve one's biography. Solomon Asch, who immigrated from Warsaw to the United States at thirteen years of age, told colleagues that the idea for his landmark experiment had emanated from his early childhood in Poland. As a boy of seven, he stayed up late for his first Passover *Seder* (a ritual service and ceremonial dinner for the first night in Israel or first two nights of Passover in the diaspora). He saw his grandmother pour an extra glass of wine in a ceremonial cup and asked whom it was for. "For the prophet Elijah" (who heralds the messiah), an uncle told him. "Will he really take a sip?" the little boy asked. "Oh, yes—you just watch when the time comes," the uncle replied. Excited with the sense of suggestion and expectation, Asch was convinced that he "saw the level of wine in the cup drop just a bit." It was this experience that sensitized him to the power of social pressure and conformity (Stout, 1996, n.p.).

Asch thus orchestrated an elegantly simple experiment to explore the extent to which social pressure from a majority group could influence a person to conform.[1] In social psychology, conformity is defined as "the convergence of individual's thoughts, feelings, or behavior toward a group norm" (Smith et al., 2015, p. 315). The original study, along with select follow-up studies, are summarized herein.

Asch used fifty male students from Swarthmore College to participate in a "'psychological experiment' in visual judgment" (Asch, 1955, p. 32). Using a line judgment task, Asch situated a naïve subject (the "real" participant) in a room with seven confederates, whom had consented, prior to the line task presentation, to what their responses would be. The naïve subject was not aware of this and was made to believe that the seven confederates were real participants like they were. Each person in the room had to articulate aloud which comparison line on the large white cards (A, B or C) was most similar to the standard line. The correct answer was always entirely obvious. The naïve subject sat at the end of the row of chairs and provided his or her answer last. There were 18 trials altogether, and the confederates gave the incorrect answer on 12 trials (i.e., the "critical trials"). Asch wanted to discern if the naïve subject would conform to the view of the majority. He also had a control condition that excluded any naïve subjects, only real participants. The results were astonishing. About one-third of the naïve subjects acquiesced and conformed to the obviously incorrect majority on the critical trials. Moreover, during the critical trials, about three-quarters of naïve subjects conformed on at least one occasion and one-quarter never conformed. In the control group, less than 1% of the naïve subjects gave the incorrect answer (Asch, 1951; McLeod, 2008).

In subsequent studies on *group size* (Asch, 1952, 1956), Asch found that the bigger the majority group of confederates, the more people conformed; however, this effect leveled off. When there was one confederate in the group, conformity was 3%, with two it was 13% and with three or more it was 32% (increasing the size of the majority group past three did not increase conformity, probably because naïve subjects would sense majority collusion). Other researchers have found that conformity achieves its maximum extent with a three to five person majority. This suggests that *group unanimity*, meaning the confederates are all in agreement, is more critical than group size. In another study, Asch (1956) compromised the total agreement of the majority group by adding a dissenting confederate into the situation. He reported that the mere presence of one confederate that opposes the majority choice is able to diminish conformity by as much as 80%. Other researchers have confirmed that the existence of an *ally* diminishes conformity, probably because there is less of an emotional need for group social approval.

Finally, Asch and others have found that when the comparison lines, such as A, B and C, were made to appear more alike in length and it was more difficult to discern the correct answer, conformity was amplified. In other words, when a person is *less certain* because the task is more difficult, they are inclined to seek out confirmation from others. Likewise, when naïve subjects were permitted to give their answer *in private* such that the remaining members of the group were unaware of their answer, there was a diminution of conformity, probably because there are fewer group and normative pressures, and anxiety about group repudiation is absent.

Social-psychological interpretations of the Asch experiments

Two main theories are typically used to interpret Asch's findings "that social forces constrain people's opinions and attitudes" (Asch, 1955, p. 31). "Normative social influence" (i.e., "going along" with others) assumes that individuals have a powerful desire to be liked or accepted by other persons, what some social psychologists believe is an instinct reflecting the need to be included in a group of some kind. This innate proclivity is triggered because when a group of people want to remain together there needs to be some degree of consensus with regards to rules, morals and behaviors, otherwise there would be high conflict among the members which undermines the integrity and continuity of the group (Fournier, 2018).

Such a source of conformity involves changing one's behavior to satisfy the expectations of others, a proclivity so strong it can override the fact that one may not truly believe the things one is doing or saying. Thus, so normative social theory claims, any circumstances that increase one's fear of rejection by others will increase one's conformity. Witnessing ridicule of others will sensitize a person to the negative consequences of not being in step with what is "acceptable" or "appropriate" to a group. As Janes and Olson (2000) noted, "jeer pressure," the fact that when we observe another person being ridiculed we fear similar rejection and failure, greatly increases conformity to social norms. Think of high school teenagers: their greatest fear is not being accepted by their peer group. Thus, paradoxically, according to normative social influence theory, conformity appears to be a rational, functional, instrumental and adaptive response to the situational forces at play (Spears, 2010). Such adaptation is not necessarily about contraction and passive accommodation but rather, to quote John Dewey in *Art as Experience*, it is "adaptation through expansion" (Phillips, 2015, p. 135). In psychoanalytic language, it is good reality testing to conform!

"Informational social influence" (i.e., being convinced by others) claims that social influence is rooted in the individual's desire to be correct, to possess accurate perceptions of the social world. In other words, other people's actions and opinions delineate social reality for us and we exploit this information to guide our own action and shape our own opinions. Put simply, we look to the behaviors of others, who are also in the same or similar circumstances, to see how they behave, then we follow their lead. We do this because we assume they know what they are doing and because we are significantly concerned about what others think about us. This gives us a protected course of action and fends off possible criticisms for our behavior. Conformity is thus based on social influence because we have a proclivity to rely on others as a repository of information about numerous aspects of the social world. This is especially the case in situations where there is less certainty about what is "correct" and "accurate" compared to those circumstances where we have more self-confidence about our decision-making. Unlike normative social influence theory that indicates that the reason people capitulate to peer pressure is to be liked or accepted by others, informational social influence theory emphasizes that people have a strong need to be validated by others, and that in many circumstances, other people are the most helpful and significant source of such validation for the person to understand and effectively negotiate the world. Since we can only discern reality by agreeing with others about what that reality is—it is rational, functional, instrumental and adaptive—it is again good reality testing to not completely trust one's own perceptions until others confirm that what we perceive is in fact true (Jetten & Hornsey, 2017).

Asch's studies have been used to understand such behavior as why Germans followed Nazi propaganda and the appeal of dictatorships, why bulimics and those with other kinds of eating disorders (and non-clinical eating issues) cannot resist the majority pressure to be thin, and football hooliganism and other kinds of crowd violence (ibid.). As Kurt Lewin, one of the pioneers of social psychology who was passionately committed to research that amalgamated the testing of theories with real-life problem solving, noted, "There is nothing so practical as good theory" (1951, p. 169). Needless to say, most people find it near impossible to resist pressures to conform to both small and large groups. When this dynamic is enacted in extremes, such conformity can have a calamitous impact on social systems and wider society.

Toward a psychoanalytic social psychology

As far as I know, there have not been any psychoanalytically informed discussions of Asch's studies or those that have derived from his path-breaking findings. In general, "mainstream" psychoanalytic theory would likely assume that the naïve subject's responses were in some way pathological, at least to some degree. This is in sync with the psychoanalytic tendency to privilege the individual over the situation (i.e., society) and emphasize the role of social groups as a port of entry into the deep structure of individuality (Haslam et al., 2012). For example, it is well known among analysts that groups can negatively impact how individuals think, including downgrading their ability to perceive what is taken to be reality and truth. Calling to mind Plato who conjectured about the "crowd mind," claiming that even the wisest of people, if gathered into a crowd, could be transformed into an irrational mob (Smith et al., 2015, p. 7), Freud wrote,

> Some of [a group's] features—the weakness of intellectual ability, the lack of emotional restraint, the incapacity for moderation and delay, the inclination to exceed every limit in the expression of emotion and to work it off completely

> in the form of actions—these and similar features ... show an unmistakable picture of a regression of mental activity to an earlier stage such as we are not surprised to find among savages or children.
>
> *(1921, p. 117)*

This includes the individual's self critical superego becoming "soluble" in, or merged with, the group, which allows him to avoid a sense of personal responsibility. While some may believe that the regression hypothesis illuminates the reasons for Asch's startling findings, for the most part, it is merely a generic re-description of the conformity phenomenon Asch identified rather than a convincing explanation. To claim that individuals conform to the norms of the group because there is a "regression of mental activity" is simply making Asch's point using psychoanalytic language.

Psychoanalysis cannot easily account for Asch's results, such as why naïve subjects modify their viewpoint when the majority does not put forth any reasoned arguments to justify their viewpoint. In this view, conformity is regarded as an irrational effect that prompts people to conform in a heedless, mechanical manner. Perhaps some useful insights can be gained from Asch's post-experimental interviews (1951) that point to a more compelling psychoanalytic explanation. Asch found three distinct motives for yielding to the pressure of the incorrect majority. First, a small number of naïve subjects actually came to perceive the majority judgements as correct, "repudiating the evidence of [their] senses" (Asch, 1955, p. 32). They report no awareness that their guesses had been influenced by the group majority. They see the incorrect matching standard line as the correct one ("distortion of perception"). In the language of moral psychology, we can say that for this group a lie becomes the truth.

Another small group of naïve subjects reported yielding to the group because of a powerful need not to appear different, inferior or foolish compared to others, largely due to their unwillingness and inability to withstand defectiveness in the eyes of the group. Some naïve subjects said they did not want to "spoil the study results" (ibid., p. 33). These people suppress their observations and parrot the majority decision with complete awareness of what they are doing ("distortion of action"). In the language of moral psychology, we can say that the lie becomes the spoken truth because of cowardice. Most naïve subjects, however, submit to group pressure because they reach the conclusion that their perceptions are inaccurate and those of the majority are correct, thinking "I am wrong, they are right" ("distortion of judgement") (ibid.). In moral psychology, we can say, the lie becomes the truth because everyone says it is.

These findings indicate how subtle changes in group structure have complicated and profound effects on people's thinking, or their ego functioning in psychoanalytic language. Groups undermine our reason, morality and agency (Haslam et al., 2012). The post-experimental interviews show that there are those naïve subjects whose actual ego functions (e.g., autonomous ego functioning) are drawn into an area of conflict that is resolved by distorting reality ("distortion of perception"). This perhaps calls to mind a psychotic-like way of being, or more commonly, the psychology of abused women. These women see themselves as powerless to make other choices and do not see the situation as it is—one from which they can break free. In these cases, the situational forces are real—"Where do I go? How can I afford to leave?," et cetera—and play into the internal forces of believing one is not lovable or deserving of a sane relationship.

A possible explanation for the second group who could not bear to appear different or defective ("distortion of action") might be rooted in exaggerated feelings of worthlessness, whereby they could not tolerate the shame or humiliation of being wrong. Perhaps this response calls to mind an avoidant personality-like way of being. The final group may have also lacked the ego strength and self-esteem necessary to uphold their view against the majority. They assume the majority is correct and comply with this view ("distortion of judgment"), perhaps calling to mind a dependent personality-like way of being. With all three groups, we sense the strong interpretive grip that affiliative needs have on individuals, and the difficulties that people have in detaching themselves even in benign situations. Anxiety, the fear of loss of affiliation, the inability to stand on one's own beliefs and even fear of betraying the group, are major psychological issues that psychoanalysts might believe are at play. Likewise, in addition to the afore-mentioned low self-esteem that may have animated naïve subjects' responses, there may be a feeling of self-betrayal at work, the type of self-undermining so often found in attachment disorders. Of course, all of these explanations are post-hoc and probably could not have been predicted using a mainstream or psychoanalytic viewpoint.

There are at least two aspects of Asch's studies that have importance to the development of a plausible psychoanalytic social psychology, one that enlarges the typical analytic lens of how psychoanalysis understands human behavior and treatment. First, once a person shows conformity in a particular group situation, he is inclined to regard it as justified, which is the case even if he is obligated to behave in ways that are in opposition to what he takes to be his true beliefs. In other words, the capacity for moral judgment can get seriously compromised by situational forces. To make matters even more complicated, in some group contexts an individual can regard conformity as rational, functional, instrumental and adaptive. Second, to recall, there was a small group of naïve subjects in Asch's experiments that resisted conformity under all conditions. Asch makes this distinction and its implications abundantly clear:

> Current thinking has stressed the power of social conditions to induce psychological changes arbitrarily. It has taken slavish submission to group forces as the general fact and neglected or implicitly denied the capacities of men for independence, for rising under certain conditions above group passion and prejudice.
> *(1952, p. 451)*

Asch is wisely claiming that there is a duality of structure and process in group life, situational forces that on the one hand tend to induce individual uniformity and passive responding in most people; on the other hand, these forces can induce difference and active responding, also known as resistance (Jetten & Hornsey, 2017, p. 88). As Camus said, "What is a rebel? A man who says no" (1991, p. 13). In this view, in terms of moral psychology, the opposite of conformity is courage. This being said, it is worth remembering that in the Asch experiments even those naïve subjects who held to their original answers were still trying to find ways to square their judgements with those of the majority when the experiment concluded. Holding one's ground against the majority opinion is no easy matter, as demonstrated by Ibsen when he famously wrote in *An Enemy of the People*, "The strongest man upon the earth is he who stands most alone" (Bigsby, 2005, p. 153). Though most scholarly renderings of the Asch "take home" point focuses on the dynamics of conformity, Asch cautions against appropriating too gloomy of a view of human behavior and potential: "We should be skeptical, however, of the suppositions that the power of social pressure necessarily implies uncritical submission to it: Independence and the capacity to rise above group passion are also open to human beings" (1955, p. 32).

Resistance to conformity

Some social psychologists view behavior, including conformity, as a product of two independent elements—the situation and the person. Situationalists hold that human behavior is determined by the totality of circumstances in which a person is lodged, rather than by personal attributes such as character/personality traits, motivations and limitations/biases of cognition. Situationalists, excluding "extreme" ones (Reicher & Haslam, 2006, p. 3), believe that there are dispositions, feelings, thoughts and prior experiences and behavior that can influence behavior; however, they insist that situations have a more commanding impact and are more predictive of what a person will do in a particular situation.

Take, for example, the clever study done by Darley et al. (1974) in which the investigators claimed that the person labeled as an "independent" in the Asch experiment was as much influenced by the experiment as the "conformer" had appeared to be, but the manner in which the Asch experiment was done did not demonstrate it. As Darley summarizes the study (Darley, in Evans, 1980), he notes that in the Asch experiment if you besiege naïve subjects with conformity pressure, but have one other person who gives the same answer that they do, then the naïve subject is inclined not to give in to conformist pressure. That is, the naïve subject in that situation remains independent. To prove their hypothesis, Darley and colleagues ran a second half to their original experiment in which they directed the "independent" naïve subject and the person who had previously given him social support to go off by themselves. The investigators then had the social supporter engage in conformity pressure on the naïve subject, and the conformity rate of the naïve subject became very high. As Darley explains,

> in the process of getting social support from the other person in the first place, which gave him the strength to stand against the entire group, he had been strongly bonded to the social supporter. The bonding showed up in the increased conformity with the social supporter on new topics in the second half of our experiment.
>
> *(Darley, in Evans, 1980, p. 222)*

The Darley and Asch studies, and others such as Milgram's obedience studies (1963) and Zimbardo's Stanford Prison Experiment (1971), strongly suggest that human behavior is largely determined by surrounding circumstances rather than by discrete personal attributes.

In contrast to the situationalists, most psychoanalytic theorizing that tries to comprehend the complicated interaction between social thoughts, social feelings and social behavior—the "stuff" of social psychology—relies mainly on trait or dispositional constructs in its explanations. That is, it points to the habitual modes of thought, feeling and action that emanate from an individual's character/personality, including his psychopathology, that are fairly stable and consistent over time and in situations, and that have been formed mainly in childhood. Of course, psychoanalysis recognizes that the outside world matters, society and culture (especially the family) impact people in important ways, but the locus of explanation tends to be the "inner" person and intra-psychic properties like desire and fantasy, rather than the "outer" world of situational forces. At its psychoanalytic worst, phenomena tend to be reduced to asocial, non-contextualized, abstract causes and motives (i.e., the variable as it functions in the world at large) such as character/personality, temperament, mood, individual differences and biological factors (Reicher & Haslam, 2006; Reynolds et al., 2010). Needless to say, there is truth, relevance and applicability to both points of view, which are dependent on the person and situation one is trying to understand. While individual idiosyncratic trajectories are always "part of the story," so are situational forces such as the "prototypicality within the group" (Reicher & Haslam, 2006, pp. 26, 27). Indeed, Asch asked after his experiment, "If consistency of independence or conformity in behavior is shown to be a fact [i.e., such behavior is constrained by social forces and influenced by situational pressures], how is it functionally related to qualities of character and personality?" (1955, p. 34). Why a particular person responds in one way or the other will depend on individual differences, or "character qualities which may be functionally connected with independence and yielding" (Asch, 1951, p. 230). In a certain sense, Asch, Darley, Milgram and Zimbardo all recognize that the mind and situation are created by and for each other (Haslam et al., 2012).

What Asch is hinting at is the need to understand conformity and independence, and most importantly, resistance, in terms of an interactionist point of view, one that does not simply allege that behavior is merely the result of two independent elements, the person and situation, what has been called a "mechanical interactionism" (Reynolds et al., 2010, p. 458). Playing off the language of psychological Gestalt theory (Asch was supervised in his graduate work by Max Wertheimer, one of the founders of Gestalt psychology), such a view assumes "that the whole is equal to the sum of its parts." What is more plausible is that "both person and situation are transformed though their interplay." Such a view assumes that the whole is something else or something different than the sum of its parts. The idea here is that personal attributes (e.g., character/personality traits and motivations) and situational forces (e.g., group pressures) "meet halfway," where they can operate alongside each other in the same direction (Haslam & Reicher, 2007, pp. 615, 619). "Dynamic interactionism" focuses on the psychological situation and the manner in which the perceiver gives the situation meaning. It is the situation-specific meaning that is regarded as most important for comprehending behavior. In this view, the person–situation relationship is mutually dependent, characterized by reciprocal interaction, and this dynamic constitutes a single assemblage of interrelated, interdependent and interactive elements (Reynolds et al., 2010, pp. 459, 461). The fact is that the naïve subjects in Asch's experiment were sometimes transformed by their group membership in highly negative ways. In other words, the mind and situation co-produced and co-potentiated each other. Such a view is in sync with conceptualizing a person as "being-in-the-world," as Heidegger called it. The human being is an individual unity of thought, feeling/kinesthetic and action engaged in the lived actuality of his everyday life.

While the issue at hand in the Asch experiment, making a line judgement, appeared to be a fairly trivial matter in terms of moral psychology (though it caused tremendous personal upheaval and therefore is quite profound), the danger of social influence impacting people on more morally important issues has confirmed Asch's findings. For example, Kassin and Kiechel (1996) showed how social influence can impact whether we judge ourselves as being innocent or guilty of a wrongful action. They asked college students to type letters either fairly quickly or in a less hurried pace on a computer keyboard, apparently to demonstrate their reflex speed. All participants were clearly warned not to press the ALT key, as doing so could crash the computer and cause serious data loss. When the computer malfunctioned shortly later, the upset experimenter blamed the student for pressing a forbidden key. The student at first denied the charge, but the experimenter turned to a confederate and asked, "Did you see anything?" In one condition, the confederate said he observed nothing, but in another condition, the confederate agreed that he had observed the student press the forbidden key, seemingly confirming the experimenter's allegation of guilt. The experimenter then demanded that the students sign a handwritten confession ("I hit the ALT key and caused the computer to crash. Data was lost."). The results were astonishing: 69% agreed to sign the confession. Even more troubling, 28% privately came to judge themselves as guilty. Participants were more likely to judge themselves guilty when the confederate agreed with the experimenter and particularly if the speed at which they were typing made them doubt what had actually occurred. In other words, as in Asch's studies, unsure participants were especially probable to accept the responses of manifold others even if it meant confessing to a "crime" they initially were all certain they hadn't committed (Smith et al., 2015, p. 315). In psychoanalytic language, "healthy" superego and ego functioning, a mindfulness of truth and reality, appears to have given way without much resistance to destructive social influence.

This "dynamic interactionism" whereby the mind and situation co-produce and co-potentiate each other with profound behavioral ramifications has been memorialized in what is called the social identity approach in social psychology. This approach incorporates at least two overlapping notions that draw from different social-psychological theories that have bearing on understanding individual resistance to conformist group pressure: First is the claim that self-categorization—how the environment, that is, the patterns of stimuli that comprise the perceiver, is given meaning—is an undeniable fact of social life. This represents a cognitive slant on understanding behavior (Reynolds et al., 2010, p. 459). Second, human beings appear to have a tendency to divide the social world into two distinct categories, an ingroup ("us"), the social group for which one perceives oneself to be a part (that increases self-esteem, pride and sense of belongingness), and numerous outgroups, any social group that one perceives as not one's own. In this view, social identity, those aspects of the self-concept that emanate from a person's knowledge and feelings about the group's membership he shares with others, also matters in terms of how the mind and situation co-produce and co-potentiate each other.[2] Most importantly for this chapter, a well-established identity, including one's beliefs and values, can serve as the self-enhancing "lynchpin" for important decisions that structure experiences in specific ways (ibid., p. 464). That is, individuals tend to try to increase their self-esteem, self-coherence and self-continuity by identifying with social groups (this can be based on religion, race, sex, sexual orientation, age, ethnic upbringing, job/ profession, income, et cetera). Such individuals, however, are prone to make the "ultimate attribution error" as it is called in social psychology, the proclivity to make positive attributions about members of one's group but not about members of other groups. As Freud noted in his notion of "the narcissism of minor differences," rather unimportant differences between people who are in other respects similar can become the foundation for hostile feelings between them, such as in ethnic conflicts. In the Asch experiments, when confederates were viewed as similar to the naïve subjects (the confederates were equals in power, status and resources) and made incorrect judgments about the length of lines, the group severely eroded the naïve subject's confidence and impacted his responses. In other words, according to self-categorization theory, others who are judged to be "like us" have a critical role in molding the psychology of the person, especially his decision-making behavior about both trivial and important matters (ibid., p. 470).

Asch claims that the presence of "pronounced individual differences" between those naïve subjects who acted independently versus those who yielded to group pressure "points to the important role of personal factors connected with the individual's character structure" (Asch, 1951, p. 229). The question that Asch does not adequately answer is what the likely "personal factors" are that contribute to individual resistance to group pressure and conformity. While offering a detailed rendering of this complex and profound subject is beyond the scope of this chapter, social psychologists and psychoanalytic thinkers have weighed in on this question. I will first briefly report some of the morally suggestive de-briefing information that Asch presents and later "spin-off" studies and discussions, followed by some psychoanalytically oriented formulations.

Asch tells us what some of the independent, resisting, naïve subjects said about their responses to the experimental conditions of intense group social pressure to conform. Among the independent persons there "were many who held fast because of staunch confidence in their own judgment" (Asch, 1955, p. 33). Though these independent naïve subjects were sensitive to the group and experience the conflict that Asch's experiment constructed, they displayed considerable "vigor" with which they withstood the group opposition. Moreover, "they show[ed] resilience in coping with it, which is expressed in their continuing reliance on their perception and the effectiveness with which they shake off the oppressive group opposition" (Asch, 1951, p. 228). That is, "the most significant fact about" independent resisters "was not absence of responsiveness to the majority but a capacity to recover from doubt and to reestablish their equilibrium." In other words, resistance requires prolonged courage, the ability to do something intimidating or frightening to oneself. Another group of independent naïve subjects came to think that the majority was correct in its judgments, "but they continued their dissent on the simple ground that it was their obligation to call the play as they saw it" (Asch, 1955, p. 33). These people resisted because they had a steadfast commitment to a principle of personal integrity, of being honest and holding to strong moral principles. So as Asch describes it, there are two clusters of independent naïve subjects, the confident/courageous ones who gave very little attention to the majority opinion, and those who believed that the majority was possibly correct, but they could not resist saying what they believed, as to do otherwise would be Sartrean "bad faith" (1951, p. 227).[3] It should be emphasized that while these resisters seemed to be more committed to being right and true to their beliefs about their own perceptions, they were also clearly troubled by the conflict they experienced. One of the naïve subjects who resisted conformity on all critical trials sojourned to the experimenter at the end of the debriefing and inquired, "Is there anything wrong with me?" (Jetten & Hornsey, 2017, p. 84). Moreover, on his way out of the room he declared, "This is unlike any experience I have had in my life, I will never forget it as long as I live" (Asch, 1952, p. 467).

The role of beliefs and values in resistance

When one lists the characteristics that Asch said were critical regarding the resisters—they "held fast because of staunch confidence in their own judgment," they displayed "vigor" in doing so, they showed "resilience in coping with group opposition," and they had the "capacity to recover from doubt to reestablish their equilibrium"—we are in the domain of personal beliefs and moral values that express and reflect one's autonomy, integration and humanity. Resisters in Asch's experiments were inclined to do what they felt they "should" do, rather than what they probably "wanted" to do, to take the psychologically easier path of conforming with the majority view. The question is how does this process of self-affirmation work, of maintaining independence and resistance within the context of an oppressive group pressure of equals? To suggest a rudimentary answer to this key question, I need to say something about how I understand the terms "self," "beliefs" and "values," for they are the constructs that help illuminate the "nuts and bolts" of the subjectivity of the resilient independent resisters.

Beliefs and values constitute the "self." Following philosopher Richard Rorty, the self is "a centerless network of beliefs [including values] and desires" (1991, p. 191), that is, "There is no self distinct from the self-reweaving web. All there is to a human self is just that web" (ibid., p. 93). Most importantly, these beliefs and desires are

> continually in process of being rewoven (with some old items dropped as new ones are added). This network is not one which is rewoven by an agent distinct from the network—a master weaver, so to speak. Rather, it reweaves itself, in response to stimuli such as the new beliefs acquired when, e.g. doors open.
>
> *(ibid., p. 123)*

Psychoanalyst Roy Schaefer formulates the "self" in a similar manner when he writes that the "self" is "an experiential phenomenon, a set of more or less stable and emotionally felt ways of telling oneself about one's being and one's continuity throughout change ... the self is a thought, not an agent ... a kind of retelling abut one's individuality" (1978, pp. 84, 86).

A belief, according to social psychologist Milton Rokeach, is "any simple proposition, conscious or unconscious, inferred from what a person says or does, capable of being preceded by the phrase 'I believe that ...'" (1968, p. 450). A belief system, Rokeach further notes, represents the total universe of a person's beliefs about the physical world, social world and the self. Most importantly, "whether or not the content of a belief is to describe, evaluate, or advocate action, or to do all three, all beliefs are predispositions to action" (ibid.).

> A value is a type of belief, centrally located within one's total belief system, about how one ought, or ought not, to behave, or about some end state of existence worth, or not worth, attaining. Values are thus abstract ideals, positive or negative, not tied to any specific attitude, object or situation, representing a person's beliefs about ideal modes of conduct and ideal terminal goals.
>
> *(ibid., p. 454)*

What needs to be emphasized is that belief systems and value systems have a behavioral component; they are "agendas for action." As philosopher Charles Peirce wrote, "the essence of a belief is the establishment of a habit; and different beliefs are distinguished by the different modes of action" (1955, p. 29). Rorty makes a similar point when he writes that beliefs are "successful rules for action" (1991, p. 65), as does philosopher S. Barry Barnes, who notes that "a value is a cluster of accepted modes of action" (1983, pp. 29–30).

Returning to the question of resisting and rejecting norms, such as oppressive group pressure, we can say that such people use their narrative of self-identity, their beliefs and values, to put "a particular face on a situation and thereby provoking a particular action" (Perry, 1974, pp. 408–409). That is, in situations of extreme pressure, the main function of beliefs and values is "acquiring habits of action for coping with reality" (Rorty, 1991, p. 10). Beliefs and values, like any kind of knowledge, help us get about in the world; they are ways of solving life's problems, of putting the causal forces of the universe to work for us; they are ways of "muddling through somehow," as the British say (Rorty, 1991, p. 69). Think of the resisters in Asch's experiment who were sensitive to the group and experienced the conflict, often doubting themselves, but who ultimately held their ground. As Rokeach noted, beliefs and values help the individual "understand the world insofar as possible, and to defend against it insofar as necessary" (1968, p. 446). Goffman made a similar point when he wrote that the individual is fundamentally "a stance taking entity," (1961, p. 66) and that steadfastly held beliefs and values can be vitally self-protective: "Strong religious and political convictions [i.e., beliefs and values] have served to insulate the true believer against the assaults of a total institution" (ibid., pp. 319–320). A total institution is a closed social system in which everyday life is governed by strict norms, rules and schedules (somewhat similar to Asch's experiment), and what occurs within it is dictated by a single authority whose will is implemented by staff who administer the rules, such as in a locked psychiatric facility (somewhat similar to the obedience studies done by Milgram and Zimbardo).

Thus, perhaps most importantly, what distinguishes the independent resisters from the conformist naïve subjects is that they have a consistent set of transcendent-pointing beliefs and values[4] that they adhered to. Remember the subject's vigorously-held conviction—"I call it the way I see it"—that maintaining courage and integrity in challenging moral situations, like group pressure to conform, is what matters most in terms of their authenticity as they judge it. This consistent set of transcending beliefs and values provides the resisters with the ability to make sense out of, and give direction to, their oppressive group situation. Further, it strengthened their autonomy and integration in the face of majority pressures. As Anthony Giddens notes, it is through a coherent narrative of self-identity that an individual has a feeling of biographical continuity which he is able to grasp reflexively and, to a greater or lesser degree, communicate to other people. A narrative, says Giddens, allows the person to have a regular interaction with others in the day-to-day world and to integrate events which occur in the external world and sort them into the ongoing "story" about the self. Moreover, a person with a coherent narrative of self-identity is better able to establish a "protective cocoon" which "filters out," in the practical conduct of day-to-day life, many of the dangers and primal anxieties which often threaten the integrity of the self. Such a person's ontological security—meaning his sense of presence in the world as real, alive, whole and temporally continuous—is more securely anchored (Laing, 1962). Finally, through a narrative of self-identity the individual is better able to accept integrity as worthwhile and justified. There is adequate self-regard to sustain a sense of the self as vitally "alive"—within the scope of reflexive control, rather than having the inert quality of things in the object world. In other words, it is through a coherent narrative of self-identity that a person is able to feel a greater sense of integration and personhood (Giddens, 1991).

What may have been occurring psychologically for the resisters in Asch's experiment is that with such an above-described belief/value narrative of self-identity they were better able to hold on to their autonomy, integration and humanity because of their inner attitude toward the oppressive group pressure. As Holocaust survivor Bruno Bettelheim noted about maintaining autonomy, integration and humanity in the concentration camps, "However restrictive or oppressive an environment may be, even then the individual still retains the freedom to evaluate it. On the basis of this evaluation he is also free to decide on his inner approval or resistance to what is forced upon him" (Bettelheim, 1960, p. 69). Such an attitude helped the inmate (and in a different way and to a lesser degree, the naïve subject) perceive

> [w]hat they had not perceived before; that they still retained the last, if not the greatest, of the human freedoms; to choose their own attitude in any given circumstances. Prisoners who understood this fully, came to know that this and only this, formed the crucial difference between retaining one's humanity (and often life itself) and accepting death as a human being (or perhaps physical death); whether one retained the freedom to choose autonomously one's attitude to extreme conditions even when they seemed totally beyond one's ability to influence them.
>
> *(ibid., pp. 158–159)*

The point Bettelheim is making, which Asch touched upon in a less extreme context, is that persons who find themselves in situations where there are powerful pressures to conform must be mindful of the fact that they have what Holocaust survivor Viktor Frankl called "a vestige of spiritual freedom, of independence of mind" (Frankl, 1963, p. 104). While everything can be taken away from them, including the familiar frames and filters that guide their everyday decision-making like in Asch's experiment, they still have "the last of the human freedoms—to choose one's attitude in any given circumstances, to choose one's own way" (ibid.). As Frankl further notes with a claim that powerfully resonates with Asch's findings about resisters, "There are always choices to make. Every day, every hour, offered the opportunity to make a decision, a decision which determined whether you could or could not submit to those powers which threatened to rob you of your very self, your inner freedom" (ibid.).

In light of the above formulations of Giddens, Bettelheim and Frankl, it is precisely this dialectical interplay between the person and situation that comprises a psychoanalytically animated, dynamic social interactionism, one that views the person–situation relationship as mutually dependent with reciprocal interaction. Resisters, whether in Asch's laboratory, in the concentration camps or in other less extreme everyday situations of social pressure, always have to have a relatively clear sense of how much of themselves, if any, they can give up to the environment, to the world of situational forces. However, while these beliefs and values have to be steadfastly maintained, they have to be creatively and flexibly applied and always critically evaluated and calibrated in a context-dependent and setting-specific manner. For while there are situations where complying as a strategic compromise may appear to be self-serving, they must judge how much of themselves they have relinquished before they give up what they judge as their moral outlook, their way of being-in-the-world that constitutes their sense of dignity. As Rorty has noted, the "self," those "webs of beliefs [values] and desires, of sentential attitudes … continually reweave themselves so as to accommodate new sentential attitudes" and thereby increase adaptation and adjustment to oppressive situations (Rorty, 1991, p. 93). The point is that a resister has the capacity to take his highly developed transcendent-pointing beliefs and values and creatively revise them as they conflict with the scope and content of the new recognized oppressive moral norms, but not in a way that he judges as significantly tainting, let alone subverting of his sense of being a dignified self who has maintained the rudiments of his autonomy, integration and humanity. Needless to say, in what appears to be a trivial situation like Asch's line judgment (despite the profound personal upheaval it caused), this process of moral reflection and judgment can be more difficult in certain contexts. For instance, Kassin and Kiechel's (1996) study mentioned earlier showed how social influence can impact whether we judge ourselves as being innocent or guilty of a wrongful action. Even more challenging are situations where there is great moral ambiguity and the stakes are very high, what Primo Levi called the "gray zone" in the Nazi concentration camp universe (1986, p. 58). In all of these contexts, there is a dynamic social interactionism at play between the person and situation, each co-producing and co-potentiating the other, creating a fertile breeding ground for the ordinary person to be governed in his decision-making by self-directed, self-regarding and self-serving considerations. This "easier" moral modus operandi, such as giving in to majority pressure, contrasts with those individuals who engage in a more "difficult" moral praxis, that of greater autonomy, integration and humanity, and display a mainly other-directed, other-regarding and other-serving outlook and behavior. As Hannah Arendt noted, "The fact that man is capable of action means the unexpected can be expected from him, that he is able to perform what is infinitely improbable" (1958, p. 178).

Implications for psychoanalytic treatment

"Analysis," said Freud, "does not set out to make pathological reactions impossible, but to give the patient's ego *freedom* to decide one way or another" (1923, p. 50). For Freud and all of the versions of psychoanalysis that he spawned, the goal of maximizing the analysand's freedom in terms of his capacity to think, feel and act is a central valuative attachment. However, what constitutes this freedom is radically perspectival in that there is no consensus among different analysts and psychoanalytic theories about what the word/concept means and how it is instantiated within the analytic setting. There are, says Jonathan Lear, "disparate images of freedom" about "what freedom might mean in a psychoanalytic context." Moreover, he notes that the analytic community is "at an early stage of thinking (working, playing) through" the concept as it operates in clinical practice. In other words, while "psychoanalysis seeks to promote some kind of freedom," such "freedom functions as an open-ended signifier" (Lear, 2017, p. 139). For the most part however, Lear speaks about freedom in terms of "freedom of mind," "freedom of speech" and "freedom to let be" (ibid., 151, 153, 154) with reference to intra-psychic processes, "the analysand's own developing ego-capacity to observe and rationally assess his own mental functioning" (ibid. p. 143), with the goal of generating "new possibilities for living" (ibid., p. 152). However laudable these intra-psychic properties are, what Lear does not adequately deal with in his notion of freedom as an "open-ended signifier" is what Asch puts into sharp focus and needs to be centrally integrated into any psychoanalytic notion of freedom: namely, the analysand should cultivate the moral armature and practical skillfulness to stand up against the wide range of dangerous situational forces that constitute his social existence. While Lear's notion of freedom advocates "independence" from "fitting any social role or social image"[5] (ibid., 155) (not being "phony" or disingenuous), he does not make the capacity to resist, reject and rebel against objectionable social norms central to his reflections about the goals of psychoanalytic treatment. As Freud noted in a letter to a colleague, "Our art consists in making it possible for people to be moral[6] and to deal with their wishes philosophically" (i.e., with rational autonomy) (Hale, 1971, p. 121). Exactly how these qualities of "mind and heart" can be developed by the analysand within the analytic dialogue is a subject that is beyond the scope of this chapter; however, a few comments seem necessary.

Social psychologists (Smith et al., 2015, pp. 383–385) have emphasized at least three straightforward, practical ways of fending off heavy-handed, unfair or objectionable social norms within a small group context of equals that an analyst can help cultivate. Such practical skillfulness is an expression of "cultural literacy," as Pierre Bourdieu called it (1977), a mindfulness of the world in which one is embedded, what amounts to the "sense of the game" that allows a person to effectively respond quasi-automatically in particular situations. More specifically, it is a developed sense of situational awareness that matters most, defined in military contexts as increased awareness of one's surroundings (time and space) and identification of potential threats and dangerous situations. For example, being mindful of how norms work and how they can be used to subvert a person is critical. Research has shown that when a person perceives how a social norm is being used to influence him, such as to conform to group pressure, it loses its power over his decision-making. Even something as simple as pointing out that one is being asked to comply helps to curtail such scheming tactics (Cialdini, 2008). Psychoanalytically speaking, such individual self-assertion and self-affirmation requires courage and moral conviction.

In general, social norms have such a strong interpretive grip on one's outlook and behavior because of the intense emotional connections between people, connections that "really matter" to a person. For example, in Asch's experiment the group was perceived as a solidified and cohesive entity, at least in the mind of the naïve subject engaged in a seemingly collective task, and such a condition influenced him toward conformity. It is a well-known observation that conformity fosters a feeling of safety and often provides concrete rewards. In general, people prefer warm consensus to their group, community and larger social environs to the distress associated with not conforming. However, when an individual is in such a group setting where social norms are being pressured, or are direct "assault[s] upon self" as Goffman called it (1961, p. 36), the self-assertion and self-affirmation of one's personal beliefs and values to the group can make a huge difference in terms of avoiding conformity. In fact, when researchers had some people reflect on their own personal beliefs and values, their behavior was less inclined to follow group norms (Binning et al., 2010). Psychoanalytically speaking, this requires understanding that within a group setting the "tools" of control, power and social governance operate to undermine individual autonomy, integration and humanity. As Michel Foucault noted, "discipline," the mechanism of power which regulates the behavior of individuals in the social body such as through normalizing judgment "may be identified neither with an institution nor with an apparatus; it is a type of power, a modality for its exercise, comprising a whole set of instruments, techniques, procedures, levels of application, targets; it is a 'physics' or an 'anatomy' of power, a technology" (1977, p. 215). In the Asch experiment, discipline was meant to bring about individual conformity through the normalizing judgment of oppressive group pressure. Conceived by Foucault, discipline is one way that power is exercised to make the individual useful and intelligible, manipulatable and analyzable. For the analysand who does not understand how he has been normalized (e.g., homogenized and individualized via a created ideal of behavior) into a strategy of disciplinary power that he does recognize as operative, he is doomed to comply and conform. If, however, he is aware of how these power relations produce different kinds of knowledge (power and knowledge always implicate each other for Foucault) that collect and combine, he has the chance to "push back" and resist conformity. While power/knowledge relations exist in every society, including in small group settings of equals like in the Asch experiment, they can be criticized and resisted in specific and changing situations in space and time. As Foucault notes, resistance is always a possibility, especially to more subtle situations of group pressure among equals, but only if one is critically aware that conformity is at play.

It is important for the analysand to cultivate a "postmodern" sensibility in the face of group pressure. By embracing an open, modifiable, reflexively monitoring notion of self-identity, one questions the possibility of any absolute truth and knowledge (e.g., metaphysical or universal truths). Therefore, the analysand hopefully recognizes that because all situations are open to multiple "storying," or to different perspectives, how one defines a situation is as credible as another person's definition or group interpretation. Using this mode of thinking, the individual has undercut, or at least questioned, the hold that the group's definition of the situation has on him. Moreover, in a group situation the faster a participant provides an alternative perspective on a situation the better, since the longer you are under the "spell" of the group, the more difficult it will be to resist group pressure to conform. In short, the faster you put forth an alternative perspective to the so-called "fact pattern," the freer you and other group members will feel to resist pressure to conform.

Final remarks

"The judges of normality are present everywhere," said Foucault, "[w]e are in the society of the teaching-judge, the doctor-judge, the educator-judge, the social worker-judge; it is on them that the universal reign of the normative is based; and each individual, wherever he may find himself, subjects to it his body, his gestures, his behavior, his aptitudes, his achievements" (1977, p. 304). Indeed, Asch's experiment dramatically demonstrates how the normalizing judgement of a small group of equals can so influence you that your sense of truth and reality gives way to what you may know is actually not true or real. Such conformity to a group, and by extension to another person, a crowd or even an authoritarian regime, evades and denies individual freedom (Cooper, 2015, p. 99). It is these considerations that in part constitute "the inescapable moral dimension to human existence" (Asch, 1990, p. 53).

The only tried and true antidote to this web of control, power and social governance is through having the will and ability to resist, which in this context means being mindful of one's freedom. As Rollo May noted, "freedom is the capacity to pause in the face of stimuli from many directions at once and, in this pause, to throw one's weight towards this response rather than that one" (1981, p. 54). Moreover, this will or agency is based on the awareness that "[t]he defiant power of the spirit" (Frankl, 1988, p. 73), his transcendent-pointing beliefs and values, can give a person the pragmatic skillfulness to stand over, above or beyond social-psychological pressures that undermine autonomy, integration and humanity. This resolutely held freedom that is the basis for actualizing the best of who one can be is what Paul Tillich calls the "courage to be" (2000). It requires vigilance and the incessant critical analysis of how power enacts behavior in specific situations. As Asch noted, "Most social acts have to be understood in their setting, and lose meaning if isolated. No error in thinking about social facts is more serious than the failure to see their place and function" (1952, p. 161). Indeed, such an "error in thinking" in the context of social pressure to conform can be lethal.

Notes

1 The renowned Stanley Milgram noted, "For me Asch's experiment rotates as a kind of permanent intellectual jewel. Focus analytic light on it, and it diffracts energy into new and interesting patterns" (Blass, 2004, p. 282).

2 Social identity theory typically involves three intra-psychic processes: social categorization, meaning we categorize ourselves and others in order to efficiently comprehend them (e.g., "blacks and whites"); social identification, meaning we embrace the identity of the ingroup (e.g., a person emotionally and practically identifies with being black or Jewish); finally, once we have categorized ourselves as part of the ingroup, and have emotionally and practically identified with that group, we then are inclined to positively compare our group with other groups (Tajfel & Turner, 1979).

3 Bad faith is Sartre's evocative term for describing a form of self-deception when a person under pressure from social forces embraces false values and renounces their inborn freedom, thus assuming an inauthentic way of being-in-the-world.

4 Self-transcending beliefs and values can reflect "vertical" or "horizontal" transcendence. For example, Gabriel Marcel, a "believer," was committed to "the transcendence, holiness, and sanctity of Christ and the martyrs." The "non-believer," Albert Camus, was committed to horizontal transcendence as manifested by charity, humanity and solidarity. Thus, for Marcel transcendence was rooted in divinity while for Camus it was rooted in history (Marcus, 2019, p. 11).

5 Lear does not seem to adequately recognize that to some extent we all need and want to "fit in," and therefore at times we assume a social role and image that is context-dependent and setting-specific. The importance is whether we choose to do this because we judge that the social role and social image is in sync with our reasoned beliefs and values or because of mindless conformity to oppressive or subtle norms. The goal is "to be what you seem" because you have chosen to do so.

6 As Freud wrote, "I consider myself a very moral human being … I believe that in a sense of justice and consideration for one's fellow men, in discomfort at making others suffer or taking advantage of them … I have never done anything shameful or malicious, nor do I find in myself the temptation to do so" (Hale, 1971, p. 189).

References

Arendt, H. (1958). *The human condition*. Chicago: University of Chicago Press.

Asch, S.E. (1951). Effects of group pressure upon the modification and distortion of judgment. In H. Guetzkow (Ed.), *Groups, leadership and men* (pp. 177–190). Pittsburgh: Carnegie Press.

Asch, S.E. (1952). *Social psychology*. Englewood Cliffs: Prentice Hall.

Asch, S.E. (1955). Opinions and social pressure. *Scientific American*, 193, 31–35.

Asch, S.E. (1956). Studies of independence and conformity: I. A minority of one against a unanimous majority. *Psychological Monographs: General and Applied*, 70(9), 1–70.

Asch, S.E. (1990). Comments on D. T. Campbell's Chapter. In I. Rock (Ed.), *The legacy of Solomon Asch: Essays in cognition and social psychology* (pp. 53–56). New York: Psychology Press.

Barnes, B. (1983). *T.S. Kuhn and social sciences*. New York: Columbia University Press.

Bettelheim, B. (1960). *The informed heart: Autonomy in a mass age*. Glencoe, IL: The Free Press.

Bigsby, C. (2005). *Arthur Miller: A critical study*. Cambridge: Cambridge University Press.

Binning, K.R., Sherman, D.K., Cohen, G.L. & Heitland, K. (2010). Seeing the other side: Reducing political partisanship via self-affirmation in the 2008 presidential election. *Analysis of Social Issues and Public Policy*, 10(1), 276–292.

Blass, T. (2004). *The man who shocked the world*. New York: Basic Books

Bourdieu, P. (1977). *Outline of a theory of practice*. Cambridge: Cambridge University Press.

Camus, A. (1991). *The rebel: An essay on man in revolt*. New York: Vintage International.

Christian, J. (2012). *Philosophy: An introduction to the art of wondering*. Boston: Wadsworth.

Cialdini, R.B. (2008). *Influence: Science and practice* (5th ed.). New York: Allyn & Bacon.

Cooper, M. (2015). *Existential psychotherapy and counselling. Contributions to a pluralistic practice*. Thousand Oaks, CA: Sage.

Darley, J.M., Moriarty, T., Darely, S. & Berscheid, E. (1974). Increased conformity to a fellow deviant as a function of prior deviation. *Journal of Experimental Social Psychology*, 10, 211–223.

Evans, R.I. (1980). *The making of social psychology: Discussions with creative contributors*. New York: Gardner Press.

Foucault, M. (1977). *Discipline and punishment: The birth of the prison*. A. Sheridan (Trans.) New York: Vintage Books.

Fournier, G. (2018). Normative social influence. *Psych Central*. https://psychcentral.com/encyclopedia/normative-social-influence/.

Frankl, V.E. (1963). *Man's search for meaning*. New York: Pocket Books.

Frankl, V.E. (1988). *The will to meaning: Foundations of and applications of logotherapy*. London: Meridian.

Freud, S. (1921) [1955]. Group psychology and the analysis of the ego. In J. Strachey (Ed. & Trans.), *The standard edition of the complete psychological works of Sigmund Freud* (Vol. 13, pp. 65–143). London: Hogarth Press.

Freud, S. (1923) [1961]. Ego and id. In J. Strachey (Ed. & Trans.), *The standard edition of the complete psychological works of Sigmund Freud* (Vol. 19, pp. 3–63). London: Hogarth Press.

Galbraith, J. K. (1971). *Economics, peace and laughter*. Boston: Houghton Mifflin.

Giddens, A. (1991). *Modernity and self-identity*. Stanford: Stanford University Press.

Goffman, E. (1961). *Asylums*. New York: Anchor Books.

Hale, N.G. (Ed.) (1971). *James Jackson Putnam and psychoanalysis: Letters between Putnam and Sigmund Freud, Ernest Jones, William James, Sandor Ferenczi and Morton Prince. 1877–1917*. J.B. Heller (Trans.). Cambridge: Cambridge University Press.

Haslam, S.A. & Reicher, S. (2007). Beyond the banality of evil: The dynamics of an interactionist social psychology of tyranny. *Personality, Social Psychology and Behavior*, 33(5), 615–622.

Haslam, S.A., Reicher, S.D. & Reynolds, K.J. (2012). Identity, influence, and change: Rediscovering John Turner's vision for social psychology. *British Journal of Social Psychology*, 51(2), 201–218.

Janes, L. & Olson, J.M. (2000). Jeer pressure: The behavioral effects of observing ridicule of others. *Personality and Social Psychology Bulletin*, 26, 474–485.

Jetten, J. & Hornsey, M.J. (2017). Conformity: Revisiting Asch's line-judgment studies. In J.R. Smith & S.A. Haslam (Eds.), *Social psychology: Revisiting the classic studies* (2nd ed., pp. 77–92). Thousand Oaks, CA: Sage.

Kassin, S.M. & Kiechel, K.L. (1996). The social psychology of false confessions: Compliance, internalization, and confabulation. *Psychological Science*, 7, 125–128.

Laing, R.D. (1962). Ontological insecurity. In H.M. Ruitenbeek (Ed.), *Psychoanalysis and existential philosophy* (pp. 41–69). New York: E.P. Dutton and Co.

Lear, J. (2017). *Wisdom won from illness: Essays in philosophy and psychoanalysis*. Cambridge: Harvard University Press.

Levi, P. (1986). *The drowned and the saved*. New York: Summit.

Lewin, K. (1951). Problems in research in social psychology. In D. Cartwright (Ed.), *Field theory is social science* (pp. 155–169). New York: Harper & Row.

McLeod, S.A. (2008). *Asch experiment*. www.simplypsychgology.org/asch-conformity.html.

Marcus, P. (2019). *The psychoanalysis of overcoming suffering: Flourishing despite pain*. Abingdon: Routledge.

May, R. (1981). *Freedom and destiny*. London: W.W. Norton and Co.

Milgram, S. (1963). Behavioural study of obedience. *Journal of Abnormal and Social Psychology*, 67, 371–378.

Moscovici, S. (1985). Social influence and conformity. In G. Lindzey & E. Aronson (Eds.), *Handbook of social psychology* (Vol. 2, pp. 347–412). New York: Random House.

Perry, R.B. (1974). *The thought and character of William James* (Vol. II). Westport, CT: Greenwood Press.

Phillips, A. (2015). *Forbidden pleasures*. New York: Farrar, Straus and Giroux.

Peirce, C. (1955). *Philosophical writings of Pierce*. J. Buchler (Ed.). New York: Dover Publications.

Reicher, S. & Haslam, S.A. (2006). Rethinking the psychology tyranny: The BBC prison study. *British Journal of Social Psychology*, 45, 1–40.

Reynolds, K.J., Turner, J.C., Branscombe, N.R., Mavor, K.I., Bizumic, B. & Subasic, E. (2010). Interactionism in personality and social psychology: An integrated approach to understanding the mind and behavior. *European Journal of Personality*, 24, 458–482.

Rokeach, M. (1968). Attitudes. In D.L. Sills (Ed.), *International encyclopedia of the social sciences* (Vol. 1, pp. 450–454). New York: Macmillan Company and the Free Press.

Rorty, R. (1991). *Objectivity, relativism, and truth: Philosophical papers*. Cambridge: Cambridge University Press.

Schaefer, R. (1978). *The analytic attitude*. New York: Basic Books.

Smith, E.R., Mackie, D.M. & Claypool, H.M. (Eds.) (2015). *Social psychology* (4th ed.). New York: Psychology Press.

Solomon, R.C. (1996). Nietzsche ad hominem: Perspectivism, personality, and resentiment revisited. In B. Magnus & K.M. Higgins (Eds.), *The Cambridge companion to Nietzsche* (pp. 218–222). Cambridge: Cambridge University Press.

Spears, R. (2010). Group rationale, collective sense: Beyond intergroup bias. *British Journal of Social Psychology*, 49, 1–20.

Stout, D. (1996). Solomon Asch is dead; a leading social psychologist. *The New York Times*, 02/29/96, n.p.

Tajfel, H. & Turner, J.C. (1979). An integrative theory of intergroup conflict. In W.G. Austin & S. Worchel (Eds.), *The social psychology of intergroup relations* (pp. 33–48). Monterey: Brooks-Cole.

Tillich, P. (2000). *The courage to be* (2nd ed.). New Haven, CT: Yale University Press.

Zimbardo, P. G. (1971). *The power and pathology of imprisonment.* Congressional Record. (Serial No. 15, 10/25/71). Hearings before Subcommittee No. 3, of the Committee on the Judiciary, House of Representatives, 92nd Congress, First Session on Corrections, Part II, Prisons, Prison Reform and Prisoners' Rights: California. Washington, DC: U.S. Government Printing Office.

3

HARMONY VERSUS DISHARMONY BETWEEN BELIEFS AND BEHAVIOR

Festinger's cognitive dissonance (1954)

"What happens to a person's private opinion if he is forced to do or say something contrary to that opinion?" This is how Leon Festinger and James M. Carlsmith (1959, p. 113) began their landmark article on cognitive dissonance, "one of the best-known and prolifically documented theories in social psychology" (Cooper, 2007, p. 6). In fact, there have been more than "a thousand research articles" written in Festinger's name (ibid., p. 29).[1] Festinger and Carlsmith's answer to their question was brilliant in its elegant simplicity: individuals hate inconsistency among their cognitions (e.g., beliefs, values and ideals) and thus, mental representations that are inconsistent with each other generate psychological stress similar to an unpleasant drive state that, like other drive states such as hunger, needs to be reduced. In addition, the more significant the cognitions to the individual, the greater the urgency to reduce any seeming inconsistency (Cooper, 2017, pp. 43–44). Put simply, Festinger and Carlsmith claimed that when a person is faced with "facts" or evidence that contradict their personal beliefs, values and ideals they will create a way to resolve the contradiction in order to reduce their stress and discomfort. This need to reduce dissonance, that which is "psychologically uncomfortable," as Festinger first described it (Festinger, 1957, p. 3), is especially salient when one engages in attitude-inconsistent behavior. As Festinger noted, "It is the idea of cognitive invention, cognitive distortion, cognitive change to make your view of the world fit with how you feel or what you are doing: That was the basic idea out of which the formulation of dissonance theory developed" (Evans, 1980, pp. 128–129).[2] For example, studies have shown that the great majority of American college students opposed cheating when they begin their studies; however, anonymous surveys indicate that many of them end up cheating in one form or another by the time they complete their undergraduate degree (Storch & Storch, 2003). How they justify their immoral behavior, or how adults rationalize ill-conceived and ill-fated behavior—like cheating on their income taxes, eating unhealthy food, engaging in cigarette smoking or taking illegal/harmful drugs—are the kinds of everyday behaviors on which cognitive dissonance theory focuses. However, dissonance processes may also have a positive function, including fostering psychotherapy effectiveness. They have also been a useful framework to understand child-rearing practices, economic and political behavior, and psychopathology (Cooper, 2007, pp. 164, 182).

While Festinger's cognitive dissonance theory assumes that in general, people are driven ("hard wired"; Cooper, 2007, p. 81) to strive for psychological consistency so as to effectively function in the real-world, and they vigorously engage in a wide range of dissonance-reducing strategies and tactics to help them live a more flourishing life, such an outlook is not wholeheartedly embraced by others who view the human condition differently. For example, Ralph Waldo Emerson wrote in his famous essay *Self Reliance*, "A foolish consistency is the hobgoblin of little minds, adored by little statesmen and philosophers and divines. With consistency a great soul has nothing to do" (2007, p. 19). Likewise, Walt Whitman noted in *Song of Myself*, "Do I contradict myself? Very well, then I contradict myself, I am large, I contain multitudes" (Reynolds, 2005, p. 88). Finally, Freud believed "neurosis had its origin in the inability to tolerate ambiguity" (Boym, 2010, p. 65). What Emerson, Whitman and especially Freud were getting at is that ambiguity and the uncertainty it evokes, particularly when it is rooted in ambivalence, characterize the human condition. The existence of contradictions in the domains of volition, such as the wish to do something and not do something, the intellect, such as believing in two contradictory ideas, and emotions, such as feeling love and hate for the same significant other, is commonplace in many social contexts (Akhtar, 2009, p. 12). In fact, for Freud and his followers, in important matters related to love, work, communal relations and faith, learning to creatively "live with" the ambiguity, uncertainty and ambivalence, rather than attempting to resolve it via a cognitive strategy the way Festinger and his followers suggest, is part of the art of living a flourishing life.[3] As well-known psychoanalysts like Jacques Lacan, Melanie Klein, Wilfred Bion and others have suggested, human subjectivity is best conceived as fragmented, decentered and discontinuous, even schizoid, as philosopher Felix Guattari and psychoanalyst Gilles Deleuze have argued, rather than being a rational, reified and substantivized entity. There is no "fixed," "true" or "deep" self in this view. The point is that Festinger's theory is built on a version of the human condition that does not adequately reckon with the fact that there are profound emotional forces at play, often unconscious ones animated by desire, phantasy, drive and affect, for human experience in our era is characterized by multiplicity, contradiction and dissolution (Frosch, 1989, p. 228).[4] This is one of the reasons that even if you make a rational choice, one that seems to be the best option given the context, you still can feel uncomfortable cognitive dissonance. Sounding like a postmodern-influenced psychoanalyst at his best, Mohandas Gandhi wisely put it, "My aim is not to be consistent with my previous statements on a given question, but to be consistent with truth as it may present itself to me at a given moment. The result has been that I have grown from truth to truth" (Jack, 1979, p. 10).[5]

Notwithstanding Festinger's oversimplified notion of human subjectivity, especially his overemphasis on the psychological importance, if not feasibility, of consistency in everyday functioning and creating a flourishing life, it is undeniable that there is much to learn from his marvelous experiments (and subsequent studies by others) on how attitude change occurs, including as it pertains to living a moral life (Festinger, 1957; Festinger, 1962; Festinger & Carlsmith, 1959; Festinger et al., 1956). It is to this topic that I now turn.

Festinger's two studies: When prophecy fails and cognitive consequences of forced compliance

In their book, *When Prophecy Fails: A Social and Psychological Study of a Modern Group that Predicted the Destruction of the World* (1956), Festinger and his colleagues (henceforth, Festinger), investigated a Chicago-based UFO cult religion Festinger named the Seekers that strongly believed that the world was going to be destroyed on December 21, 1955. The inspiration for the study came when Festinger had read in a local newspaper, "Prophecy from Planet Clarion Call to City: Flee that Flood. It'll Swamp Us on Dec.21, Outer Space Tells Suburbanite." The Seekers, who usually shunned the public, had utterly prepared for the apocalyptic day. They resigned from their employment, left college, and gave away their possessions and savings, all before they would leave on a flying saucer that was to rescue this band of die-hard, true believers. The leader, Marian Keech, a housewife who had dabbled with automatic writing (the claimed psychic ability that permits a person to generate written words without consciously writing), allegedly received a message from an imaginary planet called Clarion that told her that at midnight on December 21, a spaceship was to land at her home to shuttle the group of true believers to safety. In particular, Festinger and his colleagues were focusing on how the spiritual aspirants "managed" their outlook and behavior when the event did not happen on the morning of December 22 and the few months after. Festinger reasoned that the discrepancy between Keech's end-of-the-world prediction/prophecy and the observation of the world still existing was a dramatic cognitive inconsistency, allowing him to investigate the dissonance that his theory claimed needed to be reduced. Indeed, Festinger's prediction was correct, the Seekers would not merely maintain their aforementioned belief system, but would become more zealous in affirming it. As Festinger wrote, "If more and more people can be persuaded that the system of beliefs is correct, then clearly it must, after all, be correct" (Festinger et al., 1956, p. 28).

On the morning of December 22, Keech had received further communications from God, the key inconsistency-reducing message being, "This little group sitting all night long had spread so much light that God had saved the world from destruction," thus explaining why the prophecy did not happen (Cooper, 2017, p. 46). In other words, the Seekers' original belief system was affirmed as correct, "A greater being—God of the Earth Himself—had tested this group of Seekers and found their goodness so overwhelming that he decided to spare the world from destruction" (ibid.). In a follow-up message shortly after, Cooper notes, God had declared his message was a Christmas one and ordered it to be disseminated to the People of Earth, which is exactly what Mrs. Keech did via the *Associated Press* and other newspapers. With this divinely affirmed belief propelling them, they became vigorous proselytizers, and by gaining additional social support from other converts, their transcendence-pointing belief-system was strengthened. The point, Festinger noted, was that through this creative dissonance-reducing strategy the Seekers had stunningly reconciled the false prediction/prophecy with reality. By resolving the inconsistency between their beliefs, behavior and reality, they maintained the integrity and viability of what sociologists Peter L. Berger and Thomas Luckmann (1966) famously called their "symbolic universe."[6] In fact, for the Seekers it was only due to their divinely inspired, die-hard, belief-driven efforts that they saved the world from destruction. As Cooper concludes, "As Festinger and his fellow researchers had surmised, if everyone believed it was so, then it must have been so" (2017, p. 47).[7]

It was from this participatory observational study[8] that Festinger generated five conditions that he claimed must be in existence for a person to become a more zealous believer after a disconfirmation of a life and identity-defining belief, such as world destruction on a particular day, or more recently, the disconfirmation of the belief that the *Rebbe,* Menachem Mendel Schneerson, of the Chabad Orthodox Jewish sect, was the Messiah, though he died of a stroke in 1994. Some Chabad members continued to believe (and still do) that the *Rebbe* would rise from the dead and return, maintaining a messianic belief despite evidence that it was clearly false (Berger, 2008). These five dissonance-reducing conditions are as follows:

1. The belief has to be maintained with strong moral commitment (e.g., the world will be destroyed on a particular day because of its sinfulness) and it has to have some pertinence to the believer's behavior, that is, to what he does in his everyday life (e.g., quit work, leave college and give away one's possessions and savings, in preparation for divinely ordained rescue).
2. The believer must have devoted himself to the belief (e.g., his life revolved around the cult, the outlook and behavior required of the Seekers). He has to engage in some significant behavior that is difficult to reverse (e.g., quit work, leave college and give away one's possessions and savings). All things being equal, the more significant such behavior is, and the more difficult it is to reverse, the greater is the believer's devotion to the belief.
3. The belief has to be adequately specific and relevant to everyday life so that events may clearly disconfirm the belief (e.g., the world not being destroyed).
4. Such undeniable disconfirmatory evidence must happen and must be identified as such by the believer maintaining the belief (e.g., world destruction did not happen on a particular day).
5. The individual believer must have robust social support in maintaining his belief (e.g., it was the view of the Seekers that it was due to their goodness and faith that the world was saved). It is improbable that a solitary believer could tolerate the kind of disconfirming evidence that has been delineated in the case of the

Seekers (e.g., the world was not destroyed). By the believer being a member of a fellowship of convinced persons that provided backing and encouragement for one another, the belief may be sustained, and, according to Festinger, the believers may engage in proselytizing or persuade nonmembers that the belief is not only accurate, but morally praise- and alliance-worthy.

While Festinger's five conditions aptly describe the dissonance-reducing strategies that people often use to grapple with disconfirmatory evidence of a life and identity-defining belief—on the way to more aggressively reaffirming their belief system—what is not adequately appreciated, despite being common knowledge among sociologists, is that people do not give up their symbolic universe easily, "a particular manner of construing the world" (Geertz, 1973, p. 10). Religion, psychoanalysis, politics and even social psychology can operate as symbolic worlds. Psychoanalysis, for example, as a life- and identity-defining narrative, has its own versions of the human condition and its own ideas of what constitutes the flourishing life (Marcus & Rosenberg, 1998). A symbolic world has its own notions of how to effectively assimilate the emotionally dissonant experiences of life, including suffering and death, "into a comprehensive explanation of reality and human destiny" (Berger & Berger, 1972, p. 352). The Seekers, like psychoanalysts and social psychologists, are attracted to the "vision of reality," to the system of meaning and metaphor that it promulgates (Schafer, 1976, p. 22).

The point is that men and women need to have a rich personal and social existence, a meaning-giving, affect-integrating, action-guiding symbolic universe, to sustain against the outrageousness of everyday life, including challenges to "core," life- and identity-defining beliefs, values and ideals, and the behavior that supports them. While specifying how individuals fashion and maintain a symbolic world for themselves is beyond the scope of this chapter, what does need to be emphasized is that in the case of the Seekers, their social construction of reality involved the creation of a way of being and living that has a "family resemblance" to what Peter L. Berger (1969) called a "sacred canopy." As Berger noted, within a socially constructed world, the main function of religion conceived as "sacred canopy" is that of theodicy, the legitimation of anomic experiences, which includes reconciling the failed prediction/prophecy of the Seekers. Another way of looking at this notion is via the often-cited Thomas theorem that affirms, "If men define situations as real, they are real in their consequences" (Thomas & Thomas, 1928, pp. 571–572). In other words, how one interprets a situation motivates the action. Like Berger and Luckmann (1966) in their description of habitualization (i.e., society as taken-for-granted habit), Thomas claims that our moral codes and social norms are created by a successive series of definitions of the situation, which was powerfully evident in the Seekers' belief system and display of dissonance-reducing actions. Likewise, sociologist Robert K. Merton's notion of self-fulfilling prophecy, a false definition of the situation that induces a new behavior, which makes the originally false notion come true, helps explain how even a false idea can become true if it is acted upon. These sociological concepts were not evidently a significant part of

Festinger's study of the Seekers, nor of cognitive dissonance theory in general (Cooper, 2007, 2017).

In the famous study, "Cognitive Consequences of Forced Compliance" (Festinger & Carlsmith, 1959), the exemplification of the "induced compliance" paradigm of cognitive dissonance, naïve subjects were offered either a dollar or twenty dollars as a reward for telling a stranger that some boring task that they had just completed was actually very interesting. One of these tasks comprised placing spools on a tray, dumping them out and repeating the process a number of times. After enacting the attitude-inconsistent behavior, that is, telling the stranger that the boring task was very interesting, naïve subjects were requested to specify their own liking for those boring tasks. As predicted, those naïve subject who were given a dollar for misleading a stranger actually reported liking the tasks more than those given the twenty dollars. In other words, the investigators demonstrated what has been called the "less-is-better effect" (Hsee, 1998): The paradoxical observation that fewer rewards for counter-attitudinal behaviors (e.g., the naïve subject telling the stranger the above-mentioned experimental task was interesting when it was boring) often generate more dissonance, and thus more attitude changes. Put simply, the fewer the rewards, reasons and justifications, the more a person will modify his attitude.

For example, in one experiment, Hsee requested that naïve subjects guesstimate how much they would pay for a specific set of dishes. The first set, option one, contained forty pieces with nine that were broken, while the second set, option two, had twenty-four pieces that were unbroken. When evaluated separately, the greater majority of naïve subjects were willing to pay more for option two, when evaluated together, the majority of the naïve subjects chose option one, rationalizing that even if there were nine broken plates, there were still thirty-one unbroken ones compared to twenty-four in the second option. In other words, the naïve subjects who were evaluated separately were happier with a twenty-four-piece set of dishes that was intact than a thirty-one-piece set in which a few dishes were broken. The fact that the thirty-one-piece set of dishes included all the pieces of the twenty-four-piece set, and all of them were intact, was not important to the naïve subjects, for all they could perceive was the loss of the broken dishes. As Hsee theorized it, the less-is-better-effect can be clarified because when evaluating an option on its own, naïve subjects are inclined to concentrate on the easy attributes to evaluate, rather than the more significant attributes.[9]

It should be noted that the less-is-better effect has been verified by countless studies, but the finding has some qualifications. For example, the less-is-better effect is only operative when the naïve subject believes that he has the freedom to perform or not perform the attitude-inconsistent behavior in the specific situation he is in. Likewise, lesser rewards induce greater attitude change only when the naïve subject believes that he is personally responsible for the chosen modus operandi and has to bear alone any undesirable impact it may have. Finally, if the naïve subject believes that the financial payment is a bribe rather than a well-earned fee for service, there will not be any attitude change. For the most part, as these conditions are often part of a decision-making context, offering a naïve subject less reward can be an effective way of getting him to say or do things that are attitude-inconsistent (Baron & Byrne, 2003, pp. 150–151).

Social-psychological explanations of cognitive dissonance

While dissonance theory is probably the most important and cited theory in social psychology, there are wide-ranging, lively disputes regarding this "general theory of human behavior" (Kenworthy et al., 2011, p. 48) that aim to comprehend "the nature of human cognition and motivation" (ibid., p. 38). This includes "the theoretical origin of dissonance arousal and empirical uncertainty about the moderating variables [e.g., choice, consequences] that identify the necessary and sufficient conditions for the arousal of dissonance" (ibid.). Even the definition of dissonance, what constitutes discomfort and whether it "is a drive" or only has "motivational characteristics" is disputed (ibid., p. 40).

There are at least four theories for explaining what the role is of cognitions pertaining to the self, in the arousal and reduction of cognitive dissonance, including making different predictions (Stone & Cooper, 2001, pp. 228, 229). By cognitions, Festinger means that any kind of knowledge is "a psychological representation," though most cognitions are not conscious (Cooper, 2007, p. 6).[10] The first theory, the self-consistency model, suggests that cognitions about the self depict standards or expectancies that evoke dissonance arousal (Aronson & Carlsmith, 1962). The second theory, the self-affirmation model, suggests that cognitions about the self act as resources for dissonance reduction (Steele et al., 1993). The third theory, the new look model, suggests that cognitions about the self are immaterial to both dissonance arousal and reduction; what matters is violation of social norms (Cooper & Fazio, 1984). The fourth theory, the self-standards model, which is a refinement of the new look model, proposes that the foundation of dissonance motivation and the role played by cognitions about the self rely on the type of self-standards made accessible in the context of inconsistent behavior (Stone & Cooper, 2001). "Accessibility" in cognitive dissonance theory refers to the ease with which a specific cognition, such as a standard of judgment, can be called into mind (Cooper, 2007, p. 108). I will briefly review these theories[11] before providing a psychoanalytic gloss on cognitive dissonance.

Self-consistency theory

Self-consistency theory (Aronson, 1968; Thibodeau & Aronson, 1992) proposes that individuals maintain self-expectancies (i.e., personal standards of conduct) for competent, rational and moral behavior that they generate from the normative morals and values in society. The self is viewed as a set of expectations. Dissonance upsurges when individuals perceive an inconsistency between the behavior, such as promulgating a counter-attitudinal belief or engaging in a dubious decision, and the self-expectancies for competence, rationality and morality. The reduction of dissonance is geared to sustain a sense of competence, rationality and morality via the justification of the inconsistent behavior. Self-consistency theory additionally asserts that it is self-esteem that curbs the dissonance arousal experience because the perception of what instantiates incompetent, irrational or immoral behavior is a consequence of the expectations an individual maintains for their behavior. For example, a person with low self-esteem who has minimalist expectations of behaving morally would be less likely to judge their behavior as immoral if they did not give back a hundred dollar bill of change that the cashier accidentally gave him instead of the correct ten dollar one. Such a person would not feel dissonance at his immoral behavior, while a person with high self-esteem who has maximalist expectations of behaving morally would experience dissonance and make efforts to self-justify, that is, return the hundred dollar bill to the cashier and reduce dissonance. Thus, when a person has more favorable self-conceptions, he is more susceptible to the upsurge of dissonance following immoral behavior.

According to Festinger's theory, a situation that generates the cognition, "water is falling from the sky and I remain dry," or, "I read information that smoking is bad for me but I continue to smoke," would generate dissonance. In self-consistency theory, only the second statement would actually do so (Cooper, 2007, pp. 95, 96). That is, the self needs to be engaged in the dissonance arousal. As Aronson succinctly put it, "At the heart of dissonance theory, where it makes its strongest predictions, we are not dealing with just any two cognitions" as in the first cognition mentioned above; "rather, we are usually dealing with the self-concept and cognitions about some behavior. If dissonance exists, it is because the individual's behavior is inconsistent with his self-concept" (1968, p. 23). In other words, in self-consistency theory, the more that one's behavior generates a reduction of self-esteem and diminution in self-concept (e.g., feeling incompetent, irrational or immoral), the more likely the person will experience dissonance and make attitudinal adjustments to reduce the inconsistency.

Self-affirmation theory

Similar to self-consistency theory, self-affirmation theory claims that dissonance is generated when individuals enact behavior that is menacing to their self-concept. Both theories view the self as a potential standard of judgment, either personal or normative, that is applied to evaluate whether a behavioral consequence is aversive or not (Cooper, 2007, p. 115). The difference between the theories is that self-affirmation theory assumes that the main objective of a dissonance reduction strategy is not to salvage the specific self-image menaced by inconsistent behavior. Rather, the goal is to reinstate the moral and adaptive integrity of the assumed global self-system. Put simply, we are motivated to view ourselves as moral people, as good and honest, and any "facts" and evidence that contradict this self-conception will subvert our psychological equipoise. In this distressing context, an individual will feel compelled to rationalize contradictory behavior, to misrepresent or add information about oneself in order to maintain the integrity of one's self-system, or, in psychoanalytic language, the coherence of one's narrative of self-identity. So, returning to the aforementioned example, if we did not return the hundred dollar bill to the cashier, there must have been a good reason, like because the corporate-run store is the only one in town, and as it has a "captive audience," it grossly overcharges its customers. Or, a person will judge his behavior as not particularly bad since everyone in this situation would keep the hundred dollars. The point is that in self-affirmation theory, the need and desire to protect the integrity of the self-system, to maintain a coherent narrative of self-identity by drawing on important values or social comparisons, is the impetus for a person's efforts to reduce cognitive dissonance (Cooper, 2007). Moreover, in this theory, the higher the self-esteem, defined as the dispositional accessibility of favorable cognitions about the self, the easier it is for a person to reduce dissonance. For instance, research has shown that when people with high self-esteem are permitted a brief period of self-reflection before an inconsistent act, they report much less self-justification (in addressing the inconsistent cognitions) compared to people with low self-esteem. Thus, self-affirmation theory posits that favorable self-directed cognitions motivate people to be less susceptible to dissonance arousal and reduction following inconsistent behavior (Stone & Cooper, 2001, p. 230).

The new look at dissonance theory

The new look at dissonance theory (Cooper & Fazio, 1984) asserts that dissonance upsurges in a person when an inconsistent behavior represents a violation of societally based, taken-for-granted, normative standards for behavior. As a result of early socialization when normative standards of competence, rationality and morality are deeply internalized, when a person perceives themselves acting in a norm-defying manner (e.g., "inappropriately"), they experience dissonance that must be reduced. This is true regardless of self-esteem or of how available and accessible positive self-attributes are (e.g., other beliefs, values and ideals about the self). What motivates individuals to reduce dissonance is not these cognitions of the self, but anxiety, shame or guilt about having defied a subjectively meaningful, accepted norm. The point is that in this model, it is posited that dissonance is not evoked by cognitive inconsistencies per se, but is understood as a condition of uncomfortable arousal when a person assumes responsibility for facilitating an undesired result. Behavior that is inconsistent with attitudes, beliefs, values or ideals usually generates dissonance because people feel that they have acted autonomously, and because inconsistent behavior usually brings an undesired event or outcome. Dissonance, in other words, is caused by the individual's perceived negative consequences of inconsistent behavior and not the inconsistency per se (Cooper, 2017, p. 54).

Self-standards theory

Stone and Cooper (2001) changed the new look theory and embraced a self-standards model. They thought that the new look theory did not explain the important problem of how an individual decides whether an action has facilitated an aversive outcome. In other words, what makes an outcome of an act undesired or unpleasant? In this revised theory, Stone and Cooper posited that people need to evaluate the consequences of their behavior against a believed standard of judgment. In some instances, the standard of judgment mainly reflects an individual's idiosyncratic trajectory and subsequent self-concept; in other instances, the standard of judgment is a societally based, normative one. In both scenarios, defying a code of conduct would be viewed as ill-conceived and ill-fated and would generate dissonance. As Cooper summarizes his position,

> Dissonance is a state of arousal that happens when a person acts responsibly to bring about an unwanted consequence. The measuring rod for deciding if a consequence is undesired can be the internalized standards of one's society, culture or family, or it can be the very personal standards that have been generated by what one thinks about oneself. Either measuring rod is possible, but the playing field is not even. It tilts towards normative standards unless something in the environment specifically makes personal standards particularly accessible.
>
> *(2007, p. 182)*

While the self-standard model draws from concepts from social cognition and posits the conditions under which different standards are made accessible to a person as it impacts in the dissonance process (Cooper, 2017, p. 55), the theory does not adequately reckon with the fact that a person draws from both "measuring rods" in a uniquely personal manner. That is, the person, conceived as being-in-the-world, does typically draw from the internalized standards of society, culture or family (especially those standards based in childhood experience), but he does so in a highly personalized manner that reflects internal processes such as unconscious desire and fantasy and drive and affect. Thus, people often act in ways that are not predicted by this theory that relies so heavily on concepts from social cognition in which "internalized standards of one's society" and "personal standards" are typically viewed as separate domains of experience in understanding how people reside in the world. From a psychoanalytic point of view, there is more occurring when a person feels and deals with cognitive dissonance on the affective level.

Psychoanalytic reflections on cognitive dissonance

While psychoanalysis has not specifically discussed cognitive dissonance paradigms per se, it has from its inception dealt with the subject of the psychological discomfort/stress that analysands suffer when subjected to contradictory information that is inconsistent with their prior beliefs, values, ideals and behavior. These are the well-known psychoanalytic defense mechanisms like rationalization.[12] Festinger, in fact, acknowledges this point in an interview when he noted that "assuming Freud is correct, and in some areas I am sure he is, people use mechanisms to protect themselves from such things as guilt. They also use mechanisms to get rid of dissonance. The mechanisms may be identical, but the basic theories involved are about different processes" (Evans, 1980, p. 129). For example, in the love domain: an analysand who consciously claims that she wants to find a man to cherish her, and yet repeatedly does things to push eligible men away; in the work domain: the analysand who consciously claims that he wants to have a reasonable work/life balance, and yet almost never says no to his boss who asks him to take on extra work; in the communal domain: the analysand who claims that she is devoted to the "high" moral standards her church promulgates, and yet she badmouths, backbites and gossips about other members; in the faith domain: a devout Christian claims that his just and merciful God "hears" his prayers and will make his cancer-ridden child well, and yet the child dies from his disease. In each of these mismatched examples, the analysand engages in dissonance reduction in order to press on despite the psychic pain he or she may consciously and/or unconsciously feel. Thus, the practicing psychoanalyst and analysand struggle daily with these and other examples of cognitive dissonance. From my clinical experience, they probably constitute the majority of the analysand's "talk time." Indeed, one experimental social psychologist has claimed that "to the extent that psychotherapy is effective, it is precisely because of the arousal and reduction of cognitive dissonance (Cooper, 2007, p. 157). While each manifestation of cognitive dissonance and related psychological discomfort/stress has its own personal genealogy, subjective context and meaning, the details of which the analyst and analysand explore in depth in treatment, there are some general points that can be made about dissonance arousal and reduction. These points raise questions about aspects of cognitive dissonance theory and its "real-life" implications, especially for a person trying to fashion a flourishing way of being-in-the-world.

Awareness of unconscious processes "really" matters in our postmodern era

Psychoanalysts are used to analysands not "owning up" to what might be their "real" motivation(s) to explain their uncomfortable/stressful behavior (i.e., thoughts, feelings, actions), at least as the analysand and analyst co-construct the explanation. In most such instances the motivation is multi-determined, that is, there are many factors that contribute to the so-called neurotic behavior, behavior that is judged by the analysand and analyst as self-defeating and self-destructive. For example, while the analysand may claim that he is consciously driven to working so much and so intensely (being a "workaholic"), mainly to better provide for his family, it turns out that the "real" or more plausible reason for his behavior has to do with an unconscious wish to prove himself as an effective, if not superior man to his highly successful, emotionally remote, judgmental father, who the analysand believed never respected or even loved him. While the analysand acknowledges that his work/life balance may be awry (a manifestation of dissonance), he consciously believes he is doing what is "right" for his family (a rationalization that reduces dissonance). However, what becomes apparent in his treatment is that what mainly propels him to nearly "work himself to death," as his wife told him (and become emotionally remote to his family, like his father), is that he is unconsciously desperately looking for respect and love from his estranged, judgmental father, whom he is also competing with and wishes to supersede (i.e., "defeat"). This inner scenario calls to mind his childhood rivalry with his father for his narcissistic mother's attention, love and loyalty.

In terms of mainstream dissonance theory, this analysand feels dissonance arousal (e.g., anxiety, reduced self-esteem) when he recognizes that his work/life balance is awry, and he is letting down his wife and children (e.g., guilt, depression). He rationalizes his workaholic behavior by telling himself and his family that he works this way for their welfare, leading to a degree of dissonance reduction. However, the matter does not end there for analytic exploration, because while the analysand claims that his workaholism is mainly other-directed, other-regarding and other-serving—for the welfare of his family—it turns out, his main motivation is self-directed, self-regarding and self-serving. As the analysand does not ever feel this desperately sought emotional "victory" (i.e., superseding/defeating his father), he continues his workaholism, causing distress to his wife and family (via his emotional remoteness and lack of physical presence), which makes him feel anxious, self-loathing, guilty and depressed. Moreover, this constellation of fantasies and feelings turns out to satisfy his need/desire for unconscious punishment, for his sense that he has not only failed at proving himself to his father, but his wife and children view him as a failure as a husband and father.

In a generic psychoanalytic model, this man's destructive, repetitive pattern of alternating dissonance arousal and reduction in the context of his workaholism is mainly driven by unconscious desires and fantasies and drives and affects.[13] These desires, fantasies, drives and affects evoke in him the feeling of being both ennobled, sacrificing for the welfare of his family, and empowered, proving himself to his father, but also sinful, working for personal aggrandizement, and punishment-worthy, for harming his family. Moreover, this man feels "brain locked" when it comes to changing his workaholic behavior. That is, he is unwilling and unable to behave otherwise, positing many reasons why he feels he is "trapped" in repeating the aforementioned self-defeating dissonance arousal/reduction pattern. Of course, from a psychoanalytic point of view, his destructive work history need not be his destiny, at least not until he "sorts out" why his unconscious desires, fantasies, drives and affects have such a powerful interpretive grip on his obsessive outlook and compulsive behavior. Only then will he be willing and able to implement reason-guided changes in terms of altering his out-of-whack work/life balance, changes that better serve both himself and those he cares about.

The point I am making is that cognitive dissonance theory, as put forth by the four aforementioned models, is lodged in a modern version of the human condition, one that strives to eradicate ambivalence, ambiguity and uncertainty, and "promote the monosemic clarity of the sameness" in everyday life (Bauman, 1991, p. 98). Such an outlook wholeheartedly embraces an animating ethos of autonomous selfhood in which self-unity, rationality and control are what matter most in bringing about dissonance arousal and reduction, the latter being the ultimate goal (Elliott, 2015, p. 31). For example, Harmon-Jones suggests that people fashion a way of comporting themselves in the world that makes them more adaptive and functional, such that they act on the world without ambivalence and conflict [i.e, "effective, unconflicted action," (1999, p. 93)]. Inconsistent cognitions obstruct our "action tendencies" that "guide action," (ibid.), and thus generate negative feelings (e.g., discomfort and stress), propelling us to jettison inconsistency. However, it is not inconsistency itself that generates discomfort and stress, but rather the way it truncates our "effective behavior" (ibid.) in the social and physical world. This point of view does not require an aversive consequence or undesired happening for dissonance to get evoked (Cooper, 2007, p. 82).

While such a version of the human condition has its usefulness as a conceptual lens in some contexts (including in some cognitive dissonance experiments), as I suggested earlier, cognitive dissonance theory does not adequately take into consideration the possibility that a stable personal self may not be doable or even desirable. That is, cognitive dissonance theory may be lodged in an ill-conceived and ill-fated modernist view of the person, in which the quest for foundations, absolutes and universals regarding human behavior guides the outlook, research and interpretations of data (Elliott, 2004, p. 21). A postmodern view, however, posits that social life and its subjective experience is more aptly characterized as pluralistic, contingent, ambiguous, ambivalent and uncertain (ibid., p. 13). Therefore, so-called cognitive dissonance, especially when it is manifest regarding matters of "ultimate concern," like in love, work, community and faith, is better decoupled from its valuative attachments to objectivity, necessity and law as the constituting features of social life in our current episteme [i.e., socio-intellectual reality (ibid.)]. Put simply, self-consistency, self-affirmation, new look and the self-standards theories of cognitive dissonance do not adequately reconcile with the fact that selfhood in our era is best conceptualized as "open ended" and "self-dislocated," and not mainly expounded via pre-given social roles. Rather it is expounded via the chaotic indeterminacy of desire, fantasy, drive and affect-driven personal and social relationships. As desire, fantasy, drive and affect always outstrip a person's capacity for self-representation and representation of others, cognitive dissonance and reduction require a mode of thought/affective processing that is geared to better metabolizing the discontinuous, dislocated and dispersed character of social reality in our era (ibid.). This is what postmodern-glossed psychoanalysis does especially well, for it rejects the view of the "fixed," "true," "deep" and "real" self that cognitive dissonance theory tends to embrace. As Richard Rorty noted, the self is best viewed "as webs of beliefs and desires, of sentential attitudes," webs that repeatedly reweave themselves in order to house new sentential attitudes (1991, p. 93). In short, the self is the reweaving web, and dissonance arousal/reduction is another way of characterizing the challenges of everyday life in our postmodern world.

Experienced dissonance is sometimes "good"

Psychoanalysis has emphasized that in certain contexts, cognitive dissonance, discomfort and stress can bring about personal growth and development in an analysand. For example, an obsessive-compulsive person may think, feel and act in a manner that justifies his comportment as reasonable, appropriate and morally praiseworthy. He experiences his behavior as ego-syntonic, meaning that in the mind of the analysand, aspects of his thoughts, feelings and actions are felt to be acceptable and consistent with the rest of the personality and outlook, and are judged as morally commendable. So, for example, the analysand who would every morning check five times to make sure the gas stove was shut off before he left did so, he told me, to assure himself that his "beloved" sleeping wife would be safe from any fire risk. Moreover, he claimed that his checking behavior ("admittedly excessive," he told me), reflected the devotion that he believed was in sync with his notion of what constitutes a "loving and protective husband." However, when this analysand's obsessive-compulsive behavior was analytically explored, and it became occasionally ego-dystonic, that is, aspects of his thoughts, feelings and actions were felt to be uncomfortable, stressful, and inconsistent with his personality and outlook,[14] he became more receptive to a counter-intuitive "interpretation." He gradually embraced the idea and its profound implications that he was checking the stove not because he was concerned about his wife's welfare, but rather, because he unconsciously wished that the stove would catch fire and incinerate his wife, a woman that in many ways he found unbearable to live with!

Dissonance can be an instrument for life-enhancing personal changes in behavior, which has been social-psychologically demonstrated in experiments related to induced hypocrisy. When hypocrisy, behaving in a way you claim you are not, or believing something you claim you do not, is experimentally induced, it can be a robust instrument for modifying people's behavior in desirable personal and prosocial ways. The assumption of these experiments is that in many instances, people have the "correct" beliefs, values and ideals, like it is "smart" and sensible to wear a condom if you do not want to get a woman pregnant or contract venereal disease ("safe sex"), and yet, many "reasonable" men (and women) do not translate what they know to be true and sensible into protective action. Social psychologists have found that if one can generate feelings of hypocrisy in an offending person, in highlighting the discrepancy between their beliefs, values, ideals and their actions, dissonance will upsurge and require reduction. The dissonance in beliefs, values and ideals should be so intense that implementing common dissonance reduction tactics like sidetracking oneself or shoring up one's ego by doing other favorably judged behaviors would not suffice. Only actions that directly eradicate the discrepancy between what one believes and does would lead to a successful outcome in terms of changed behavior.

Stone et al. (1994) asked naïve subjects to make a videotape promoting the use of condoms to stop the transmission of HIV. Then naïve subjects were requested to reflect on the reasons why they themselves hadn't used condoms in the past (condition one: personal reasons), or, provide reasons why people typically occasionally fail to use condoms (condition two: normative reasons that didn't focus on their own personal behavior). The experimenters predicted that hypocrisy would be maximized in the personal reasons condition, in which naïve subjects had to confront, head-on, their own hypocrisy. All naïve subjects were offered a choice between a direct means of dissonance reduction, buying condoms at a cheaper price, and an indirect means of dissonance reduction, giving a donation to a program intended to assist homeless persons. The results of the study were telling: when naïve subjects had been requested to concentrate on the reasons why they personally hadn't engaged in safe sex in the past, the greater majority chose to buy condoms, the direct approach to dissonance reduction. On the other hand, when requested to reflect on their reasons why people in general didn't engage in safe sex, more naïve subjects chose the indirect approach to dissonance reduction, a donation to the assist-the-homeless project.

As Baron and Byrne (2003) note, for such interventions to be most effective, the person being considered must publicly promote the desired behavior, like using condoms. He also must be induced to reflect on his own personal failures to enact this sensible behavior in the past, and he must be provided access to direct means for dissonance reduction. Such considerations are broadly in sync with how psychoanalytic "insight" works, at least when conceived as a developing and dynamic process, "the condition, catalyst and consequence of the analytic process" (Blum, 1979, p. 66). First, insight emanates from the reciprocal interaction between the analyst and analysand, rather than from "god's-eye" knowledge of the analyst qua authority to the "sick" analysand. Second, insight involves assimilation and integration of beliefs, values and ideals into one's lived life, and is not simply the ultimate curative intellectual goal (e.g., the analysand must emotionally "reflect" on his behavior and enact his new "truths" in "real life"). Third, while insight is one of the important healing factors in psychoanalysis (Akhtar, 2009), so called "cure" also typically involves a "holding environment" (i.e., the supportive psychotherapeutic relationship) and "an average expectable environment" (i.e., "external" reality must not be too traumatically disruptive of the analytic process). These conditions are optimum so that the analysand can do the "heavy-lifting" of reconfiguring his emotional infrastructure related to his childhood traumas. The analyst must provide access to dissonance reduction via the analysand's containing, but also thought-provoking, relationship with the analysand.

Implications for treatment

To summarize, Festinger and his cohort have brilliantly studied one of the most important aspects of everyday functioning, including striving to live a flourishing life—namely, reconciling with the fact that conflict upsurges when there is a perceived discrepancy between one's behavior and prior attitude. This is especially the case when the perceived discrepancy pertains to matters that "really" matter to people, like love, work, community and faith. Based on accrued research (Smith et al., 2015, pp. 283–284), dissonance arousal typically occurs under four conditions:

1. When the individual perceives the behavior as inconsistent with a favorable sense of himself. That is, anxiety-generating inconsistency tends to upsurge when behavior is inconsistent with views of ourselves that matter to our important beliefs, values and ideals connected to our narrative of self-identity. For example, when I view myself as a caring and loving husband but my wife demonstrates that I treated her meanly.
2. When the individual perceives the behavior as freely chosen, dissonance is generated. Coercion of any type in which the person can externalize responsibility for his discrepant behavior, like a financial reward or a threat, does not bring about dissonance. For instance, seduction in the sexual context will not bring

about dissonance because the person judges his compliant behavior as self-chosen. Yet in the prior husband/wife example, I freely made the choice to treat my wife in a mean manner, therefore dissonance was generated.

3. When an individual feels unpleasant physiological arousal (e.g., increased blood pressure, respiration) in the context of a discrepancy between belief and behavior, dissonance is often experienced in the form of anxiety and guilt. However, such physiologically anchored arousal can enhance performance on simple tasks but not on challenging ones. It is well-known that a manageable amount of experienced physiological arousal, typically called stress, can be enabling of effective behavior, like how an actor feels before going on stage. In the above husband/wife example, I feel physiologically anchored guilt, depression and anxiety because I treated my wife in such an undeservedly mean manner, a woman who has always been caring and loving toward me and our children.
4. When the individual believes that the unpleasant physiological arousal and experienced discomfort/stress is due to the discrepancy between his belief and behavior, he feels dissonance. This has been proven when naïve subjects were hoodwinked into believing that the discomfort/stress they experienced was not due to the mismatch between belief and behavior, but due to something else, like fluorescent lights that did not work properly, a pill they swallowed, electric shocks that they anticipated receiving or prison goggles they had to put on. In the above example, when I reflect on my freely chosen behavior toward my innocent wife, despite my view of myself as a man who could and should do better, I feel reduced self-esteem, if not self-loathing. I apologize to my wife and promise to do better.[15]

Dissonance reduction typically includes the following:

1. *The insufficient justification effect.* As Festinger and Carlsmith (1959) showed, the insufficient justification effect occurs when an individual generates an internal reason for an explanation to a behavior because there isn't an external reason. This effect reduces cognitive dissonance via justifying a behavior internally when there is inadequate external justification. In the above example, I believe that I am a flawed and limited husband who mistreated his innocent wife in this specific instance, though generally I am a caring and loving husband.
2. *The effort justification effect.* As Aronson and Mills (1959) showed, an individual will believe a goal is worth striving for if they have exerted considerable effort to get there. Thus, even if they do not achieve their goal, they will justify their actions as being worth the effort. In the above example, I tell myself that I try very hard to be a caring and loving husband, and while I sometimes fail, I am working to improve myself.
3. *Post-decisional regret effect.* An individual's belief will change to diminish the dissonance (e.g., the worry or anxiety) caused by the freely made choice or decision executed. Cognitive dissonance theory predicts that the dissonance will be correlated with the net desirability of the chosen and unchosen options and the

> significance of the decision to the individual. In the example above, while I regret that I have freely chosen to treat my wife in a nasty way in this one instance, I try to and usually succeed at behaving otherwise. When I think about it, she has occasionally been mean to me, so I am not as "bad" as I thought.

It should be stressed that justification processes have a long-term psychological and pragmatic payoff. When an individual experiences dissonance he engages in labor-intensive and high-maintenance thinking and emotional processing. For example, he may attempt to reconcile discrepant beliefs and behavior by entertaining arguments that he had overlooked or previously disregarded, he may seek out new self-serving facts or evidence, he may interpret his behavior in creative and novel ways, he may engage in consequential thinking regarding his discrepant behavior, and overall he may critically reflect on what he feels and how he behaves. Such labor-intensive cognitive and affective processing can lead to belief, value and ideal change that is long-lived. In one study, business students were experimentally asked to provide hypothetical decisions between vacation spots and then rate the spots again. As predicted by cognitive dissonance theory, their chosen spot was rated much more favorably than the rejected destination. Even more remarkably, the outcome was identical when the students rated the same vacation spots about 2.5 to 3 years later (Smith et al., 2015, p. 289).

What are the psychoanalytic implications of cognitive dissonance findings for analysands in treatment who are struggling to live a flourishing life? Dissonance is a ubiquitous experience in Western society. Every time a person makes a choice or exerts effort to achieve an objective, there is a degree of "uncomfortable tension," as Festinger called it (Cooper, 2007 pp. 7, 117). As such, learning to accept a degree of dissonance is essential.[16] As some scholars have noted, the experience of dissonance both as background and foreground to everyday experience seems to be frequently evoked in our postmodern world, in part because so many of the affect-integrating, meaning-giving and action-guiding social structures and practices appear to be giving way to something felt to be ambiguous, uncertain and ambivalent. That said, what constitutes dissonance on the personal level is radically philosophical, meaning it is rooted in the person's idiosyncratic psychological trajectory. One person's constraining dissonance is another person's enabling dissonance. This is how it unfolds in the psychoanalytic conversation between analysand and analyst.[17]

Learning to "live with" a modicum of dissonance requires embracing a way of thinking and emotionally processing experience so that the dissonance arousal does not become debilitating. While there are no "quick fix" dissonance-reducing strategies or tactics that can inoculate a person from the deleterious effects of too much dissonance, as each dissonance-arousing experience has its own characteristic arc, there are at least two points relevant to one's existential orientation that are worth considering.

First, as I have repeatedly argued in this book, to the extent that one has strongly felt, flexibly and creatively applied transcendent-pointing moral beliefs and values, he is more likely to deal with his everyday existence in a manner that reflects reasonable consistency in outlook and behavior. This usually means experiencing less self-defeating and self-destructive dissonance while still allowing for appropriate context-dependent, setting-specific guilt and anxiety. These beliefs and values tend to enhance one's sense of self-coherence, self-continuity and self-esteem that emanates from efficacious functioning (future behavior that is made consistent with one's attitude). This approach is the most direct route to dissonance reduction (Cooper, 2007). Such beliefs and values are like a frame and filter that serve as an emotional "shock absorber" when one's actions seriously disagree with one's outlook. More profoundly, what such beliefs and values give a person is a more robust capacity to maintain autonomy and integration because he has a more attuned ability to balance the needs of the self and the demands of the external world. In other words, a person needs to be more informed about how far he is willing and able to go to reduce dissonance at the expense of his autonomy and dignity. With strongly felt, flexibly and creatively applied, transcendent-pointing moral beliefs and values, a person is more willing and able to test the vast number of choices which have to be made in one's life against their beliefs and values and interests, and thereby cut the wide range of problems down to a manageable size. In such a situation, a person will feel less overpowered than others by any new need for judging how much of themselves they can surrender to the external world and still maintain their autonomy and integration (Bettelheim, 1960).

In the psychoanalytic context, dissonance arousal is often associated with experienced ambivalence, which is not the same as having mixed feelings toward someone. Ambivalence is psychoanalytically defined as "an underlying emotional attitude in which the contradictory attitudes derive from a common source and are interdependent, whereas mixed feelings may be based upon a realistic assessment of the imperfect nature of the object" (i.e., the significant other) (Rycroft, 1995, p. 6). Ambivalence, what can be roughly described as a subsect of cognitive dissonance, "refers to affective states in which intrinsically contradictory or mutually exclusive desires or ideas are each invested with intense emotional energy. Although one cannot have both simultaneously, one cannot abandon either of them" (Flax, 1990, p. 50).

What is most important about ambivalence conceived as an exemplar of dissonance arousal is that to achieve dissonance reduction, one needs to learn how to "live with" the discomfort and stress, at least until one has sufficiently explored and made peace with the dissonance:

> According to analytic theory, ambivalence is an appropriate response to an inherently conflictual situation. The problem lies not in the ambivalence, but in the premature attempts to resolve or deny conflicts. The lack of coherence or closure in a situation and existence of contradictory wishes or ideas too often generate anxiety so intense that aspects of the ambivalence and its sources are repressed. It is often better in such a situation to analyze the sources of the ambivalence and one's inability to tolerate it. It is equally important to examine why, when lacking absolute certainty, the will becomes paralyzed.
>
> *(ibid., p. 11)*

Given the aforementioned role of ambivalence in psychic and practical life, the goal of psychoanalysis is not, as cognitive dissonance theory implies, the permanent reduction of the "uncomfortable tension" (though when this happens it is not to be pooh-poohed). Rather, as Flax further notes, the goal of psychoanalysis

> is not to achieve closure of a final truth [e.g., about ambivalence] that renders further investigation unnecessary. Rather the analyst hopes that in and through the process of analysis a patient will overcome some of the internal barriers to the desire for self-understanding. Although the analysis will be "terminated," the analytic process will continue with the former patient now able to be her own analyst. For the termination process and hence the analysis to be successful, both analyst and patient must accept that closure is to some extent arbitrary, temporary, and conventional.
>
> *(ibid., p. 13)*

Put differently, when one cannot learn to creatively "live with" ambivalence, and thus engages in massive efforts at self-justification for jarring disconfirmatory evidence, the danger of ambivalence morphing into feelings of destructive certainty, or neurotic guilt that becomes fury, is quite likely (Tavris & Aronson, 2015, p. 232).

Finally, it should be emphasized that the aforementioned psychoanalytic perspective on ambivalence and other open-ended, self-dislocated psychoanalytic renderings about human subjectivity that emphasize the role of desire, fantasy, drive and affect, are in sync with certain social-psychological claims about cognitive dissonance. For example, Cooper says that cognitive dissonance may well be "a learned secondary drive" that can be reversed (2007, p. 88). A secondary drive is one that is acquired, like the desire to acquire money, that is probably connected to an innate drive: "There is some evidence that dissonance can be unlearned and that by using principles of secondary learning, people can learn to become less aroused by dissonance procedures" (ibid., p. 89). Moreover, cultural factors appear to have a role in dissonance arousal, suggesting that it may be a socially constructed, acquired behavior. Dissonance is impacted differently in different cultures, suggesting that inconsistency is not what matters most. What creates dissonance is how freely chosen behavior diverges from personal and normative standards (ibid., p. 149). For example, in Western society, self-identity is connected to individual choices and actions, whereas in Asian societies, self-identity is strongly connected to roles and status, emphasizing an individual's location in society and obligations that it requires. As Heine and Lehman (1997) noted, because of these considerations, post-decision dissonance may be more robust for individuals from Western societies compared to many Asian ones.

While Cooper (2007) points to the usefulness of cognitive behavior therapy in reducing dissonance in very specific clinical and other social-psychologically studied contexts, the fact that dissonance arousal may be a learned phenomenon raises the possibility for something more far-reaching and important for someone in pursuit of a flourishing life: Namely, the creation of a self-identity that does not regard most contradictions, ambiguities and ambivalences as problematic, but rather as the way the world "hangs together." Indeed, from my clinical experience, much of a person's felt worries and troubles are about happenings that have no reasonable, effective, sustained dissonance-reducing intervention. In this view, the best response is to "manage" these challenges by learning to live with the unavoidable existential contradictions about love, work, community and faith. This may be better than the outlook that dissonance theory inadvertently suggests, imposing a totalizing and harmonizing outlook and way of living. Such an outlook tends to undermine individual autonomy, integration and humanity in the long term. This does not mean that one does not try to make things better, but one does so knowing that the options for morally animated, effective intervention are limited and incomplete, especially in matters that "really" matter to people. Building an expanded and deeper capacity for tolerating inconsistency is crucial to achieve a modicum of spiritual equipoise. This means having a better understanding of how dissonance arousal/reduction operates in one's everyday life. Moreover, what is phenomenologically true about happiness—namely, the greater the perceived congruence between one's expectations and one's fate, the greater the experienced happiness—is conversely true about dissonance arousal. The greater the inconsistency between one's expectations and one's experience, the greater the dissonance.

This being said, the "new subjectivity" that I am suggesting is in a certain way also an "old" one, as it posits a person who is always mindful of both the intentional and unintentional ways we harm others. Genuine guilt is the consequence of injured relations between people about which the perpetrator is consciously or unconsciously aware and for which they feel deeply regretful. "Existential guilt" occurs "when someone injures an order of the human world whose foundations he knows and recognizes as those of his own existence and of all common existence" (Buber, 1965, p. 127). Guilt, conceived as dissonance arousal, is only reduced via acts of internal, and most importantly, external reparation.

Such a view is perfectly in sync with research findings in cognitive dissonance theory. As Kenworthy et al. (2011) pointed out in their trans-paradigm synthesis of cognitive dissonance theory, none of the aforementioned theories "supported Festinger's notion that discomfort mediates dissonance effects" (p. 36). However, only guilt, conceived as "the drive component of dissonance theory, strongly predicted dissonance effect sizes, virtually irrespective of which model was tested" (ibid.). Moreover, "a theory integrating the guilt and dissonance theories is stronger than either set of theories in isolation" (ibid.).

Thus, psychoanalytic and cognitive dissonance theory agree in terms of what matters most with regards to avoiding destructive dissonance and engaging in living a flourishing life. Dissonance is a motivational state that is most powerfully brought about when a person's cognitions involve a serious discrepancy between current behavior and personally held standards of conduct. It is self-identity and one's standards, beliefs, values and ideals that are the crucial determinants of the importance of cognitions. Cognitions are important to the extent that they are pertinent to moral values and standards for personal conduct, which almost always implicates others. What most mediates and moderates[18] experiences of dissonance is the magnitude of self-awareness of guilt, of taking personal responsibility for one's acts of omission and commission,[19] though behavior is rarely governed by one variable in isolation from the rest of personality and social context (ibid., pp. 91, 94). Thus, one of the important "take home" points about living a flourishing life is to follow Socrates's advice about the way to gain a good reputation, "endeavor to be what you desire to appear".[20] By being what you seem to be, especially by engaging in counter-guilt-inducing behavior, being other-directed, other-regarding and other-serving in your overall comportment in the world, you will be less susceptible to the upsurge of emotional storms associated with morally serious dissonance arousal.

Notes

1 Tavris and Aronson (2015, p. 16) have indicated that the theory has inspired greater than three thousand experiments.

2 By way of contextualizing Festinger in the history of psychology, when he began his work on cognitive dissonance, behaviorism was in ascendance, a theory that emphasized external behavior and its effects. Festinger was one of the theorists who initiated what became known as the "cognitive revolution," a perspective that emphasized internal mental states and processes. Festinger, a student of the founder of social psychology, Kurt Lewin, was also influenced by Fritz Heider who developed Balance Theory. Balance Theory emphasized the human predilection for cognitive consistency, specifically feelings toward others and opinions of objects (Morvan & O'Connor, 2017, pp. 10, 12, 73). In 1954, Festinger also did path-breaking work in what he called social comparison theory, which claimed there is an innate drive within people to attain accurate self-evaluations by comparing their personal qualities to others.

3 There are some social psychologists who acknowledge that in some relational contexts, "learn to live with it" is the best one can do, such as how high-functioning couples manage their conflicts (Tavris & Aronson, 2015).

4 To be fair, there are some cognitive dissonance theorists (Tavris & Aronson, 2015) who give a marginal role to unconscious processes in self-justification processes. Likewise, such formulations are applied in ways that significantly diverge from psychoanalytic notions of unconscious processes. Bem (1967), in his self-perception theory, claimed that when individuals have undeveloped cognitions (i.e., they are unclear or not accessible), they are inclined to infer their attitudes by observing their actual own behavior.

5 Similar to psychoanalysis, cognitive dissonance theories are meditations on how much truth a person can tolerate about his flawed and limited way of being-in-the-world, especially before he makes efforts to protect himself from "fessing up." Similar to psychoanalytic defense mechanisms, the forms of self-justification that cognitive dissonance theorists have described about how people cope with their mistakes and failings resonate with the main thrust of psychoanalytic values and clinical practice. As is well-known, people will resort to astonishing conscious and unconscious self-justifying strategies and tactics to avoid facing the "harsh" truths about their deficiencies. This is especially the case when others are implicated. As Tavris and Aronson noted, "self-justification is designed to protect our feelings of self-worth, of being loved, of being a good and respected person" (2015, p. 223). Sometimes self-justifications can permit a person to engage in evil behavior, like "killing in the name of healing," as was the case of the Nazi doctors who participated in the extermination of Jews and other groups. In this situation, "doubling," dividing the self into two functioning wholes, so that a specific self acts as a complete self, and splitting or dividing beliefs, actions, objects or persons into good and bad by concentrating discriminatively on their positive or negative characteristics, were in play.

6 A "symbolic universe," roughly, is a worldview, "a set of beliefs and assumptions that describe reality" (Koltko-Rivera, 2004, p. 3) that is created to legitimize the created institutional structure (Berger & Luckmann, 1966). Symbolic universes are conceptualized as set of beliefs "everybody knows" that strive to render the institutionalized structure plausible and acceptable for the individual, who possibly would not then

comprehend or concur with the fundamental logic of the institution. As an ideological framework, the symbolic universe "puts everything in its right place." It furnishes explanations for why people do things in a particular manner. A symbolic universe includes, for example, proverbs, moral maxims, wise sayings, mythology, religions and other theological reflections, metaphysical traditions and other value systems.

A worldview, says Koltko-Rivera, is defined as "a way of describing the universe and life within it, both in terms of what is and what ought to be. A given worldview is a set of beliefs that includes limiting statements and assumptions regarding what exists and what does not (either in actuality, or in principle), what objects or experiences are good or bad, and what objectives, behaviors and relationships are desirable or undesirable. A worldview defines what can be known or done in the world, and how it can be known or done. In addition to defining what goals can be sought in life, a worldview defines what goals should be pursued. Worldviews include assumptions that may be unproven, and even improvable, but these assumptions are super ordinate, in that they provide the epistemic and ontological foundations for other beliefs within a belief system" (2004, p. 4).

7 After Keech's prediction/prophecy did not materialize, she fled Chicago after being imperiled with arrest and involuntary commitment in a psychiatric hospital. Not deterred, Keech subsequently founded the Association of Sananda and Sanat Kumara, which is still active. Renaming herself Sister Thedra, she carried on practicing channeling (a person's body being taken over by a spirit for the purpose of communication) and other psychic practices until she died in 1992.

8 Festinger and his colleagues were first denied entry into the Seekers, but once it was deemed by a senior member that the investigators were dispatched by the heavenly beings the Seekers were in contact with, they were permitted to join the group (Cooper, 2017, p. 45).

9 https://thedecisonlab.com/bias/less-is-better-effect/ retrieved 12/12/18.

10 By cognition Festinger meant "any knowledge, opinion, or belief about the environment, about oneself, or about one's behavior" (1957, p. 3).

11 I have liberally relied on Stone and Cooper (2001) and Cooper (2007) in my summaries of the four theories.

12 Social psychologists have described other ways that people cope with disconfirming evidence like the "confirmation bias," the proclivity to interpret new evidence as confirmation of one's prior beliefs or theories. If you are buying a new car, don't ask someone who has bought the car you are considering, ask someone who is still researching the matter. Once people make an important decision, they are inclined to maintain their bias after the decision (e.g., buying the car was a good decision even if it subsequently has some mechanical problems).

13 In contrast, a social psychologist might consider personality style and situational variables, such as income, health and level of stress in the household, to understand this man's workaholism. What both perspectives are suggesting is that dissonance awareness, being mindful of the contrast and general relationship between the situational and unconscious processes, is what matters most in terms of sorting out a serious problem.

14 Some people, like psychopaths, often do not feel much, if any, dissonance about their morally objectionable behavior. Reduced dissonance allows them to maintain their troubling way of being-in-the-world. Conversely, there are people who cannot let go of their dissonance, that is, no attempts at self-justifying can reduce their discomfort/stress; for example, an analysand who cannot tolerate his career success because it does not allow him to view himself as a pity-worthy "loser." Such "masochistic" people are wedded to a devalued self-conception that no "good news" can positively impact, let alone in a sustained manner. Other analysands are not willing or able to "forgive" themselves for various real or imagined misdeeds.

15 Cooper (2007) has summarized the limiting conditions of cognitive dissonance: inconsistent behavior brings about dissonance when decision freedom is high, people are committed to their behavior, the behavior leads to aversive results, and those results are predictable.

16 Whether cognitive dissonance is a universal phenomenon, as Festinger claimed, is still an open question; however, authorities on the theory believe it probably is (Cooper, 2007; Tavris & Aronson, 2015).
17 Festinger was aware that there were differences in how individuals experienced and responded to dissonance. Some people can tolerate more dissonance than others; why this is the case has not been researched in much depth by subsequent investigators (Festinger, 1957; Morvan & O'Connor, 2017).
18 A moderator is a variable that can negate or reverse the usual effects reported with a phenomenon. In other words, there are limiting conditions to the formation of dissonance and discomfort (Morvan & O'Connor, 2017).
19 What constitutes personal responsibility is a complex and ambiguous philosophical and psychological subject, but Cooper aptly defined personal responsibility as it pertains to cognitive dissonance. It is "the attribution that the locus of causation for an event is internal. Informally, it's the conclusion that, 'I did it; I brought it about'" (2007, p. 76).
20 samples.jbpub.com/9781284155594/9781284155594_CH01_Stanford.pdf, retrieved 12/25/18.

References

Akhtar, S. (2009). *Comprehensive dictionary of psychoanalysis*. London: Karnac.

Aronson, E. (1968). Dissonance theory: progress and problems. In R.P. Abelson, E. Aronson, W.J. McGuire, T.M. Newcomb, M.J. Rosenberg & P.H. Tannenbaum (Eds.), *Theories of cognitive consistency: A sourcebook* (pp. 5–27). Chicago: Rand McNally.

Aronson, E. & Carlsmith, J.M. (1962). The effect of the severity of the threat on the devaluation of forbidden behavior. *Journal of Abnormal and Social Psychology*, 66, 884–888.

Aronson, E. & Mills, J. (1959). The effect of severity of initiation on liking of a group. *Journal of Abnormal and Social Psychology*, 59(2), 177–181.

Baron, R.A. & Byrne, D. (Eds.) (2003). *Social psychology* (10th ed.). Boston: Pearson Education.

Bauman, Z. (1991). *Modernity and ambivalence*. Cambridge: Polity Press.

Bem, D.J. (1967). Self-perception: An alternative interpretation of cognitive dissonance phenomena. *Psychological Review*, 74(3), 183–200.

Berger, D. (2008). *The Rebbe, the Messiah, and the Scandal of Orthodox Indifference*. Portland: Littman Library of Jewish Civilization.

Berger, P.L. (1969). *The sacred canopy: Elements of a sociological theory of religion*. New York: Anchor.

Berger, P.L. & Berger, B. (1972). *Sociology: A biographical approach*. New York: Basic Books.

Berger, P.L. & Luckmann, T. (1966). *The social construction of reality: A treatise in the sociology of knowledge*. New York: Anchor.

Bettelheim, B. (1960). *The informed heart: Autonomy in a mass age*. Glencoe, IL: The Free Press.

Blum, H. (1979). The curative and creative aspects of insight. *Journal of the American Psychoanalytic Association*, 27(Suppl.), 41–69.

Boym, S. (2010). *Another freedom: The alternative history of an idea*. Chicago: University of Chicago Press.

Buber, M. (1965). *The knowledge of man: Selected essays*. M.S. Friedman (Ed.). New York: Harper & Row.

Cooper, J. (2007). *Cognitive dissonance: Fifty years of a classic theory*. Los Angeles: Sage.

Cooper, J. (2017). Cognitive dissonance: Revisiting Festinger's End of the World study. In J.R. Smith & S.A. Haslam (Eds.), *Social psychology: Revisiting the classic studies* (2nd ed., pp. 43–57). Thousand Oaks, CA: Sage.

Cooper, J. & Fazio, R. (1984). A new look at dissonance theory. In L. Berkowtiz (Ed.), *Advances in experimental social psychology* (Vol. 17, pp. 229–264). Orlando: Academic Press.

Elliott, A. (2004). *Subject to ourselves: Social theory, psychoanalysis and postmodernity*. Boulder: Paradigm.

Elliott, A. (2015). *Psychoanalytic theory: An introduction* (3rd ed.). New York: Palgrave.

Emerson, R.W. (2007). *Self-reliance*. Rockville: Arc Manor.

Evans, R.I. (1980). *The making of social psychology: Discussions with creative contributors*. New York: Gardner Press.

Festinger, L. (1957). *A theory of cognitive dissonance*. Stanford: Stanford University Press.

Festinger, L. (1962). Cognitive dissonance. *Scientific American*, 207(4), 93–107.

Festinger, L. & Carlsmith, J.M. (1959). Cognitive consequences of forced compliance. *Journal of Abnormal and Social Psychology*, 58, 203–210.

Festinger, L., Riecken, H.W. & Schachter, S. (1956). *When prophecy fails*. Minneapolis: University of Minnesota Press.

Flax, J. (1990). *Thinking fragments: Psychoanalysis, feminism, and postmodernism in the contemporary west*. Berkeley: University of Berkeley.

Frosch, S. (1989). *Psychoanalysis and psychology: Minding the gap*. New York: New York University Press.

Geertz, C. (1973). *Interpretations of culture*. New York: Basic Books.

Harmon-Jones, E. (1999). Toward an understanding of the motivation underlying dissonance effects: Is the production of aversive consequences necessary? In E. Harmon-Jones & J. Mills (Eds.), *Cognitive dissonance: Progress on a pivotal theory in social psychology* (pp. 71–103). Washington, DC: American Psychological Association.

Heine, S.J. & Lehman, D.R. (1997). Culture, dissonance, and self-affirmation. *Personality and Social Psychology Bulletin*, 23, 389–400.

Hsee, C.K. (1998). Less is better: when low-value options are valued more highly than high-value options. *Journal of Behavioral Decision Making*, 11(2), 107–121.

Jack, H.A. (Ed.) (1979). *The wit and wisdom of Gandhi*. Mineola: Dover.

Kenworthy, J.B., Miller, N., Collins, B.E., Read, S.J. & Earleywine, M. (2011). A trans-paradigm theoretical synthesis of cognitive dissonance theory: Illuminating the nature of discomfort. *European Review of Social Psychology*, 22(1), 36–113.

Koltko-Rivera, M.E. (2004). The psychology of worldviews. *Review of General Psychology*, 8 (1), 3–58.

Marcus, P. & Rosenberg, A. (Eds.) (1998). *Psychoanalytic versions of the human condition: Philosophies of life and their impact on practice*. New York: New York University Press.

Morvan, C. & O'Connor, A.J. (2017). *An analysis of Leon Festinger's a theory of cognitive dissonance*. London: Routledge.

Reynolds, D.S. (Ed.) (2005). *Walt Whitman's Leaves of Grass*. Oxford: Oxford University Press.

Rorty, R. (1991). *Objectivity, relativism, and truth: Philosophical papers*. Cambridge: Cambridge University Press.

Rycroft, C. (1995). *A critical dictionary of psychoanalysis*. London: Penguin.

Schafer, R. (1976). *A new language for psychoanalysis*. New Haven: Yale University Press.

Smith, R., Mackie, D.M. & Claypool, H.M. (Eds.) (2015). *Social psychology* (4th ed.). New York: Psychology Press.

Steele, C.M., Spencer, S.J. & Lynch, M. (1993). Self-image resilience and dissonance: The role of affirmational resources. *Journal of Personality and Social Psychology*, 64, 885–896.

Stone, J., Aronson, E., Crain, A.L., Winslow, M.P. & Fried, C.B. (1994). Inducing hypocrisy as a means of encouraging young adults to use condoms. *Personality and Social Psychology Bulletin*, 20, 116–128.

Stone, J. & Cooper, J. (2001). A self-standards model of cognitive dissonance. *Journal of Experimental Social Psychology*, 37, 228–243.
Storch, E.A. & Storch, J.B. (2003). Academic dishonesty and attitudes towards academic dishonest acts: Support for cognitive dissonance theory. *Psychological Reports*, 92, 174–176.
Tavris, C. & Aronson, E. (2015). *Mistakes were made (but not by me): Why we justify foolish beliefs, bad decisions, and hurtful acts*. Boston: Mariner Books.
Thibodeau, R. & Aronson, E. (1992). Take a close look: reasserting the role of the self-concept in dissonance theory. *Personality and Social Psychology Bulletin*, 18, 591–602.
Thomas, W.I. & Thomas, D.S. (1928). *The child in America: Behavior problems and programs*. New York: Knopf.

Internet sources

https://thedecisonlab.com/bias/less-is-better-effect/, retrieved 12/12/18.
samples.jbpub.com/9781284155594/9781284155594_CH01_Stanford.pdf, retrieved 12/25/18.

4

INTERGROUP CONFLICT VERSUS COOPERATION

Sherif's Robbers Cave experiment (1954)

"Civilized society," said Freud in *Civilization and its Discontents*, "is perpetually menaced with disintegration through this primary hostility of men towards one another" (1961, p. 112). In the last paragraph of his essay, Freud observed, "Men have gained control over the forces of nature to such an extent that with their help they would have no difficulty in exterminating one another to the last man" (ibid., p. 145). Indeed, Freud's troubling words written in 1930 are incredibly timely. As of 2011, there were 37 armed conflicts throughout the world (Themner & Wallensteen, 2012), and there are currently about 25 armed conflicts and nuclear threats from North Korea and Iran that have serious bearing on American foreign policy and world stability.[1] Taken together, wars and genocides have led to about 200 million deaths in the twentieth century (Bohm et al., in press, p. 1). It is within this ominous context that the pioneering intergroup relations and conflict studies of Muzafer Sherif and his colleagues (henceforth, Sherif) from the early 1950s[2] should be appreciated (Sherif et al., 1988). For as the late Harvard social psychologist Roger Brown noted, the Robbers Cave study, the most famous of the Boys' Camp studies, as they are collectively known[3], was "the most successful field experiment ever conducted on intergroup conflict" (Platow & Hunter, 2017, p. 147).[4] What makes Sherif's experiments so important is that they demonstrate to what extent real-life group behavior is context-dependent and setting-specific, compared to individual dispositional/personality factors, biological considerations or ingroup dynamics (ibid., p. 146). Specifically, Sherif demonstrated that intergroup conflict and hostility surfaces when there is competition for limited resources, prompting group members to think and behave negatively toward the other group. Conversely, as Carolyn W. Sherif, one of Sherif's co-authors (and wife) noted, the reduction of group conflict and hostility occurred when the contact between equals included interdependence of a type that necessitated the sharing of resources and energies of all the members of both groups. Moreover, this contact had to be in pursuit of a goal that everyone needed and wanted to engage in, what were called "superordinate goals" (Evans, 1980, p. 48). While psychoanalysis at the time of the study tended to emphasize the unconscious processes that animated individual and group pathology, which caused intergroup conflict and hostility, Sherif's study showed that intergroup conflict and hostility were mainly "products of social structure, including the very organization of persons into discrete and potentially competing social groups" (Campbell, 1988, pp. xviii–xix). In other words, in Sherif's view, it was not personality characteristics that mattered most, whether pathological or otherwise, but rather, "the locus of the person in the intergroup social structure" (ibid., p. xix).

While these findings appear to be taken for granted in some scholarly arenas now, at the time of publication they were groundbreaking, in part because they dramatically affirmed "realistic conflict theory,"[5] a mid-twentieth-century perspective that claims that intergroup conflict and hostility comes about from the competition among groups for scarce though valued material resources (e.g., money, political power, military protection, social status). Sherif's work was a seminal contribution to understanding social identity, common ingroup identity and leadership (Platow & Hunter, 2017, pp. 157–159), as well as group prejudice, discrimination and aggression.

Finally, as with many of the influential social psychologists referred to in this book, it deserves mention that Sherif's passionate interest in intergroup conflict and cooperation should not be entirely surprising given his troubling childhood and later experiences while in Turkey: He was born in Turkey in 1906, he went to Harvard for a second masters in 1929, he returned to Turkey in 1937 and emigrated to the United States in 1945. Sherif had witnessed warfare at about age eight when European armies tried to invade Turkey during World War I, and he was "exasperated by the needless death of numerous innocent civilians" (Brannigan, 1967, p. xi). Moreover, at the end of the war, Turkey was thrust into a civil war among political groups fighting for power and this too left a residue of insecurity in Sherif's outlook. He also barely escaped being killed by Greek soldiers (Platow & Hunter, 2017, p. 146). As a result of his political activism against the Turkish government that was politically sympathetic with the Nazis, Sherif was detained in 1944 without trial by Turkish authorities and kept in solitary confinement for about four months. He was only freed after the intervention of the U.S. State Department acting at the request of his previous American professors and graduate students. Sherif returned to the United States in 1945, where he joined the faculty at Princeton as a fellow of the U.S. State Department (Brannigan, 1967, p. x). As sociologist Augustine Brannigan implied, the aforementioned traumatic experiences left an indelible mark on Sherif's psyche, for his "primary purpose of studying social psychology was to confront the darkest aspects of human societies, conflict and politically grounded misery" (ibid., p. xi). Perhaps, most of all, Sherif hoped that social psychology would surmount political conflict via scientific analysis of social interaction and develop morally guided public policies to lessen conflict and suffering (ibid.).

The Robbers Cave experiment

In the summer of 1954, Sherif investigated two groups of eleven- and twelve-year-old boys (twenty-two in total) who were attending camp in the Sans Bois Mountains, close to Oklahoma City. The children were vetted[6] and found to be "normal" and homogenous (Sherif et al., 1988, p. 53), "healthy, socially well-adjusted, somewhat above average in intelligence, and from stable White middle-class Protestant homes" (Sherif, 1956, p. 54). None of the children knew each other prior to their camp experience, nor did they know that they were part of an experiment (though their parents knew and gave consent). The counselors and director were social psychologists and research assistants.[7] They also did not know that there was another group of children sharing the campsite. Sherif says that he deliberately chose informal groups of children "where group organization and attitude would evolve naturally and spontaneously, without formal direction or external pressures" (ibid.).

In the first week (phase one: "formation of ingroups"), the boys were involved in activities that were geared to facilitate group cohesion, such that norms were generated and leaders took power. For example, the groups assigned themselves names, the Eagles and the Rattlers, and they designed their own flag. Toughness became a norm while homesickness was viewed as a sign of weakness. The boys engaged in activities that required group cooperation like constructing dams and lean-tos or did treasure hunts that involved a collective reward, as well as the usual summer activities like swimming, boating and hiking. Competitive activities, such as baseball, were avoided.

However, by the end of the first week, the two groups accidentally noticed each other. Seeing "those guys" using "our ball field" and "our hiking trails" incited demands for competition. In fact, importantly, even prior to the boys actually competing with each other there was an ingroup bias, as they had developed a negative outlook on the other group, characterized by an upsurge of territoriality and prejudicial attitudes toward the group that they had no actual intergroup contact with (one Eagle called the Rattlers "nigger campers") (Platow & Hunter, 2017, p. 151). The counselors and director were delighted to organize a four-day tournament that included competitive activities such as baseball, touch football, tug-of-war and other such spirited activities (phase two: "production of negative attitudes"). It should be noted that the experimenters chose some competitive activities, such as song and skits, for which they could rig the outcome as the judges (ibid.). Most importantly, the counselors and director promised the victorious group a trophy, medals and four-bladed pocketknives. As a result of these experimentally choreographed conditions for limited and valued resources, the boys practiced with great effort, cheered their fellow-group members, and severely booed and insulted their competition. In fact, the antagonism between the groups became so extreme as the tournament proceeded that it culminated in a flag burning when the Eagles were defeated in the tug-of-war. As Sherif noted, "From that time on, name calling (e.g., 'bums' and 'cowards'), scuffles and raids were the rule of the day" (Sherif, 1956, p. 57). It is clear that the goals and efforts of the boys during the competition had become intensely meaningful to them on the personal level.

Sherif tells us that the Eagles were ultimately victorious in the tournament (though the tournament was rigged for practical reasons related to sustaining the experiment), and were awarded the trophy, medals and coveted pocketknives. However, while the Eagles were participating in a celebratory swim, the Rattlers raided their cabins: they overturned beds, tore out mosquito netting, snatched personal property and, significantly, stole their prizes. As a result of this raid, the rivalry had turned into a full-scale war, and the counselors and director were occupied with suppressing name calling, breaking up fist fights and tidying up after cabin raids and food fights. After two weeks, the experiment had taken these "normal" boys with no history of school, psychological or behavioral difficulties, and converted them into fighting firebrands, full of aggression and highly motivated to seek out revenge for every real or imagined insult. As Sherif noted, "experimental assessment of intergroup attitudes showed unmistakable attribution of derogatory stereotypes to the villainous outgroup and of favorable qualities to the ingroup" (Sherif et al., 1988, p. 210).

In the final phase of the experiment (phase three: "reduction of friction"), Sherif tried to reduce the aforementioned demonizing thoughts, aggressive feelings and negative behavior displayed by both groups of boys. While at first it would appear that increasing the amount of contact between the groups would improve their bellicose relationship [e.g., "to communicate accurate and favorable information about one group to the other" (Sherif, 1956, p. 58).][8] it actually made matters worse. For instance, the fact that the boys were asked to eat together only led to more food fights. Rather, what made the positive difference was that when the groups recognized that it was essential to work together, to cooperate with each other to reach superordinate goals—ones they greatly desired—there were dramatic improvements in their relationship. After the boys worked together to repair their water supply (deliberately damaged by the counselors and director), amalgamated their money to rent a movie that neither group could afford alone and collectively fixed a broken-down truck (they restarted the truck by pulling on a rope attached to its bumper, the opposite of the tug-of-war competition), the tensions and hostilities between the groups gradually dissipated, and many cross-group friendships were established. Intergroup ratings supported this finding.

It should be emphasized that while superordinate goals reduce intergroup tensions and hostilities, they do not do so quickly. For example, after the boys fixed the water supply and the two groups amicably mingled together, they still had a food fight at the end of the day. Likewise, while the two groups amalgamated their money to pay for the movie, when they viewed the movie they sat on opposite sides of the dining hall. It took about six days before the prior tensions and hostilities were significantly diminished (though, as expected, there was some residual ingroup favoritism). Rather encouragingly, when it was time for the boys to travel home from the camp, the two groups requested that they travel on the same bus, and the boys seated themselves without distinguishing their Eagle or Rattler preference.[9]

The Boys' Camp studies demonstrated three important ideas that are well accepted today, though in need of further study. First, "that groups have a material reality that includes interdependencies, and role and status relationships, but that these vary dynamically as a function of the nature of the intragroup and intergroups relations" (Platow & Hunter, 2017, p. 154). In other words, rather than believe, as was the case at the time of his study, that only individuals have a scientifically credible material reality, Sherif showed that a variety of social-psychological variables are in play only at the conceptual level of the group. For example, the leader's effectiveness qua leader is not simply a question of his individual disposition, but is dependent on the group that he leads (ibid.). In fact, each co-potentiate the other in a dynamic interaction and enactment.

Second, the Boys' Camp studies showed "that groups have substantive psychological meaning and significance for their members" (ibid.). That is, as Sherif noted, the boys in his studies very much identified with their groups and felt a sense of belonging. The fate of the group, its successes and failures, animated their sense of individual self-identity. It is also worth mentioning that prior to their intergroup contact, the group had established identity-defining qualities that included negative intergroup attitudes, and thus they created domains and objects reflecting ingroup territoriality, like "our baseball diamond," "our Upper Camp" and "our fish" (Sherif et al., 1988, pp. 94, 92, 128, respectively). Prior to Sherif's Boys' Camp studies, stereotyping, prejudice and discrimination were explained in terms of individual psychological dispositions or cognitive error,[10] more or less isolated from social context (e.g., religious, political and ideological attachments that generate social organization that impact the person), or as reflecting an intragroup characteristic (Platow & Hunter, 2017). However, despite Sherif designing his studies to invalidate such an explanatory approach, by choosing a homogenous group of "normal" boys who had no alleged psychological deficits, subsequent studies continued to argue otherwise (ibid., pp. 154–155). For example, as Bohm et al. (in press, pp. 4–5) noted, personality theories of intergroup conflict, like T.W. Adorno's *The Authoritarian Personality* (Adorno et al., 1950), claimed that fascistic potential was lodged in a pathological personality constellation, which negatively impacted thinking (e.g., stereotyping, prejudice), feeling (e.g., fear and hate) and behavior (e.g., discrimination and aggression). Likewise, based on psychometric findings, "right-wing authoritarianism" (Altemeyer, 1998) that further developed Adorno's concepts claimed that those individuals who fit into this category are more endorsing of punishment and control of norm deviators, and are geared to prejudice against ethnic and racial minorities.

Third, the Boys' Camp studies demonstrated "that intergroup impressions [i.e., stereotypes], attitudes, and behavior are both (a) a consequence of intergroup relations (as opposed to causes) and also (b) psychologically meaningful for group members" (Platow & Hunter, 2017, p. 155). That is, stereotypes, defined as those mental representations of a social group that individuals fashion by connecting specific characteristics and emotions with the group, had a strong interpretive grip on the groups of boys in terms of content and valence, thus reflecting modifications in the competitive and cooperative interactions between the two groups. The take home point is that interaction between rival and hostile groups cannot be improved by mere contact as a way to find out they are similar to each other. Though this is important, in addition, any intervention must modify the actual relationships between the actual group members from which the stereotyping emanates (ibid.).

There have been some important methodological criticisms of Sherif's research, despite the elegant simplicity of his experimental design, the compelling findings, and the numerous field and experimental replications in a variety of settings, cultures and social categories (ibid., p. 157). For example, some have argued that Sherif's mode of hypothesis testing was not properly scientific and was self-serving. Sherif began his study believing in the contact hypothesis (i.e., the theory that particular kinds of direct contact between members of hostile groups will diminish stereotyping and prejudice). For example, Carolyn W. Sherif noted, "one hypothesis would say, let it be contact in which both groups are doing something they want to do very much and their pleasure at these activities will spread to their relationship" (Evans, 1980, p. 47). However, "for about three days this hypothesis was tested, and in a total of thirteen different situations in which the groups were together, they continued to fight and call each other nasty names" (ibid., p. 48). In other words, intergroup relations were "not improved simply by developing cooperative and friendly attitudes and habits within groups" (Sherif et al., 1988, p. 207). It was only late in Sherif's study that he then developed the hypothesis that ameliorative contact had to have superordinate goals that conflicting groups jointly solved, thus, say the critics, implying that Sherif was biased to empirically verify rather than test his hypothesis (Platow & Hunter, 2017, p. 155). In my view this criticism is something of a "straw dog" argument. Sherif was revising his hypothesis in sync with the emerging fact pattern as the experiment proceeded, which was entirely in accordance with his "main focus of study—the flow of interaction within groups and between groups under varying conditions" (Sherif et al., 1988, p. 121). Such a methodology exemplifies scientific field study at its best, what O.J. Harvey (1988, p. xxiii) called "experimental anthropology," and to be criticized for doing what he set out to do is a disingenuous criticism rooted in an extremely narrow definition of science. Sherif's critics have no compelling evidence that Sherif was pre-meditatively trying to verify rather than test his evolving hypothesis.[11]

Another criticism of the Boys' Camp study was that it only encompassed two weeks of the boys' lives, a relatively short period of time, and the summer camp setting has its own unique characteristics and ambience.[12] Also, two of the boys from the Eagles got so homesick they were sent home, which means that the Rattlers, viewed by the boys to be tougher, evolved into the numerical majority group. Thus, as Sherif noted (Sherif et al., 1988, p. 100), the experimenters believed that they had to engineer the ultimate result of the tournament because other homesick Eagles were susceptible to becoming too disorganized (e.g., shift status positions) and downhearted if they were defeated. Similarly, while like any field study that involves participant observation, some critics have alleged that the experimenters may have been too enmeshed in the experiment and influenced some of the group behavior related to competition and cooperation. For example, there is a photograph of the counselors photographing one of the group raids, implying to the raiders that their behavior was acceptable. To some extent, the counselors and director qua group had an undertheorized interfering role in bringing about Sherif's findings. While Sherif mentions that some of these unplanned interferences by the experimenters may have influenced group behavior (Sherif et al., 1988, p. 32), these considerations are not factored into Sherif's overall explanation of his findings (Platow & Hunter, 2017, p. 156).

Also worth mentioning is that some critics have claimed that Sherif did not distinguish between competition that was based on material competition, say for water or food, and more symbolic competition, such as that which is lodged in values, prestige and social status, or in the case of the Eagles and Rattlers, competition for an elaborate trophy and other paraphernalia (ibid., p. 156). Thus, these critics claim, the consequences of these two forms of competition may have different outcomes. The problem with this criticism is that it is lodged in a category mistake rooted in a questionable understanding of human being-in-the-world, for as Heidegger showed, material and symbolic competition are always enmeshed, just as thinking, feeling and action are the constituent interrelated, interdependent and interactive elements of *Dasein* (human existence).

Despite the criticisms of Sherif's study, most of which are insubstantial in my view, he has given us "a chilling picture of how rational competition over scarce resources can quickly escalate into full-scale conflict which then, in turn, fosters the accompanying negative attitudes toward opponents that form the core of prejudice" (Baron & Byrne, 2003, p. 217).

Psychoanalytic reflections on the Robbers Cave experiment

Not only was Freud fairly pessimistic about the role of psychoanalysis in preventing or stopping wars or conflicts (Freud, 1964), but so are most contemporary psychoanalytically oriented theorists of politics and international relations (Volkan, 2005). While there have been some interesting contributions to understanding large-group conflicts (Volkan, 2006), for the most part, psychoanalysis has been of limited value to "'curing' large-group conflicts, taming aggression and destruction, and diminishing the derivatives of aggression within human nature" (Volkan, 2005, p. 528).[13] However, as Volkan further notes, "I am optimistic about using psychoanalytic insights and concepts to deal with and modify certain specific and limited political and international situations," always in collaboration with an interdisciplinary team (ibid.). That is, while psychoanalytic insights and concepts can illuminate some of the psychological issues that may have bearing on the sources of intergroup conflict and its reduction, each political, international and other conflict has its own idiosyncratic history and trajectory that cannot be easily, if at all, generalized to other situations, let alone scientifically tested.[14] Likewise, while many analysts are familiar with the psychology of small groups in the therapeutic and organizational/industrial context, mainly intragroup dynamics, such as in the work of Wilfred R. Bion, Elliott Jaques and M.F.R. Kets de Vries (Marcus, 2017), none of these writers have applied their theories to Sherif's landmark study, or for that matter systematically to other social-psychological theories and findings in the psychology of intergroup conflict (e.g., social identity theory, integrated threat theory and the theory of bounded generalized reciprocity) (Bohm et al., in press). This being said, it should be stated that Sherif lodged his study in "actual small groups in social life"[15] (Sherif et al., 1988, p. xxix), though as D.T. Campbell notes in his introduction to Sherif's book, he quite clearly wanted his work to be useful to "anyone specializing in the interdisciplinary and multidisciplinary areas of intergroup and international conflict" (ibid., p. xx). With these conceptual and practical drawbacks in mind, what "limited" contributions, to quote Volkan, can psychoanalysis offer by way of understanding the kind of intergroup conflict and cooperation that Sherif so brilliantly demonstrated?

The narcissism of minor differences

Intergroup conflict, says Freud, involves the "narcissism of minor differences" (1957, p. 199). The idea here is that it is often seemingly unimportant differences between people, like the Sunnis and the Shiites, Eagles and Rattlers, or the Freudians and Relationalists, who are otherwise similar, that generate the basis of the enacted hostility and aggression between them. For example, while the Sunnis and Shiites maintain somewhat different religious beliefs, they are Muslims who have lived together as neighbors with shared ancestry and similar customs, yet some of the bloodiest conflicts have been between them. Likewise, Werman (1986) has pointed out how the narcissism of minor differences has destructively played out in psychoanalytic organizations and treatment, such as in internecine theoretical disputes that have fragmented the field and profession. Freud further commented on this dynamic, noting that it is frequently "communities with adjoining territories, and related to each other in other ways as well, who are engaged in constant feuds and in ridiculing each other" (1961, p. 114). Elsewhere he notes that the phenomenon is not limited to ethnic or religious peoples either: "Every time two families become connected by a marriage, each of them thinks itself superior to or of better birth than the other. Of two neighboring towns each is the other's most jealous rival; every little canton looks down upon the others with contempt" (Freud, 1955, p. 101).

Freud explained the narcissism of minor differences as an expression of the inborn human tendency for aggression and the wish to assert a distinctive identity. If one were to view one's neighbor as the same, then one's sense of unique self-identity and imagined superiority would be undermined, creating disturbing cognitive/affective dissonance. Thus, by asserting one's difference as opposed to one's similarity to the other, one diminishes narcissistic injury, that is, one shores up one's self-esteem and enhances one's self-concept. Indeed, Freud's linking of minor differences to identity assertion/distinctiveness is a theme that is the basis of social identity theory (Tajfel et al., 1971). This theory claims that individuals are motivated to derive self-esteem via their group membership, which largely accounts for ingroup bias, including the sense of "weness." In other words, favoring the ingroup over the outgroup becomes a mode of conveying regard for the ingroup, and is thus a way of increasing self-regard, of esteeming me and mine. As Freud noted, "It is always possible to bind together a considerable number of people in love, so long as there are other people left over to receive the manifestations of their aggressiveness" (1961, p. 114). With the aforementioned dissonance-reducing dynamic in play, it is not difficult to see how divergences between individuals and groups can be expanded and intensified into near insurmountable ruptures between groups, as was the case between the Eagles and the Rattlers. As Freud noted in his personal "confession" in the *Interpretation of Dreams*, he always required a close friend and a hated enemy in his life (Akhtar, 2009, p. 184). Likewise, as large-group psychoanalytic theoretician Vamık D. Volkan claims, all human beings have a need for allies and enemies (1999).

Indeed, the Eagles and the Rattlers kept their distinctiveness as a group self (i.e., thinking and feeling themselves to be intensely committed to their respective groups) by assuming a negative identity. That is, they defined themselves by what they were not, and thus focused on fairly unimportant differences. In this way, they vigorously shielded themselves from any subversion of their unique individual and group identity. For example, by the groups naming themselves Eagles or Rattlers, giving themselves their own flag, and referring to places and things as "ours," they accentuated their unique identity. The aggressive aspect of their negative identity was expressed in flag burning, name-calling, fist fights and raids. Chances are these hostile actions in part reflected unconscious externalizations and projections[16] onto, and into, the adversarial group of qualities that they felt about themselves. The overall purpose of these externalizations and projections was group protection, the group with which the self is utterly narcissistically enmeshed.

The problem with generating a social identity that is a negative identity, that is, one that is based on what they were not, an Eagle or Rattler, is that one does not actually stand for anything that is lodged in one's own dearly held beliefs or values and correlated effective actions. For example, choosing a career or significant other based on what you don't like or don't want is hardly an approach that will generate a long-term favorable outcome. Rather, one has to engage in the psychological "heavy lifting" of clarifying what one wants and why. Put colloquially, "Being opposed to something is simple," but courageously affirming, "This is what I stand for" is a lot more difficult.

The role of the leader in intergroup conflict

Sherif makes it clear that his study was not mainly about leader/group relations. In fact, he notes that theories of intergroup relations that theorize single variables such as the type of "leadership, national character, or individual frustrations, as sovereign determinants of intergroup conflict or harmony," have clarified only selectively chosen examples (Sherif et al., 1988, p. 201). However, Sherif was well aware that leadership is important, as are the prevailing norms of social distance, the structure and practices within the groups, and the personal frustrations of individual group members. That is, in Sherif's view, none of these single variables determine the trend of intergroup behavior at a particular time; rather, they all make their contribution with dissimilar weights at dissimilar times: "Intergroup behavior at a given time can be explained only in terms of the entire frame of reference in which all these various factors function interdependently," this being the "starting point of our experiments on intergroup relations" (ibid.). A frame of reference is composed "of the totality of functionally related factors, external and internal, that operate interdependently to determine the psychological reaction at any given time" (ibid., p. 141). In light of Sherif's holistic point of view, in which the whole is different than the sum of the parts, he made a few observations about leaders that are worth highlighting, for they can be connected to psychoanalytic understandings of small intergroup conflict.

The hierarchical group structures of the Eagles and the Rattlers were influenced not only by the particular experimental problem the experimenters created, but also the kind of leadership that emerged (i.e., a pyramidal hierarchy with the leader at the apex). Most importantly, this hierarchy developed within the context of the specific set of values or norms that were dominant in the group along with the character of the values and norms of the general sociocultural setting in which the group was ensconced (ibid., p. 33). Put colloquially, every group gets the leader it not only needs but deserves. For example, "in no instance did an ingroup engage, as a group, in aggressive action toward the outgroup if doing so had not been approved by the leader" (ibid., p. 126). One of the Rattlers' retaliatory raids, in "true commando style (darkening faces, arms, etc.)" was led by "Mills," who was viewed as "especially heroic because he jumped in a window and secured comic books and a pair of blue jeans which, much to the Rattlers' delight, turned out to be Mason's," the Eagles' leader (ibid., p. 112). The retaliatory raid by the Eagles was led by "Mason," during which they seriously "messed up the Rattler's cabin" (ibid.).

Unfortunately, Sherif does not tell us much about the psychological particulars of Mills or Mason, though he does mention that "the frustrations, deprivations, and gratifications in the histories of the individual member" should be factored into any theory of intergroup conflict (ibid., p. 201). In general, many members throughout the three phases of the experiment—formation of ingroups, production of negative attitudes and reduction of friction—performed leadership functions such as initiating activities, offering suggestions, and implementing tasks in various situations; however, each group had only one "leader," Mills and Mason [the latter of whom had replaced "Craig," see p. 76 (ibid., p. 89)]. About Mills we learn that he perpetuated a "'toughness' norm," though he also maintained his leadership standing by playing the "'clown' role" which kept him "in the center of activity" (ibid., p. 71). Rather important to twelve-year old boys was the fact that Mills was a superior athlete, including in baseball, which was especially important to these boys at the time of the experiment (ibid., p. 129). About Mason, Sherif noted that he came to the leadership position in the early days of intergroup competition and rivalry in the tournament. He was intensely involved with the group effort to win and was identified with its victory, and he tended to avoid contact with the Rattlers in the friction reduction phase of the experiment, which was not replicated by his fellow Eagles (ibid., p. 191).

A psychoanalytic lens on Sherif's experiment might focus in on phase one, the formation of the ingroup, by suggesting that in some sense the Eagles and the Rattlers, qua small groups, unconsciously represented an idealized mother, that is, a psychological parent that symbolized nurturance and stability. As a result, the members had an intense narcissistic attachment to their group/mother. In social-psychological language, this means an individual's membership in a group is a critically important part of self-identity. For example, a group provides a feeling of belongingness and value, of being affirmed on one's own terms; it allows one to enjoy the reflected glory of the group's accomplishments other than one's own; it gives one a feeling of being "at home" in a sheltering place of similarity and understanding. Group membership links one to others as the foundation of one's involvement in social life; it reinforces one's needs and desires for mastery and connectedness. Groups can provide support and confidence in one's ways of comprehending and navigating the world. Finally, they can act as an emotional shock absorber and in other ways amplify a sense of being psychologically intact, and, in some instances, enhance physical safety (Smith et al., 2015, p. 191).

Psychoanalysts have highlighted the fact that a group demarcates itself by creating boundaries and borders that generate an intense feeling of "we-ness," "sameness" and "togetherness" compared to outgroups that can become the "other," an adversary or enemy. This process of identification with the group self involves giving up one's individual self-identity, though some have argued that the self-identity always includes a relationship to small and large groups and only involves a modification of feelings, perceptions and actions that are largely context-dependent and setting-specific. In terms of the leaders of the Eagles and the Rattlers, an analyst might suggest that they were related to by the other group members as if they were similar to a protective and guiding father.[17]

With regards to the second phase of the experiment, the production of negative attitudes, a psychoanalyst might analogize the bellicose behavior of the Eagles and the Rattlers as a reflection of a regressed group, the main focus of Freud's study of group psychology. As Freud wrote,

> Some of [a group's] features—the weaknesses of intellectual ability, the lack of emotional restraint, the incapacity for moderation and delay, the inclination to exceed every limit in the expression of emotion and to work it off completely in the form of actions—these and similar features ... show an unmistakable picture of a regression of mental activity to an earlier stage such as we are not surprised to find among savages or children.
>
> *(1955, p. 117)*

Group regression was clearly manifested by introducing situations that were "competitive and reciprocally frustrating" (Sherif et al., 1988, p. 96). Such situations created unfavorable stereotypes, manifested by name calling, derogation of the outgroup and the clearly stated wish to avoid any contact with the outgroup. As the intergroup friction escalated, there were fights, raids and a flag burning, what in psychoanalytic language are regressive behaviors. When the experimentally induced competition and frustration between the Eagles and the Rattlers increased, each group held tighter to their group affiliation while at the same time devalued the adversarial group through negative stereotyping and the like. Defeats, such as in the tournament, further inflamed the losers and emboldened the victors. This made each group more vulnerable to conscious or unconscious manipulation by the leaders, who, in the case of the Eagles and the Rattlers, were primed to engage in the kind of degraded thought processes (e.g., impaired judgment and consequential thinking), and compromised emotional processing (e.g., lack of self-control and holding on to negative emotions) that are typical of intergroup conflict, especially in large-group psychology (Volkan, 2014).

Finally, the third phase of Sherif's experiment is reducing friction. Psychoanalysts would wholeheartedly agree that joint ventures that demand cooperation are an effective way to reduce friction between two small or even large groups. However, before this can be achieved in a lasting way, psychoanalysts would focus on the often "extreme" perceptions and expectations that are the basis of intergroup conflict. These are animated by high-intensity emotions, such as inordinate pride and entitlement, shame and humiliation, and other kinds of narcissistic injury that can lead to rage-filed expressions and horrendous behavior against the "enemy." Indeed, when the ingroup believes it can do no wrong and the outgroup can do no right, high-intensity conflict is nearly inevitable. For example, group polarization occurs when group members discuss issues with each other, a process that tends to provoke them to more passionately and rigidly maintain their point of view and become more attached to their ideas. When group polarization occurs, the group members are largely impervious to critical reflection, modulation and self-correction of what may be unreasonable positions. Similarly, in competitive and frustrating situations like with the Eagles and the Rattlers, each group generated what amounted to rules of non-engagement in which they did not associate with the enemy, or else ingroup members were guilty of "'betrayal' or 'treason'" (Sherif et al., 1988, p. 213). The use of threats and counter-threats, often rooted in some real or imagined need for revenge, are other tactics that groups use, especially their leaders, which need deconstruction and modulation before the reduction of friction can take place and have lasting psychological and practical traction.[18] These are the "usual suspects" associated with most forms of psychoanalytically informed conflict resolution approaches that need to be addressed. To some extent, these are touched upon by other psychologically minded conflict-resolution approaches. The work of W. R. Bion (1959) on small-group behavior, for example, is especially important. While it mainly focused on intragroup processes (Sherif's first phase, formation of ingroups), it has some bearing on understanding aspects of the Eagles' and the Rattlers' behavior during all three phases of the experiment.

Bion's view of small group behavior

Bion defines his famous basic group assumptions as "the capacity of the individual for instantaneous combination with other individuals in an established pattern of behavior" (1959, p. 160). Basic assumptions are the unconscious group dynamics, the "common, agreed upon, and anonymous obedience prevalent in a group at a given time" (Akhtar, 2009, p. 33). When a group is lodged in a basic assumption, its capacity to work efficiently and effectively is seriously compromised, which often leads to more primitive, archaic and infantile modes of behavior that make the realistic business of the small group, say a team in the workplace, or the Eagles and the Rattlers enjoying a tournament in camp, impossible to engage in. Bion describes three types of basic assumption: dependency, fight-flight and pairing, though others have formulated fourth, fifth and sixth assumptions.[19]

Dependency

The first assumption, dependency, "is that the group is met in order to be sustained by a leader on whom it depends for nourishment, material and spiritual, and protection" (Bion, 1959, p. 132). This basic assumption thus postulates a "collective belief in a protective deity, leader, or organization that will always provide security for the group" (Akhtar, 2009, p. 33). For example, the group leader on a team in the workplace may ask a thought-provoking question, only to be received by the members with passive silence, as if he had not spoken at all. The leader may be idealized into something of an omnipotent and omniscient god who can perfectly look after his docile children, a role that certain types of zealous leaders may assume. Mills and Mason, the leaders of the Rattlers and the Eagles, respectively, each in their own way and at different times, displayed behavior that calls to mind aspects of what Bion described. Likewise, the typical boy's enmeshment with the Eagles or the Rattlers qua group provided him with a strong sense of security and self-value. However, says Bion, resentment at being dependent on the god-like leader may gradually stimulate the wish to depose the leader, if not "kill" him off, and then look for a new leader, only to repeat the destructive process.[20] Indeed, Mason, the Eagles' leader, replaced Craig not only due to resentment of his dependency on the god-like leader, but also from Craig's gradual drop in status due to his defection at a number of critical points of the tournament. For example, when the group was losing the first tug-of-war, Craig simply walked away from the rope prior to the contest's conclusion. Craig then tried to blame other group members for the defeat. "He's quit on us *again*," one boy said about their leader. Even worse, perhaps, Craig pretended to be asleep during the first Rattler raid and stayed in the background during the second (Sherif et al., 1988, p. 129). In other words, Craig had displayed cowardice, irresponsibility and lack of motivation as a leader. The group replaced him with Mason to fill the power vacuum.

As Kets de Vries (2011) points out, groups that are under the sway of the dependency assumption seek out a charismatic leader because, like small children, they feel helpless, inadequate, needy and fearful of the external world. In such groups one frequently hears such statements in the workplace as, "What do you want me/us to do?" Or, "I can't take this kind of decision; you'll have to talk to my boss." While group cohesion and goal-directedness may be present in such groups, for the most part the group is not capable of autonomy, criticality or creativity. Even when the leader has left the group and they can independently grow and develop, groups under the dependency assumption tend to reside in a retrospective consciousness, fantasizing about what the long-lost leader/parent would have done in a decision-making situation. In such instances, the group may fall back on bureaucratic inactivity and apathy and, thus, function without a trace of initiative or innovation (Kets de Vries, 2011, p. 33). It is interesting to note that Mason displaced Craig as the Eagles' leader in part due to the fact that Craig would not make important decisions, leaving the group on its own (i.e., frustrating their dependency needs), often ultimately submitting to Mason, the superior athlete. Mason had enlisted another boy, Wilson, to support his leadership grab. Wilson became his lieutenant, and as such was increasingly important to the group since he was a good athlete, was devoted to maintaining joint efforts to win the tournament and he supported Mason's decisions (Sherif et al., 1988, p. 129). The larger point about leadership is that effective leadership is not simply about having a specific cluster of leadership characteristics the way many analysts and personality theorists would view it; rather, the required characteristics of a leader are correlated with changes in social context and setting, especially to the extent that the ingroup's interests can be promoted (Platow & Hunter, 2017, pp. 152, 158).

Fight-flight

The fight-flight group assumption "is that the group has met to fight something or to run away from it. It is prepared to do either indifferently" (Bion, 1959, p. 138). In other words, the group believes in "the existence of an external enemy who one must vanquish or avoid" (Akhtar, 2009, p. 33). This assumption has obvious applicability to the Eagles' and the Rattlers' intergroup conflict, as I have earlier pointed out. An important characteristic of this group culture is that it puts into sharp focus the individual with "paranoid trends," causing the work world to be divided into those who are beloved friends and hated enemies, an "us-versus-them" outlook (Bion, 1959, p. 63; Kets de Vries, 2011, p. 33). As Kets de Vries notes, fight responses are expressed in aggressive behavior against colleagues, bosses or the self. "Envy, jealousy, competition, elimination, boycotting, sibling rivalry, fighting for a position in the groups and privileged relationships with authority figures" are typical reactions in this group culture (2011, p. 33), and indeed emerged in the Eagles and the Rattlers. Flight reactions in the work context may include avoidance of colleagues, managers and bosses, absenteeism and an overall comportment of having given up caring. Common remarks of such groups are, "Let's not give those updated figures to the contracts department; they'll just try to take all the credit," and "This company would be in good shape if it weren't for the so-and-sos who run the place." In addition, there is a lack of embracing of individual responsibility; rather, there is a marked tendency to project and externalize, blaming others for one's mistakes or for the team's lack of success. This latter response was manifest at different times in both the Eagles and the Rattlers. In such groups there is an inevitable strengthening of group cohesion and identity and increased dependence on a strong, charismatic leader who self-righteously fosters the "you are either with us, or against us" way of thinking, which further "fires up" group members to adhere to their irrational group mentality (ibid.). This too was evident in the behavior of the Eagles and Rattlers.

Pairing

Finally, we come to the pairing group assumption, "the opposite pole to feelings of hatred, destructiveness, and despair" that may exist in fight-flight group cultures, what Bion describes as "the air of the hopeful expectation" (1959, p. 136). The function of the pairing group "is to provide an outlet for feelings centered on ideas of breeding and birth, that is to say for Messianic hope, … a precursor to sexual desire," and "without ever arousing the fear that such feelings will give rise to an event that will demand development …" (ibid., pp. 136, 143). Thus, the pairing basic assumption expresses "the messianic hope that someone from the future generations will solve the problems of the group" (Akhtar, 2009, p. 33). As Kets de Vries notes, the pairing assumption is a way for an individual group member to connect to a perceived powerful other and assist him in effectively managing his "anxiety, alienation and loneliness" (2011, pp. 33, 34). In the workplace this powerful individual can be a colleague, manager or boss. Not only does such a tactic provide a modicum of safety and security, it satisfies the fantasy that by connecting with a powerful other, individual and collective creativity will magically upsurge. In the case of the Eagles and the Rattlers, it was the experimenters, qua leadership group, that functioned in the boys' unconscious minds as a modulating bridge between the second phase (production of negative attitudes) and the third phase (reduction of friction) that became the healing experience to their intergroup conflict. In this context, both groups of boys unconsciously identified with the hopeful aspirations of the experimenters that by engaging in joint problem-solving activities they would no longer be adversaries but would gradually become friends, which is what happened. Moreover, in a certain sense, the reduction of friction phase gave the groups an opportunity to diminish their narcissistic investment in their respective group culture and identify with a common goal of similarity and understanding that was experimentally induced by their participation in activities that had superordinate goals.

The main thrust of Bion's psychoanalytic contribution to the psychology of small-group process, including its applicability to the Eagles and the Rattlers, is that when the group is under the sway of one of the basic assumptions, it cannot reasonably think, so it becomes "psychotic, albeit temporarily" (Bain & Gould, 1996, p. 119) and engages in "patterns of psychotic behavior" (Bion, 1959, p. 165). For example, there are severe impairments in representing, mentalizing, remembering and acknowledging, mainly because the group's tendencies for direct hallucinatory gratification of early developmental wishes for safety and security have a strong interpretive grip on the group process (Roth, 2013, pp. 535, 527). That is, Bion's brilliant two-tier psychology of the small group shows how the internal mental state of the group, the "group culture," resonates with particular primordial unconscious anxieties and fantasies that greatly hinder and obstruct the efficient and effective "surface" work of productivity of rationally-conceived group function (ibid., p. 526). Bion calls the standard, normative group structures that promote adaptation to reality, are instantiated by the accomplishment of realistic group goals and that gratify the members' reasonable needs the "work group culture." In Sherif's experiment, the reduction of fiction phase, in which the groups came together to cooperatively problem-solve and develop lasting friendships, personifies the work group culture.

Implications for treatment

Sherif's three-phased experiment, including formation of ingroups, production of negative attitudes and reduction of friction, has significant bearing on how ordinary people, whether in psychoanalytic treatment or not, can be better able to create a morally animated, flourishing life.

In terms of formation of ingroups, it is indisputable that having a small (and large) group identity can be a beneficial addition to one's everyday life. Indeed, while group identity is formed by the members establishing roles, status, norms and cohesiveness, the sense of belongingness and empowerment that comes from inclusion and feeling accepted is a powerful need and desire. It may even be "hardwired," as evolutionary psychologists have alleged. However, the main problem with a small-group affiliation, Sherif's primary concern, is that such groups hold powerful sway over one's individual outlook and behavior, which can become highly problematic for the individual trying to live life according to strongly felt, flexibly and creatively applied, transcendent-pointing moral beliefs and values. That is, there is always a danger that an individual's autonomy, integration and humanity can be subverted through his group affiliation. Such a person becomes so wedded to the group's roles, status, norms and cohesiveness, that he denies, rationalizes or reconstitutes his own personal needs, desires and, most importantly, moral beliefs and values, in order to comply with the conscious and unconscious demands of the group. If Bion is right that all small groups have a psychotic potential, then the question for the ordinary person who resides in a small-group culture is where to "draw the line" between what one chooses to give to the group, and what one affirms to oneself, "from here I will not retreat."

This is no easy matter, because in most circumstances there is no actual "line in the sand" to be drawn once and for all. There is more so a constant, creative recalibration of one's beliefs and values in accordance with the vague and unsure demand characteristics of the context and setting of the particular decision to be made. Put differently, what one has to do to sustain a modicum of autonomy, integration and humanity is never static or fixed. However, as long as one has an intact sense of self that is lodged in strongly felt, flexibly and creatively applied, transcendent-pointing moral beliefs and values, a wide range of behavior may be necessary for a person to maintain his autonomy, integration and humanity, as the circumstances of many small groups are often morally ambiguous and ambivalent. One of the important take home points regarding Sherif's formation of group phase is that one has to know what beliefs and values "really" matter and be willing and able to stand up for them, even though this can lead to ostracism and other types of social devaluation that can operate in both obvious and subtle ways in small groups. While it may sound polemical, it is helpful to keep in mind that one is constantly fighting a moral battle with forms of power-relations, and one has to use one's moral beliefs and values to animate one's decisions.

When a person becomes utterly ensconced in the small-group culture, as were the Eagles and the Rattlers during the production of negative attitudes phase, the situation can become very "nasty and mean." Analysts call this group regression, which calls to mind aspects of Bion's three basic group assumptions (especially "fight-flight"). Group regression can lead to the full-scale conflict that the Eagles and the Rattlers engaged in, like the fist fights, raids and avoidance of the other group. One of the main take home points about Sherif's second phase is that one has to be mindful to what extent one is inclined to use externalization and projection as a basis for capitulating to the worst aspects of small-group functioning, the "them" (outgroup) and "us" (ingroup) orientation, as well as over-identifying with a questionable leader. This is especially important when one understands that groups generally tend to select leaders who personify the group's stereotypes, norms or main identity-defining characteristics (Hogg, 2012). Without understanding why one follows a leader, without continual critical evaluation of what they stand for and to what in the follower they appeal, the chances of capitulating to the dark side of leadership remains a strong possibility. This is yet another reason to be guided by transcendent-pointing moral beliefs and values. In fact, if, as Bion and others have noted, small groups are prone to primitive defenses, object relations and anxieties that can implode a group's high-level functioning, it is imperative that one be highly critical of leaders, many of whom are narcissistic personality types who know exactly how to use their interpersonal wizardry to exploit individual and group psychological vulnerabilities to bring about conformity to their irrational wishes and desire to dominate.

Finally, Sherif's third phase, reduction of friction, wherein the Eagles and the Rattlers engaged in cooperative problem-solving activities for superordinate goals, emphasizes the opposite of polarized perceptions of ingroups and outgroups that guided the production of negative attitudes. The idea is that if you change perceptions, you change aggressive and hostile reactions between small groups. It is well-known that aggression and hostility can be reduced by generating different norms, those of non-aggression in both the ingroup and outgroup context. Likewise, Sherif suggests, and later research has shown, that when you eradicate the typical cues of aggressive and hostile behavior, for instance, firearms, there is a reduction of violence. Of course, the capacity for morally infused critical thinking combined with the ability to metabolize complex and strong emotions associated with intergroup conflict (e.g., anger, hatred, territoriality) make it less likely that one will engage in aggressive, hostile or violent behavior. Such behavior is often rooted in simplistic and stereotypical thinking about and lack of empathy for the outgroup, as well as biased attributions and favoritism for the ingroup.

In closing, Sherif's Boys' Camp studies masterfully attempted to battle the upsurge of individualistic and reductionist accounts of human behavior, the kind that the psychoanalysis of the time tended to put forth. Rather, Sherif claimed that what mattered most was "the social structuration of the human mind" (Kayaoğlu et al., 2014, p. 833). While the Boys' Camp studies have a seemingly simple take home point, "psychological relations between group members reflect functional relations between groups" (ibid.), there is a much more profound message: Group behavior should not be reflexively reduced to intrapersonal proclivities or interpersonal conflicts. Rather, it mainly depends on social structural considerations, those that reflect the social makeup of mind. Thus, "group behavior must be studied in its context, and we must employ rich methods that make this possible" (ibid.).

Notes

1 www.cfr.org/interactives/global-conflict-tracker, retrieved 1/8/19
2 Sherif did two earlier studies in 1949 and 1953 which were further refined and culminated in the book publication of *The Robbers Cave Experiment: Intergroup Conflict and Cooperation* in 1961, which was reissued in 1988.
3 They were named after the Oklahoma park where the study was done in 1954, the former hideout of Jesse James and Belle Starr.
4 As Platow and Hunter note, Brown's quotation was reproduced in Sherif's *New York Times* obituary when he died in 1988 of coronary disease (2017, p. 147).
5 The theory was first officially named by social scientist Donald T. Campbell (1965), who wrote a new introduction to the 1988 reissuance of Sherif's 1961 study.
6 Each boy's family, teachers and school officials were interviewed. His school and medical records were carefully reviewed, as were his scores on personality and intelligence tests, and he was observed in his classroom and at play with his fellow schoolmates (Sherif, 1956, p. 54).
7 Data was systematically collected using, for example, written observations, sociometric scores and status ratings by participant observers, tape recordings, photographs, et cetera. Sherif also asked the boys to rate their own and the other group on such positive traits as "brave," "tough" and "friendly" and negative traits like "smart alecks" and "stinkers." This technique added a degree of experimental rigor to the study (Platow & Hunter, 2017, p. 152).
8 It is well-known that positive interaction between disparate groups can enhance intergroup attitudes and diminish prejudice, in part by encouraging members to view themselves as part of a common group that shares similarities. However, in some contexts this means underplaying or ignoring important real-life differences, such as a group's social disadvantage, and thus truncating efforts to bring about policy and practical change (Smith et al., 2015, pp. 223–224). It was G.W. Allport (1979) who first developed the important "intergroup contact hypothesis," which posits that if a group has more actual contact with a group of a dissimilar race, ethnicity, gender or religion, then the group will have diminished prejudice toward those dissimilar members. The contact situation required four elements: the groups had to have equal status in the situation; they had to have common goals; there had to be intergroup cooperation; and they required the support of the authorities, law or custom (O'Connor, 2017, p. 60). This being said, Allport recognized that "it would be fair to conclude that contact, as a situational variable, cannot always overcome the person variable in prejudice. This is true whenever the inner strain within the person is too tense, too insistent, to permit him to profit from the structure of the outer situation" (1979, p. 267). It is also important to note that two antagonistic groups can cooperate against a "common enemy" (Sherif et al., 1988, pp. 45–46).
9 Exactly how "us" versus "them" becomes "we" is not detailed by Sherif except in terms of the superordinate goal notion. However, other theorists lodged in the "common ingroup identity" approach of Samuel L. Gaertner and John F. Dovidio (a view derived from the social identity theory) emphasize how individuals create and sustain group boundaries (i.e., social categorizations). Other social-psychological perspectives have been posited on this problem, including those lodged in psychoanalytic theory.
10 For example, Allport noted that "that the dynamics of prejudice tend to parallel the dynamics of cognition … the style of thinking that is characteristic of prejudice is a reflection, by and large, of the prejudiced person's way of thinking about anything" (1979, pp. 376–377).
11 There have been longstanding criticisms of field studies like Sherif's, including the fact that there were so many variables at work at the same time that it is nearly impossible to discern which variable had what impact and to what degree. This being said, experimental studies are methodologically limited in that they do not reflect real life in real-time effects, among other criticisms.
12 Sherif has been criticized because all of the group members in the study were boys, and perhaps most importantly, the boys were from a homogenous background that by definition may not be generalizable to other types of racial, ethnic, religious or social groups. This may be true to some extent. However, this criticism appears to be disingenuous

because Sherif clearly indicates that he chose a homogenous group of boys so that he had a sample population about which he could make some generalizations. In my view, to criticize him for doing what he said he would do for good reason is precisely the kind of post-hoc criticisms that occur when critics are "looking to" unfairly criticize a brilliant piece of social-psychological research.

13 This conclusion has been reiterated by psychoanalyst Howard B. Levine, "Attempts to apply psychoanalytic insights to politics, large social groups and the interactions between large groups and their leaders have met with little success" (2014, p. xi).

14 Volkan thinks otherwise, though he does not in any way substantiate his claim beyond his personal experiences: "Otherwise, working in many parts of the world, I have come to the firm conclusion that individual and large-group psychology of human beings, whatever large-group identity they may have, [is] the same everywhere" (2014, p. 102). Volkan's sweeping conclusion may in part be lodged in his modernist notion of what he calls "human nature" (2006, p. 14). Needless to say, as someone lodged in a postmodern outlook, I disagree with these claims.

15 Exactly what constitutes a "small group" is not agreed upon by social psychologists or psychoanalysts (nor is what constitutes intergroup relations). Sherif, however, defines a group as "a social unit that consists of a number of individuals who, at a given time, stand in more or less definite interdependent status and role relationships with one another, and that explicitly or implicitly possess a set of norms or values regulating the behavior of the individual members, at least in matters of consequence to the group" (Sherif et al., 1988, p. 200).

16 Depending on one's psychoanalytic theory, there are differences, even hairsplitting ones, between externalization and projection. For example, one author confusingly claims "Projection signifies placing impulses or parts of the self into external objects whereas externalization involves creating or finding a reality to support the defences, including projecting" (Giovacchini, 1977, p. 289). Volkan refers to "*externalisations* of unwanted self-and object images/*projections* of unacceptable thoughts and affects" (2014, p. 63). While I am not going to sort out this controversy, I want to alert the reader that, along with projective identification, there is no consensus of terms among analysts. None of these concepts have been adequately experimentally studied as far as I know.

17 I am aware that using the terms mother and father, and assigning certain "conventional" symbolic meanings to them, presupposes certain stereotypical notions, and that in our modern current society these terms can be used more or less interchangeably given the changing roles that mothers and fathers have in the way families are constituted and operate.

18 Volkan, who has mainly written about large-group psychology, has described regression in terms of the collective sense of victimization within a large group (a kind of identity indicator) that may get stirred up again by an attack of the enemy or some other disaster, like an economic one, which may revive a sense of past shared historical trauma and grievances ("chosen traumas") wherein the past and present get powerfully merged and acted upon in violent ways ("time collapse"). An "us against them" dynamic is in play. Large groups can be further inflamed and geared toward violence when they draw from "chosen glories," those collective mental representations of historical events and the heroes and heroines connected to these events that are powerfully mythologized over time and transmitted to the next generation (Volkan, 2014). One can see how these large-group formulations have some "family resemblance," mainly in terms of the "feel" of Sherif's observations about the production of friction phase of his experiment, even if it was only a two-week study with boys who did not know each other from the onset. Volkan's Tree Model, a psychoanalytically animated methodology that tries to foster coexistence of opposing large groups, heavily uses a workshop model that takes years of implementation: "During the workshops there are plenary sessions, but most of the work is done in small groups led by members of the facilitating interdisciplinary team," a small-group approach that resonates with Sherif's experiment and findings (ibid., p. 126). As far as I know, none of Volkan's observations and formulations have been experimentally tested, though they appear to be plausible from my

clinical experience in high-conflict resolution work, particularly in terms of "custody wars" (Helmreich & Marcus, 2008).

19 Namely "oneness" (Turquet, 1975), further elaborated as "incohesion: aggregation/massification" (Hopper, 2003); "Me-ness" (Bain & Gould, 1996); and "violent destructive aggression" mainly expressed in large groups (Roth, 2013, p. 527). These latter three assumptions have not "caught on" in small-group theory the way Bion's three assumptions have, and Nitsun raises the criticism that any conceptualization of basic assumptions tends to create "confusion and overlap … between different versions of assumptions" as well as arbitrary "fixed polarities" that do not do justice to the real-life complexity and fluidity of group process (Nitsun, 2015, p. 243), including intergroup relations and conflict.

20 http://achakra.com/2013/11/30/wilfred-bion-group-dynamics-the-basic-assumptions-from-wikipedia/, retrieved 4/27/15.

References

Adorno, T.W., Frenkel-Brunswick, E., Levinson, D.J. & Sanford, R.N. (1950). *The authoritarian personality*. New York: Harper & Row.

Akhtar, S. (2009). *Comprehensive dictionary in psychoanalysis*. London: Karnac.

Allport, G.W. (1979). *The nature of prejudice*. New: Basic Books.

Altemeyer, B. (1998). The other "authoritarian personality." *Advances in Experimental Social Psychology*, 30, 47–92.

Bain, A. & Gould, L.J. (1996). The fifth assumption. *Free Associations*, 6:1(37), 1–20.

Baron, R.A. & Byrne, D. (Eds.) (2003). *Social psychology* (10th ed.). Boston: Pearson Education.

Bion, W.R. (1959). *Experiences in groups*. New York: Ballantine Books.

Bohm, R., Rusch, H. & Baron, J. (in press). The psychology of intergroup conflict: A review of theories and measures. *Journal of Economic Behavior and Organization*, https://doi.org/10.1016/j.jebo.2018.01.020.

Brannigan, A. (1967). Introduction. In M. Sherif (Ed.), *Social interaction: Process and products* (pp. ix–xvi). New Brunswick: Transaction.

Campbell, D.T. (1965). *Ethnocentric and other altruistic motives*. Lincoln, NE: University of Nebraska Press.

Campbell, D.T. (1988). Introduction to the Wesleyan edition. In M. Sherif, O.J. Harvey, B. J. White, W.R. Hood & C.W. Sherif (Eds.), *The Robbers Cave Experiment: Intergroup conflict and cooperation* (pp. xxiii–xxi). Middletown, CT: Wesleyan University Press (Original work published 1961).

Evans, R.L. (1980). *The making of social psychology: Discussions with creative contributors*. New York: Gardner Press.

Freud, S. (1955). Group psychology and the analysis of the ego. In J. Strachey (Trans. and Ed.), *Standard edition of the complete psychological works of Sigmund Freud* (Vol. 18, pp. 61–143). London: Hogarth Press (Original work published 1921).

Freud, S. (1957). Taboo of virginity. In J. Strachey (Trans. and Ed.), *Standard edition of the complete psychological works of Sigmund Freud* (Vol. 22, pp. 191–208). London: Hogarth Press (Original work published 1917).

Freud, S. (1961). Civilization and its discontents. In J. Strachey (Trans. and Ed.), *Standard edition of the complete psychological works of Sigmund Freud* (Vol. 21, pp. 59–151). London: Hogarth Press (Original work published 1930).

Freud, S. (1964) Why war? In J. Strachey (Trans. and Ed.), *Standard edition of the complete psychological works of Sigmund Freud* (Vol. 22, pp. 199–215). London: Hogarth Press (Original work published 1933).

Giovacchini, P.L. (1977). Alienation: character neuroses and narcissistic disorders. *International Journal of Psychoanalytic Psychotherapy*, 6, 289–314.
Harvey, O.J. (1988). Preface to the Wesleyan edition. In M. Sherif, O.J. Harvey, B.J. White, W.R. Hood & C.W. Sherif (Eds.), *The Robbers Cave Experiment: Intergroup conflict and cooperation* (pp. xxiii–xxv). Middletown, CT: Wesleyan University Press (Original work published 1961).
Helmreich, J. & Marcus, P. (2008). *Warring parents, wounded children and the wretched world of child custody: Cautionary tales*. Westport, CT: Praeger.
Hogg, M.A. (2012). Social identity and the psychology of groups. In M.R. Leary & J.P. Tangney (Eds.), *Handbooks of self and identity* (2nd ed., pp. 502–519). New York: Guilford.
Hopper, E. (2003). Traumatic experience in the unconscious life of groups: The fourth basic assumption: Incohesion: Aggregation/Massification or (ba) I:A/M. In M. Pines (Ed.), *International library of group analysis* (Book #23). London: Jessica Kingsley.
Kayaoğlu, A., Batur, S. & Aslıtürk, E. (2014). The unknown Muzafer Sherif. *The Psychologist. British Psychological Society*, 27, 880–883.
Kets de Vries, M.F.R. (2011). *Reflections on groups and organizations*. San Francisco: Jossey Bass.
Levine, H.B. (2014). Foreword: Psychoanalysis and political conflict: Is psychoanalysis relevant? In V.D. Volkan, *Psychoanalysis, international relations and diplomacy: A sourcebook on large-group psychology* (pp. ix–xvi). London: Karnac.
Marcus, P. (2017). *The psychoanalysis of career choice, job performance, and satisfaction: How to flourish in the workplace*. London: Routledge.
Nitsun, M. (2015). *Beyond the anti-group: Survival and transformation*. East Sussex, UK: Routledge.
O'Connor, A. (2017). *An analysis of Gordon Allport's* The Nature of Prejudice. London: Routledge.
Platow, M.J. & Hunter, J.A. (2017). Intergroup relations and conflict: Reviewing Sherif's Boys Camp studies. In J.R. Smith & S.A. Haslam (Eds.), *Social psychology: Revisiting the classic studies* (2nd ed., pp. 146–163). Los Angeles: Sage.
Roth, B. (2013). Bion, basic assumptions, and violence: A corrective reappraisal. *International Journal of Group Psychotherapy*, 63, 525–543.
Sherif, M. (1956). Experiments in group conflict. *Scientific American*, 195, 54–58.
Sherif, M., Harvey, O.J., White, B.J., Hood, W.R. & Sherif, C.W. (1988). *The Robbers Cave Experiment: Intergroup conflict and cooperation*. Middletown: Wesleyan University Press (Original work published 1961).
Smith, R., Mackie, D.M. & Claypool, H.M. (Eds.) (2015). *Social psychology* (4th ed.). New York: Psychology Press.
Tajfel, H., Billig, M.G., Bundy, R.P. & Flament, C. (1971). Social categorization and intergroup behavior. *European Journal of Social Psychology*, 1, 149–178.
Themner, L. & Wallensteen, P. (2012). Armed conflicts, 1846–2011. *Journal of Peace Research*, 49, 1565–1585.
Turquet, P. (1975). Threats to identity in the large group. In L. Kreeger (Ed.), *The large group: Dynamics and therapy* (pp. 57–86). London: Constable.
Volkan, V.D. (1999). Psychoanalysis and diplomacy, Part I: Individual and large-group identity. *Journal of Applied Psychoanalytic Studies*, 1, 29–55.
Volkan, V.D. (2005). Politics and international relations. In E.S. Person, A.M. Cooper & G. O. Gabbard (Eds.), *Textbook of psychoanalysis* (pp. 525–534). Washington, DC: American Psychiatric Publishing.
Volkan, V.D. (2006). *Killing in the name of identity: A study of bloody conflicts*. Charlottesville: Pitchstone Publishing.

Volkan, V.D. (2014) *Psychoanalysis, international relations and diplomacy: A sourcebook on large-group psychology*. London: Karnac.
Werman, D.S. (1986). Freud's "narcissism of minor differences": Review and reassessment. *Journal of the American Academy of Psychoanalysis*, 16(4), 451–459.

Internet sources

http://achakra.com/2013/11/30/wilfred-bion-group-dynamics-the-basic-assumptions-from-wikipedia/, retrieved 4/27/15.
www.cfr.org/interactives/global-conflict-tracker, retrieved 1/8/19.

5

OBEDIENCE VERSUS RESISTANCE

Milgram's obedience to authority experiments (1961)

"Rebellion against tyrants," said Benjamin Franklin, "is obedience to God" (White, 1922, p. 438). Indeed, obedience to authority, in this case to divine authority, had motivating and liberating effects during the American Revolution, a war that is usually judged positively in our era. In this case, obedience was a "virtue," reflecting the best of "conscience," as Milgram called it (1974).[1] However, from the British point of view of the time, and from others now, such obedience was judged as "destructive" (ibid.), highlighting the fact that what constitutes destructive obedience to authority, even "heinous sin" (ibid.), is in the eye of the beholder. There are countless examples of obedience to divine authority, or its secular equivalent, that have been judged as diabolical by most "decent" and "reasonable" people [one only has to think of the followers of Islamic State in Iraq and Syria (ISIS) or Bashar al-Assad's Syrian regime as examples]. Put simply, when it comes to judging what is, and is not, destructive obedience to authority, one man's freedom fighter is another man's terrorist. To make matters even more complicated, who would deny that in some circumstances, such as military battle, obedience to authority, even so-called "blind" obedience, can save your skin and those of your fellow warriors; it can also be life-saving when a fireman instructs you to follow his lead as he rescues you from a burning building. Even in everyday life, obedience to authority can be a life-affirming and sensible response from ordinary people. We stop at red lights to avoid killing ourselves or someone else, and we pay our utility bills to avoid them being turned off and us being prosecuted for non-payment. However, such seemingly benign compliance with authority can, depending on context, become destructive. I am reminded of the Holocaust survivor whom I treated years ago (the only survivor in his family) who told me that he would never forget that when he, his parents and three siblings were deported from Nazi Germany to Auschwitz, and they were told by the Nazis that they had two hours to gather their essential belongings and report to the railroad station, his mother was dawdling because she insisted on paying the electricity bill before going to the railroad station! While his mother's behavior may have been an unconscious attempt to deny the horror of what was happening by carrying on with a "business as usual" attitude, it nevertheless suggests to what extent obedience to authority, whether conceived as positive or negative behavior, is as much a complex and ambiguous moral category and process, saturated by personal moral beliefs and values, as it is a conventionally conceived social-psychological one originating from situational forces.[2]

Stanley Milgram, the son of two Eastern European Jewish immigrants, born the year that Hitler became chancellor of Germany (1933), described his interest in obedience as emanating from his childhood identification with the Jewish people and his struggle to reckon with the Holocaust. He made this point explicitly in *Individual in a Social World,*

> [My] laboratory paradigm ... gave scientific expression to a more general concern about authority, a concern forced upon members of my generation, in particular upon Jews such as myself, by the atrocities of World War II ... The impact of the Holocaust on my own psyche energized my interest in obedience and shaped the particular form in which it was examined.
>
> *(quoted in Blass, 2004, p. 62)*

Milgram's landmark studies on obedience to authority (1963, 1965, 1974) were particularly impacted by Hannah Arendt's controversial "banality of evil" thesis about Adolph Eichmann and the higher echelons of the Nazi leadership. She suggests that rather than being ideologically driven evil warriors or sadistic monsters,[3] they were ordinary-looking, unexceptional functionaries, "desk killers" who were thoroughly engaged in thoughtless and inattentive bureaucratic banality that made Nazi genocide and warmongering possible. As Arendt wrote, Eichmann "had no motives at all. He merely, to put the matter colloquially, never realized what he was doing" (1963, p. 287).[4] Milgram's findings, described in the next section on "The obedience shock experiments", concurred with Arendt's formulation,

> After witnessing hundreds of ordinary people submit to the authority in our experiments, I must conclude that Arendt's conception of the *banality of evil* comes closer to the truth than one might dare imagine. The ordinary person who shocked the victim did so out of a sense of obligation—a conception of his duties as a subject—and not from any particular aggressive tendencies. This is, perhaps, the most fundamental lesson of our study: ordinary people, simply doing their jobs, and without any particular hostility on their part, can become agents in a terrible destructive process.
>
> *(Milgram, 1974, pp. 5–6)*

It is mainly within the psychosocial context of trying to fathom the Holocaust that Milgram designed a series of obedience to authority experiments that provided "evidence of probably the most compelling phenomenon ever uncovered by social psychology" (Reicher & Haslam, 2017, p. 125). Indeed, researchers and scholars are still debating Milgram's fifty-year-old findings and analyses, though the obedience to authority phenomenon "still lacks a compelling explanation" (ibid.).

The obedience shock experiments

In Experiment 5, the most famous of the eighteen variations, Milgram informed naïve subjects in the all-males study that they were engaged in a scientific investigation of the effects of punishment on learning [all were "decent and courteous" in real-life says Milgram (1974, p. 132)]. One of the men in each participant pair would act as the "Learner" and would attempt to do a simple task involving memory by supplying a word. The other man was the "Teacher" who was requested to read the words to the Learner and would punish mistakes through an electric shock if the Learner did not provide the second word in each pair. The shocks were delivered by an imposing, realistic-looking machine (henceforth, the shock generator) that contained thirty numbered switches spanning from 15 volts ("slight shock") through 450 volts ("XXX"; the descriptor for 375 volts read, "danger severe shock"), reflecting the first to the thirtieth switch. The two participants involved in the study, the naïve subject (the Teacher) and a research assistant (the Learner) then drew slips of paper from a hat to decide who would assume each role. The drawing was rigged so that the naïve subject always assumed the role of the Teacher. The Teacher was then instructed by the scientific-looking authority in a white coat to give a shock to the Learner whenever he made an error on the memory task. Most importantly, the Teacher was instructed that they had to increase the strength of the shock each time the Learner made a mistake. What this meant was that when the Learner made numerous mistakes, he would soon be getting strong and seemingly painful jolts of electricity. It is vital to understand that the Learner, who was actually a research assistant, never received any shocks during the experiment. The only time a shock was ever used was a mild pulse from switch number three to persuade naïve subjects that the shock generator was in fact real.

During the experimental session, the Learner, who complied with previously-agreed-upon instructions, made many mistakes. Therefore, naïve subjects soon found themselves confronted with a stressful moral quandary: Should they continue punishing this Learner with what appeared to be increasingly painful shocks, or should they refuse to carry on? If the naïve subjects hesitated in administering the shocks, the Experimenter pressured them to carry on with a graded series of "prods": "Please continue;" "The experiment requires that you continue;" "It is absolutely essential that you continue;" and the most controlling command, "You have no choice—you must go on." If the Teacher still wished to stop after the four successive verbal prods, the experiment was halted. Otherwise, it was halted after the Teacher had given the maximum 450-volt shock three times in a row. These prods are best viewed as Milgram's way of defining the situation in a particular manner, such that the Teachers would have to respond via obedience or disobedience.

The results were surprising. Though all of the naïve subjects were volunteers and were paid prior to the investigation, one would expect that they would refuse the

Experimenter's orders, as harming an innocent person would go against their moral sense and conscience. However, 65% of the naïve subjects showed total obedience; that is, they administered the entire series of graded shocks, including what they thought were life-threatening shocks to an innocent person (450 volts). In another study, Milgram found that the level of obedience for women was virtually the same as it was for men.

As I will describe shortly, there were many naïve subjects who protested and requested that the session be concluded, though the majority of naïve subjects gave in to the Experimenter's influence and carried on obeying his orders. Indeed, the naïve subjects were so engaged in their role as Teacher, paid to do a job that was defined by the authority figure, that they carried on shocking even when the Learner pounded on the wall screaming in protest from the very painful shocks at the 300-volt level. At 150 volts the Learner said, "Get me out of here, please! My heart's starting to bother me. I refuse to go on. Let me out." At 300 volts he screamed, "I absolutely refuse to answer any more!" After 330 volts the Learner no longer responded, as if he had fainted. The Experimenter instructed the Teacher to regard failure to answer as mistakes, so that from then on, many naïve subjects thought they were administering dangerous, if not lethal shocks to someone who might have been unconscious.[5]

Social-psychological interpretations of Milgram's experiments

Social psychologist Muzafer Sherif, who headed the classic Robbers Cave experiment (1961), noted that "Milgram's obedience experiment is the single greatest contribution to human knowledge ever made by the field of social psychology, perhaps psychology in general" (Reicher & Haslam, 2017, p. 111). If Sherif's exalted characterization of Milgram's obedience experiments is plausible, how did Milgram and later researchers explain his deeply troubling findings?

By obedience, Milgram meant "the action of the subject who complies with authority,"[6] while its cousin term, conformity, as described in the Asch line judgment experiments, refers to "the action of a subjects when he goes along with his peers, people of his own status, who have no special right to direct his behavior" (Milgram, 1974, p. 113).[7] There have been mainly two social-psychological explanations of obedience to authority, the one given by Milgram, called the "agentic shift" account (1974), and the other, called the "engaged followership" account (Haslam et al., 2015b). While there have been hundreds of studies investigating Milgram's experiments, including those that have made methodological advances (Hollander & Maynard, 2016), and those lodged in recent information gathered from Milgram's personal archive at Yale University (Jetten & Mols, 2014), the challenge of satisfactorily explaining the obedience to authority effect has not been resolved. It has, in part, been used to explain behavior during the Holocaust, the My Lai massacre, Abu Ghraib prisoner abuses, terrorism (Gibson, 2014, p. 436), and other toxic social phenomena.

As Milgram describes it, the individual, upon entering the laboratory, becomes integrated into a situation that carries its own psychological momentum and drama. The naïve subject's struggle is whether to stay engaged in the ugly destructive direction and harm another human being or resolve the struggle by disobeying orders. The naïve subjects, reasons Milgram, have entered into an "agentic state" in which the individual no longer views himself as responsible for his own actions but defines himself as an instrument for carrying out the wishes of others (somewhat like Zimbardo's deindividuation). The agentic state is not just a replacement term for obedience; rather, it is a "mental organization which enhances the likelihood of obedience" (Milgram, 1974, p. 148). According to Milgram, a major alteration of moral consciousness occurs such that the "person becomes something different from his former self, with new properties not easily traced to his usual personality" (ibid., p. 3). A transformation of moral thinking occurs so that naïve subjects feel more obligated to the Experimenter than they do the Learner/victim they are allegedly painfully shocking. As Milgram puts it, "Although a person acting under authority performs actions that seem to violate standards of conscience, it would not be true to say that he loses his moral sense. Instead, it acquires a radically different focus," namely, "living up to the expectations that the authority has of him" (ibid., p. 8). Once in this state of agency, certain powerful "binding factors" cement the individual into a role that is not easily reversed. The recurrent nature of the action demanded of the Teacher/naïve subject during the experiment itself creates binding forces. As the Teacher/naïve subject delivers more, increasingly painful shocks, he must seek to justify what he has done. One form of justification is to continue shocking to the highest level on the shock generator. By doing so, the subject reassures himself that what he has done before and what he continues to do now is correct and acceptable.

Another binding factor is the etiquette that plays a part in regulating behavior. The Teacher/naïve subject has made an initial agreement to aid the Experimenter in the name of science and feels awkward, if not anxious, about reneging on this commitment. Milgram has noted that, to the outsider, the act of refusing to shock stems from moral considerations rooted in their personality structure and personal convictions. The action, however, is experienced by the Teacher/naïve subject as renouncing an obligation to the Experimenter. This repudiation is dramatic and not undertaken lightly. Since the Teachers/naïve subjects perceive themselves as locked into a hierarchical situation, any attempts to alter the defined structure "will be experienced as a moral transgression and will evoke anxiety, shame, embarrassment, and diminished feelings of self-worth" (ibid., p. 152).[8]

Furthermore, Milgram, like Erich Fromm (as we shall see, the only psychoanalyst to seriously comment on Milgram's experiments), believes that the intense anxiety reaction experienced by the obedient Teacher/naïve subject merits explanation. Fromm believes that the anxiety reaction may be interpreted as a positive sign of the respondent's empathic response to their victims. Milgram does not totally disagree. He certainly agrees that respondent's obvious signs of distress—the sweating, the trembling, the uncontrollable fits of nervous laughter—are preferable to expression of indifference, happiness or enthusiasm. Milgram adds, however, that expression of these emotions alone is inadequate in terms of moral process and decision-making. Those emotional experiences are useful only to the extent to which they become translated into action—which in this case is to break with authority and refuse to administer another shock. The reason most respondents do not defy the orders of the Experimenter, according to Milgram, lies more so in understanding the interplay between the subjects and the context in which they are behaving, and less so in their alleged "pent-up anger or aggression" or other personality/dispositional factors (ibid., p. 168).

While the ethics of Milgram's early research has been questioned, the key findings of the study have been partially replicated by Burger (2009), with changes in the methodology that comply with current professional ethical rules. Indeed, Milgram's study in its original form has never been replicated due to ethical guidelines that were imposed after the experiment received so much attention and criticism.[9] In Burger's sample of men and women, 70% obeyed beyond the 150-volt level ("strong shock"), including 67% of the men. These reported rates are lower than the 80% of Milgram's male Teacher/naïve subjects who went to that level, but the result is still astonishingly high. Another troubling "real-life" Milgramesque study took place in a hospital setting (Hofling et al., 1966). Researchers investigated registered nurses' responses when a "doctor" (the authority figure) gave an obviously ill-conceived and ill-fated patient prescription order. A researcher posing as a doctor telephoned twenty-two different nurses' stations at a number of hospitals, describing himself as a doctor at the hospital. He directed the nurse, who was alone at the station, to give 20 milligrams of a fictitious drug called Astroten to a particular patient. Such directions went against hospital policy in many ways. Prescriptions were supposed to be given in person, not over the telephone; the drug had not been cleared for use on the specific ward; the instructed dosage was twice the amount listed as allowable on the container; and the doctor giving the order was unknown to the nurse. Despite these danger signs, only one nurse did not immediately prepare to obey the doctor's order to give an overdose to the patient. In other words, the norm of obedience to authority, to professional standards, overrode their extensive medical training, clinical knowledge and experience. In another study conducted by Krackow and Blass (1995), 46% of nurses complied with an order from a doctor they thought would hurt the patient, highlighting the extraordinary force of the obedience effect, especially in organizational contexts that are probably the central aspect of modernity (Blass, 2004; Smith et al., 2015).

The "engaged followership" account challenges Milgram's claim that destructive behavior was largely the result of an intrinsic tendency to passively conform to the demands of those in authority (roughly, "I was only following orders"). That is, the behavior that Milgram observed was a consequence of the structure of his experimental paradigm in that it generated a compelling sense of obligation to, and identification with, the Experimenter, and depended on and communicated setting-specific behavioral norms. Thus, rather than Milgram's agentic account which stresses passive obedience, the behavior that Milgram observed is better comprehended as "engaged followership." Drawing from the social identity point of view on social influence and leadership, these researchers claim that a person's willingness and ability to give in to the requests of others is based upon social identification with them and a related sense that they are legitimate representatives of shared group goals, values and aspirations (Haslam et al., 2015b, p. 60). As Haslam and colleagues further elaborate,

> In other words, and in line with Milgram's own assertions in his 1963 study ["the subjects have come to the laboratory to form a relationship with the experimenter"],[10] those who administered shocks were aware of the consequences of their actions. Indeed, they continued shocking precisely because their actions were construed to be contributing to a moral, worthy, and progressive cause.
>
> *(ibid.)*

Haslam and colleagues have described the mounting evidence that their reconceptualization of Milgram's obedience phenomena, in which identification acquires a central significance, is more plausible than Milgram's agentic account. For example, as previously mentioned, Milgram relied on Arendt's "banality of evil" thesis to construct his experiment and explanation, and this view has been challenged by historians. Eichmann and other likeminded perpetrators were not motivated by a lack of consequential thinking about the nature of their atrocities, or "blind obedience" ("I was only following orders"), but rather they were willing and able participants in genocide ("I chose to follow orders"). As engaged followers, they knew exactly what they were doing, and they felt and thought it was right. As the Eichmann prosecutor Gideon Hausner noted, Eichmann didn't only round up Jews and others for deportation to death camps, "but had gone about his work with extraordinary zeal and initiative" (Haslam et al., 2015a, p. 2).

The engaged followership account has also received some support after researchers recognized the effort that Milgram went to in order to guarantee that naïve subjects understood his project as a well-intentioned, commendable, scientific experiment, and thus, became cognitively and emotionally connected to its apparent objectives. For example, Milgram, who had a talent for dramatic brilliance and used "technical illusions" (Milgram, 1974, p. 193), gave exacting attention to the design of the shock generator, the laboratory ambience, and the way he enlisted and greeted participants, in addition to "major departures from the experimental scripts that positioned Teachers as ingroup collaborators rather than detached actors" (Haslam et al., 2015a, p. 61).

As Haslam et al. (2015b) further point out, a meta-analysis of Milgram's findings suggested that the two key moments where naïve subjects stop administering shocks were at 150 volts ("strong shock") and 315 volts ("extreme intensity shock"). This is when the Learner/victim first requests to be released from the experiment and then articulates his most resolute objections, and thus they are the stages at which identification with the Experimenter is contested by, and must be reconciled with, another source of identification, this being the key psychological process to understand the obedience effect from the "engaged followership" point of view.

When Teachers are given a prod which orders them to carry on shocking, especially, "You have no choice—you must go on," they are powerfully motivated to disobey the order. This further supports the "engaged followership" account. In other words, it may be that orders stimulate reactance, but not obedience, and this may be due to the fact that they compromise the Teacher/naïve subject's sense that the Experimenter/authority is behaving in terms of an identity that they have in common, less an agentic shift process.

A final finding that challenges Milgram's agentic account and supports the "engaged followership" one is that identification and obedience are greatly reduced when two Experimenters controvert each other, when the Experimenter is not present in the laboratory during the experiment, or when the Experimenter's role is played by someone who appears to be another naïve subject. As Haslam and colleagues conclude in support of their "engaged followership" account, across the many variations of Milgram's paradigm,

> the willingness of the Teachers to administer the maximum level of shock can be predicted with a high degree of accuracy by observers' estimates of the degree to which a given variant encourages participants to identify with the Experimenter and the science that he represents rather than with the Learner and the general community that he represents.
>
> *(Haslam et al., 2015b, p. 62)*

In summary, the "agentic state" notion, that "the condition a person is in when he sees himself as an agent for carrying out another person's wishes," rather than as an autonomous being, "when a person sees himself as acting on his own," was Milgram's main explanatory framework to account for obedience to destructive authority (1974, p. 133). Milgram's agentic shift was not a compelling account to explain his findings, as he "fails to use these insights as building blocks for a theory of obedience" (Jetten & Mols, 2014, p. 594). Following Reicher and Haslam (2011) and others, Jetten and Mols argue for an identity-based engaged followership model, which claims that by comprehending the manner in which the experimental setup animates the Teacher's identification with the Learner/victim and Experimenter (i.e., Teachers embrace the Experimenter's scientific objectives and the leadership that he displays in pursuing them), "we are able to predict quite accurately when participants will display obedience" (2014, p. 594). While Milgram tends to see destructive obedience as an underlying human proclivity that, once activated by situational forces, leads to a loss of agency and "blind-like obedience,"[11] and Haslam and colleagues view obedience as an identity-based affirmation of agency and engaged followership, both theorists view destructive obedience in terms of individual choice (Milgram, 1974, p. 197). A partial reconciliation of these two explanations is suggested below.

Psychoanalytic reflections on the obedience effect

Milgram was well aware that he was only pinpointing one crucial aspect of the complex obedience effect. He noted that the "implicit model" of his "experimental work" was

> a social psychology of the reactive individual, the recipient of forces and pressures emanating from outside oneself. This represents, of course, only one side of the

> coin of social life, for we as individuals also initiate action out of internal needs and actively construct the social world we inhabit. But I have left to other investigators the task of examining the complimentary side of our natures.
>
> *(quoted in Blass, 2004, p. 290)*[12]

In fact, Milgram speculated what may constitute these "internal needs," having written, "I am certain that there is a complex personality basis to obedience and disobedience. But I know we have not found it" (1974, p. 205). Milgram mentions that psychological tests he had administered by Alan Elms indicated "that there was a relationship between obedience in the experiment and score on the *F* scale" [authoritarianism], though the relationship was at best "suggestive" and "not very strong" (1974, pp. 204, 205). Likewise, he reports that Lawrence Kohlberg, a colleague of Milgram's at Yale University, who used his "scale of moral development" during Milgram's pilot studies, "found that those who broke off were at a higher level of moral development than those who remained obedient" (ibid., p. 205). However, as Milgram notes again, "the findings were suggestive, though not very strong" (ibid.).

In light of Milgram's aforementioned comment suggesting there may be "a complex personality basis to obedience and disobedience," there are recent social psychologists who found suggestive evidence between personality and obedience. For example, Burger (2009, p. 10) tentatively noted in his partial replication of Milgram's experiment that those naïve subjects who were high in "empathic concern" displayed an unwillingness to continue with the experiment earlier than those who were low on the trait; however, this early unwillingness did not translate into a greater likelihood of refusing to administer the shock. Similarly, for those naïve subjects who had "a high desire for control" that Burger hypothesized would be most likely to act independently rather than obey the Experimenter, this effect was found only in the base condition. As Burger concluded, "although I found evidence that personality traits play a role in participants' responses to the situation, the relationship between personality and obedience remains speculative" (ibid.). Thus, to date, there does not appear to be any experimentally verifiable personality type or characteristic that clearly distinguishes naïve subjects who were obedient versus disobedient. This has maddened psychologists who have been determined to find predictive factors that are internal rather than situational.

A psychoanalytic interpretation

A conventional psychoanalytic interpretation of Milgram's experiment would presume that the respondents who shocked the participants were flawed psychologically. Perhaps they had serious ego deficits or superego lacunae which prevented them from refusing to hurt an innocent person. In this view, a weakness in character structure renders the subject vulnerable to a faulty decision-making process. Erich Fromm (1973), for example, has argued that about 65% of the respondents in Milgram's experiment obeyed because they were "narcissistic people" who insulated against the pain they were inflicting. Another reason Fromm suggested to account for the high level of obedience involved the supposed "psychopathic" nature of these respondents and their lack of capacity for genuine guilt. He described such respondents as possibly having a "sadistic and destructive character" (ibid., p. 52). Fromm also argued that Milgram misconstrued his results by not focusing on the fact that most subjects experienced considerable conflict during the experiment, thereby showing that they, in fact, find cruel behavior intolerable. Although Fromm's interpretations of why subjects obeyed are interesting and perhaps even somewhat accurate, they are also open to criticism. For example, while narcissism and psychopathy, both hard to clearly define and instantiate even among psychoanalysts, may be factors that animate some of the naïve subjects' responses, there is no credible scientific evidence that these factors are determinative in the Milgram studies, let alone for the majority of naïve subjects. Fromm's interpretations are at best incomplete and fail to grasp the main point of Milgram's analysis of obedient behavior to destructive authority. Namely, "the disposition a person brings to the experiment is probably less important a cause of his behavior" than typically assumed; rather, "it is not so much the kind of person a man is as the kind of situation in which he finds himself [that] determines how he will act" (Milgram, 1974, p. 205). Ambivalence about obeying destructive authority is not what most counts theoretically and practically, as Fromm suggests. It is whether that ambivalence leads the person to be disobedient, which requires understanding the context-dependent, setting-specific, situational forces at play because they are emotionally and intellectually metabolized by the person into action.[13]

Perhaps a way to build a modulating bridge between the thrust of Milgram's agentic shift and Haslam and colleagues' engaged followership accounts is to understand naïve subjects' obedience to destructive authority as the typical consequence of what psychoanalysts call "ego regression." Ego regression, mainly as a result of felt anxiety, is when primitive methods of expression subsume more advanced ones in which there is lowered anxiety tolerance and reduced impulse control. The defense mechanism of ego regression means that there is a loss of ego functions, like thinking, perception, reality testing, attachment, internalization and, most importantly in our context, a kind of "superego" backsliding, in which parental injunctions and prohibitions, the basis of moral emotions such as guilt and shame, give way to more sinister motives, the result of biopsychosocial stress (Akhtar, 2009, pp. 243, 90, 89). Indeed, biopsychosocial stress is exactly what Milgram's experimental design intentionally tried to induce in naïve subjects by creating a conflict between conscience and authority.

Naïve subjects responded to what they felt was an "extreme" psychological situation in which adult authority (e.g., the commanding, stern and intellectual Experimenter), the oppressive laboratory environment (e.g., the shock generator, the loud protests of the Learner) and the moral conflict that Milgram deliberately created were dramatically geared to break the naïve subject's individuality, mature sense of self, and personal moral beliefs and values. In other words, naïve subjects had quickly become adjusted to their laboratory context, a "way of life" in microcosm, and they temporarily lost their sense of adult autonomy, integration and pre-experimental moral world of meanings. This regression, characterized by taking on the perceived scientific beliefs and values of the destructive authority figure by identifying with the Experimenter, allowed naïve subjects, after experiencing anxiety (e.g., sweating, trembling, uncontrollable fits of nervous laughter), to justify their alliance with the perceived scientific beliefs and values of the destructive Experimenter. In other words, the naïve subjects felt like they were "forced" into a regressive state via their intense identification with the authoritative Experimenter. In this process they mainly unconsciously "chose" to jettison their adult sense of themselves, their autonomy and integration and their pre-experimental moral world of meanings, and become docile and "child-like." By capitulating to the harsh demands of the "parental-like" Experimenter, they relinquished any summoning sense of adult responsibility for their moral decision-making and behavior. In this context, the likelihood of exercising counter-will and counter-conduct, as Foucault calls practices of adult freedom, was minimized if not absent by the time the Teachers were well into administering the punitive shocks to the Learner.

Thus, the obedient naïve subject can be described as having been induced by the Experimenter and overall experimental setup into regressive self-experience and behavior characterized by dependency, helplessness and powerlessness. This is the opposite of self-coherence, agency, self-control and moral decision-making, the lattermost being correlated with an "intact" superego, the socially generated conscience that offsets the id with moral and ethical prohibitions. As is well-known, in circumstances where one's world has been undermined or destroyed, as in Milgram's experimental paradigm, the individual tends to display a heightened suggestibility or vulnerability to the promptings of others, especially others perceived to be more powerful, such as the imposing Experimenter. I am calling this regression, and like many forms of ego regression (especially when there is superego backsliding), a person's capacity to engage in autonomous, morally principled reasoning, judgment and behavior, and "do no harm" to an innocent person, gives way to truncated ties to empathy, aggressive behavior and worse.

This ego regression explanation is plausible when one considers the key factors of social influence that the agentic shift and engaged followership accounts point to (Baron & Byrne, 2003, pp. 378–379). For example, in an obedience to destructive authority context, the naïve subject allows himself to jettison responsibility for his own decisions and actions. In Milgram's experiment, the transfer of authority was explicitly operative. That is, from the onset of the experiment, naïve subjects were told that the Experimenter would be solely responsible for the Learner's safety. Put colloquially, at least on the surface level of conscious experience, Learners could say to themselves, "I am completely off the hook regarding the outcome of my actions," and without too much anxiety, obey the Experimenter's orders to administer the final punitive shock in a subservient, child-like manner.

Another social influence consideration that emanates from these obedience studies is that the individual in authority, the Experimenter, was emanating symbolic signs of his higher status such as wearing a white coat and conducting research associated with Yale University (though another experiment that used a less auspicious setting had the same results). In other words, informational social influence, an important component of conformity to social norms, was operative in Milgram's study. Such a context calls to mind the child-like injunction, "obey the person in charge," for to do otherwise is to do something wrong that will get you into trouble.

Another form of social influence that tends to lead to obedience relates to the graduated escalation of the authority figure's orders. In the Milgram experiment, the first administered shocks to the Learner were fairly benign "punishments," but as the experiment continued, the intensity of the inflicted punishments gradually became greater and more painful. Such a "foot in the door" compliance technique assumes that agreeing to a small request increases the likelihood of agreeing to a second, larger request, which can induce people to do harmful things to innocent others without sufficiently reckoning with the deleterious meanings of their actions.[14] Such a lack of adequate consequential thinking is not only a tell-tale sign of ego regression, but it is the basis for the radical blunting of moral emotions and moral reasoning often associated with child-like, self-centric ways of being in the world.

Lastly, it is well-known that in high-stress social situations like Milgram's experiment, things move very quickly and are disorienting, thus the naïve subject has little opportunity to critically reflect on what is occurring. Participants had little time to metabolize the moral meaning and consequences for the Learner of the Experimenter's verbal demands. Milgram thus characterizes the obedient act as "perseverative" (Blass, 2004, p. 278). Within a few minutes of entering the laboratory, Milgram's naïve subjects found themselves being requested—and by prompt number four, ordered—to administer punitive electric shocks to the Learner, what must have felt surreal and overwhelming to their usual sense of themselves as morally feeling and reasoning agents. In such a fast-paced, disorienting, biopsychosocially stressful context, child-like obedience to authority is often the outcome.

Disobedience to destructive authority

Milgram was very interested in the naïve subjects who were disobedient to the four prods, especially the last one, "You have no choice—you must go on."[15] Milgram discusses what he calls "strain," the "experience of tension" in naïve subjects that shows the weakness of the power of authority, in that it only partially transformed the naïve subjects into the agentic state of profound submersion in their roles (1974, pp. 154, 155). Milgram mentions that "residues of selfhood, remaining in varying degrees outside the experimenter's authority, keep personal values alive in the subject and lead to strain, which, if sufficiently powerful, can result in disobedience" (ibid., p. 155). In other words, it is through personal moral beliefs and values that the disobedient naïve subject maintains his sense of agency, the bedrock of his narrative of self-identity, such that his moral judgments and decisions are lodged in his relatively autonomous inner center of gravity, and not disrupted by the orders of imposing authority and other situational forces that are powerfully bearing down on him. How this works in real-life is complicated, but a few comments on what Milgram calls "sources of strain" and the "resolution of strain" on the way to "disobedience" are worthy of review.

Milgram notes that he designed his experiment recognizing that "nothing is more dangerous to human survival than malevolent authority combined with dehumanizing effects of buffers," like the variables of "distance, time, and physical barriers" that he skillfully manipulated to "neutralize the moral sense" (1974, p. 157). Most of Milgram's Teachers gave way to the infliction of punishment to the innocent Learner by drawing on defensive maneuvers such as avoidance, denial and subterfuge. Using avoidance, the Teacher shielded himself from the sensory consequences of his pain-inflicting actions (e.g., awkwardly turning his head to avoid viewing the victim suffer). Denial was manifest in naïve subjects who convinced themselves that the punitive shocks they were administering were not as painful as they seemed, or that the innocent Learner was not suffering. Subterfuge refers to the ways that Teachers undermined the cruel significance of their behavior during the experiment (e.g., trying to prompt the Learners by signaling the correct response to them, but never to a degree where they chose to stop the experiment). In all these defensive maneuvers, Milgram claims, the goal is the same: the "abrogation of personal responsibility" which "is the major psychological effect of yielding to authority." Such defensive variations allow the "psychological closeness" between the naïve subject's perceived actions and the consequence of his actions to be diminished. In this way, they permit the naïve subject's relationship to authority to stay intact by lessening their moral conflict to a bearable level. That is, personal responsibility is abdicated, even to the point of blaming the victim for volunteering for the experiment, or in more extreme responses, for the Learners' "stupidity and obstinacy." In this last defensive permutation, the Learner is made into a devalued person who does not deserve empathy, and the administration of pain feels acceptable (Milgram, 1974, pp. 157–161).

While there are no personality/character profiles that would guarantee disobedience in a Milgramesque experiment, or more importantly, in its real-life analogues, Milgram and others have suggested what may be some of the personal factors at play that appear to be associated with greater levels of disobedience. Put differently, how does the naïve subject reconceptualize his relationship to authority so that he is more likely to become disobedient?

Milgram notes that the naïve subjects might think or fantasize that disobedience to authority carries a price. For instance, the Experimenter might retaliate in some form, like taking legal action for non-compliance to their agreement (some Teachers wanted to give the $4.50 back they received for participating in the experiment as a way of getting out of the perceived contract). This kind of retaliating fantasy is often seen in children who are anxious about disobeying a parent's orders. Milgram describes this process as beginning in "inner doubt," the internal tension that eventually gets externalized on to the Experimenter, such that the Teacher expresses his apprehension or points to the Learner's suffering as a basis to end the experiment. When the Teacher experiences the Experimenter as not having the same moral sensibility and outlook, he "dissents" by trying to convince the Experimenter that his authoritative behavior is ill-fated and the Teacher should be released from the experiment. When his attempts to convince the Experimenter of his misguided behavior fail, he engages in a "threat" to refuse the Experimenter's orders. Finally, after the process of inner doubt, externalization of doubt, dissent and threat, the naïve subject comes to a culminating point of inner "victory" and he becomes disobedient. It should be emphasized that disobedience is difficult—the Teacher no longer is shifting responsibility for administering punitive shocks on to the Experimenter, but instead takes responsibility for destroying the experiment. He is frustrating the purposes of the scientist and appears not to be "up to snuff" to complete the task he was given. However, most importantly, "At that very moment he," the Teacher, "has provided the measure we sought and an affirmation of humanistic values" (ibid., p. 164). In other words, the disobedient naïve subjects assign "primary personal responsibility to themselves," (ibid., p. 204). As I have argued in earlier chapters, this affirmation appears to be lodged in strongly felt, flexibly and creatively applied, transcendent-pointing moral beliefs and values that are primarily other-directed, other-regarding and other-serving. In fact, conversational analysis from 117 audio recordings of Milgram's original experimental sessions found that defiant Teachers implemented two "other-attentive" practices never implemented by obedient Teachers: the "Golden Rule" based on empathetic identification with the Learner, and "letting the Learner decide," based on their conviction that it is the Learner who should decide whether to continue with the experiment (Hollander & Maynard, 2016). I will conclude this chapter with a few comments on how these transcendent-pointing moral beliefs and values can animate the way of being of the individual who chooses to disobey destructive authority.

The role of moral beliefs and values

In his *Nicomachean Ethics*, Aristotle highlighted one of the main "take home" points of Milgram's experiments—that the goal of studying ethics (or in our case, social and moral psychology) "is not, as in other inquires, the attainment of theoretical knowledge: we are not conducting this inquiry in order to know what virtue is, but in order to become good" (Aristotle, 1962, p. 1103b). While what constitutes "good" is historically situated and perspectival, at least from a postmodern point of view, the fact is that the psychology of goodness, of striving to create the conditions of possibility for bringing out what is "best" or even "sacred" (i.e., judged as having infinite moral significance), seems like an existentially worthwhile, valuative attachment to live one's everyday life. Indeed, like Emmanuel Levinas, I regard goodness as being for the other before oneself, or at least as much as for oneself. My claim is that those disobedient naïve subjects, mainly by virtue of their moral beliefs and values, have the capacity to transcend their regressive, self-centric, morally truncated outlook and behavior, the deleterious way of being that autonomous adults often associate with an obedient, child-like state of mind that was brilliantly induced in Milgram's experimental paradigm.

As Milton Rokeach, the great social psychologist of human values noted, there are three kinds of beliefs: descriptive beliefs, which are capable of being true or false; evaluative beliefs, in which the object of the belief is judged to be either good or bad; and most importantly for this chapter, prescriptive beliefs, in which "some means or end of action is judged to be desirable or undesirable" (Koltko-Rivera, 2004, p. 5). According to Rokeach, a value is this third kind of belief. Such values function as a lens and filter through which experiences are perceived and comprehended. There is no way of having a "gods-eye" perception of reality, as all humans are embedded in some kind of hermeneutic angle of vison or symbolic world (ibid., pp. 8, 20).

It is important to note that moral beliefs and values as I am using the terms are not merely intellectual or philosophical reflections about morality, the kind of cognition often associated with ethics professors, who, one would think, due to their explicit moral reasoning, would be more inclined to moral behavior. However, this is not what I have in mind. For as philosopher Eric Schwitzgebel (2009) found in his study of ethics professors, classic pre-1900 ethics books were twice as likely to be missing/presumed stolen from leading academic libraries compared to other philosophy books similar in age and popularity. Moreover, fairly obscure, contemporary ethics books of the kind likely to be borrowed by professors and advanced students of philosophy were about 50% more likely to be missing. As Schwitzgebel concluded, while it would be premature to draw general conclusions about ethics professors without investigating more diverse moral behavior, "in one domain in which ethicists could have displayed superior conscientiousness, honesty, and concern for other's property, they failed to do so" (ibid., p. 723). In other studies, Schwitzgebel found that moral philosophers were in no way better than other philosophers or professors in terms of giving to charity, voting, calling their mothers, donating blood or organs, or cleaning up after themselves. Thus, the capacity for moral reasoning in no way means that one will be more prone to act morally, and it may actually make things worse since the ethical philosopher may be more willing and able to rationalize his objectionable behavior (Haidt, 2012, p. 104).

While there are many recent examples of people with the demonstrated capacity for great intellectual and philosophical cognition, including moral reasoning and the like, who have behaved deplorably in real-life—Martin Heidegger's Nazi affiliation during World War II comes to mind—there are other examples taken from the accounts of death camp survivors who have confirmed this point while in the *lager*. They have observed that such intellectual and philosophical moral cognition, when not lodged in transcendent religious or moral convictions, especially an ethics of being-for-the-other, was not enough to significantly help inmates maintain a modicum of their autonomy, integration and humanity during the Nazi onslaught. As Elie Wiesel noted,

> Within the system of the concentration camp … the first to give in, the first to collaborate—to save their lives—were the intellectuals, the liberals, the humanists, the professors of sociology, and the like. Because suddenly their whole concept of the universe broke down … Very few Communists [secular believers] gave in … They were the resisters … Even fewer to give in were the Catholic priests … yet there were exceptions. But you could not have found one single rabbi—I dare you—among all the kapos or among any of the others who held positions of power in the camps.
>
> *(1974, p. 273)*[16]

By drawing from these extreme Holocaust examples that are applicable to Milgram's experiment of disobedience to destructive authority, I demonstrate that it is not simply enough to maintain intellectual and philosophical positions on morality that allows a person to "remain human." Rather, these moral beliefs and values must be deeply internalized and enacted in real-life being-in-the-world. These moral beliefs and values are the basis of one's self-respect and therefore are non-negotiable. As Natan Sharansky repeatedly told himself until it "stuck" while incarcerated in the gulag, "Nothing they do can humiliate me. I alone can humiliate myself" (1988, p. 8). As Wiesel (and Auschwitz survivors Primo Levi, Jean Amery and Viktor Frankl) observed, whether Communists, Catholic priests or rabbis, what is common among these "believers" was that they had strongly felt, flexibly and creatively applied, transcendent-pointing moral beliefs and values that animated their everyday existence. Along with likeminded inmates, this constituted a moral community in which being-for-the-other was paramount. Indeed, the key to understanding those who were disobedient to authority in Milgram's experiments is structurally similar. There is a "family resemblance" to the death camp inmates who resisted Nazi domination, and by doing so, maintained a modicum of their pre-incarceration autonomy, integration and humanity. In both cases, they applied their individual freedom enacted through their moral beliefs and values. In this way, they resisted becoming regressed, self-centric, and morally truncated (in short, obedient) as Milgram (albeit, for ennobling reasons) and the Nazis wanted.[17] Indeed, Milgram ironically (considering what I have despairingly reported about ethical philosophers) describes a professor of the Old Testament who displayed disobedience:

EXPERIMENTER: It's absolutely essential to the experiment that we continue.
SUBJECT: I understand that statement, but I don't understand why this experiment is placed above the person's life.
EXPERIMENTER: There is no permanent tissue damage.
SUBJECT: Well, that's your opinion. If he doesn't want to continue, I'm taking order from him.
EXPERIMENTER: You have no other choice, sir, you must go on.
SUBJECT: If this were Russia maybe, but not in America.

(The experiment was terminated) (Milgram, 1974, p. 48)

During the debriefing, Milgram asked the subject, "What in your opinion is the most effective way of strengthening resistance to inhuman authority?" The subject replied, "If one had as one's authority God, then it trivializes human authority."[18] Milgram concludes that the subject's response does not so much repudiate authority, "but in the substitution of the good—that is, divine—authority for the bad" (ibid.). While religiously inspired moral beliefs and values can lead to perpetrating terrible inhumanity in certain contexts, the aforementioned points in a life-affirming, morally praiseworthy direction.

Implications for treatment

Resisting the impact of destructive obedience to authority is challenging, especially in the ebb and flow of everyday life. In some social contexts, like facing a dictatorship, disobedience can be dangerous, if not life threatening. This being said, psychoanalysts can help cultivate qualities of mind and heart in analysands that counteract such harmful social influence. Research has suggested a few strategies that may be helpful, strategies that both emanate from, and reinforce, individual autonomy, integration and humanity (Baron & Byrne, 2003).

For example, when individuals are simply reminded that they, and not authority figures, are ultimately responsible for any harmful consequences of their actions, there have been marked decreases in compliant behavior. As Milgram has noted, culture has for the most part failed to inculcate effective internal controls and actions that are originally lodged in childhood relations to parental authority. One strategy for resisting destructive authority is to adequately teach children when they are young how to distinguish between "good" and "bad" authority, rather than just tell them that authority must be obeyed regardless, simply because it *is* authority. The analyst and analysand need to be ever mindful of this often deeply internalized, child-like social tendency when in the context of authority (e.g., in a work setting) and call upon their adult, deeply felt moral beliefs and values to guide their critical interrogation of destructive authority. This will encourage counte-decisions that reflect those "higher" moral beliefs and values rather than regressive self-experience. As Percy Bysshe Shelley aptly put it, "Obedience indeed is only the pitiful and cowardly egotism of him who thinks that he can do something better than reason" (1998, p. 92).

A second strategy for resisting destructive authority involves being mindful of the findings on obedience to destructive authority. Some research suggests that by simply being knowledgeable of this research, studies can contribute to changing behavior in terms of sensitizing people to the dynamics of obedience to destructive authority. As Milgram demonstrated, obedience was maximized when the Experimenter's commands were given by an authority figure rather than another volunteer, when the experiments were carried out at a prestigious institution, when the authority figure remained in the room with the naïve subject, when the Learner was in another room, and when the naïve subject did not view other subjects disobeying commands. Such findings are ideally the basis for greater situational awareness in the face of powerful situational forces.

Lastly, it is a well-known research finding that destructive compliance to authority can be reduced when individuals are exposed to disobedient role models, as Milgram found in one of his experimental variations. This is especially the case in a group context: when others disobey destructive authority, we feel more willing and able to follow suit, thus undercutting authority's hold on us. As Milgram noted, "the mutual support provided by men for each other [when defying destructive authority] is the strongest bulwark we have against the excesses of authority" (Blass, 2004, p. 108). The point is that, to the extent that the analyst displays such autonomous moral feeling, reasoning and behavior to the analysand—the analysand's all-important, transferentially-tinged role model—the more likely that the analysand will internalize this moral outlook and behavior and reproduce it in his own flourishing life.

Indeed, it is well-known that positive role models are exceedingly important in child development, but they are also valuable in adulthood, though adults don't like to admit this to others. Research has shown that via a process known as vicarious reinforcement, there's a proclivity to imitate the behavior of someone who acquires praise or attention as if you were acquiring the rewards of that behavior yourself. In light of this finding, I will close this chapter by recalling a visualization of one of my adult role models, one that I often return to for inspiration when I feel like I am up against oppressive authority and the like. It is from Natan Sharansky's memoir, *Fear No Evil* (1988), the story of the Jewish refusenik in the USSR in the 1970s, his show trial on fabricated charges of espionage, his brutal incarceration for nine years in the worst of the gulags by the KGB, and his liberation to freedom in Israel. I quote from an American newspaper summary, after his KGB tormentors ordered him to walk across the Glienicke Bridge:

> Sharansky marched across the bridge like a deranged crab … It was a last gesture of defiance toward a regime that had tried to silence his protest. They had told him to "walk straight." … He was not, by God, going to start following their orders now, not on his final steps to freedom.
>
> *(Phillips, 1991)*

Notes

1 "Conscience" is a contested notion by most philosophers and psychologists, but it was Darwin who aptly captured the evolutionary basis of the term that is worth thinking about. He said, "Ultimately our moral sense or conscience becomes a highly complex sentiment—originating in the social instincts, largely guided by the approbation of our fellow-men, ruled by reason, self-interest, and in later times by deep religious feelings, and confirmed by instruction and habit" (Darwin, 1998, p. 137).

2 As we shall see, Milgram defines obedience in a specific manner that somewhat differs from how the word is usually understood. However, he says that it is the "ideological abrogation to the authority that constitutes the principal cognitive basis of obedience," that is, "the world or the situation is as the authority defines it," which leads to a certain set of actions (1974, p. 145).

3 As Milgram noted, in this view, "if a person is placed in a situation where he has complete power over another individual, who he may punish as much as he likes, all that is sadistic and bestial in man comes to the fore" (1974, p. 70).

4 Arendt's characterization has been vigorously rejected by those who believe that Eichmann was a pathological individual who never took meaningful responsibility for his heinous actions, let alone felt guilt or remorse about his role in the Final Solution. For example, psychological testing of Eichmann revealed that his Rorschach projective responses and drawings (the Bender-Gestalt Test and the House-Tree-Person Test) were not those of a "normal" person. This being said, some believe that the tests do not have credible scientific validity. Likewise, there is considerable evidence that many of the perpetrators and Nazi functionaries were not simply "blindly following orders" but were

aware, highly motivated, and creatively and emotionally engaged participants in conceptualizing and implementing their genocidal program (Seltzer, 1977).

5 Milgram gave a detailed rendering of the experiment to Yale University seniors, middle class adults and a group of psychiatrists to get their prediction of Teacher compliance. They confirmed that his findings were radically unexpected. He did the prediction exercise with a group of psychiatric residents at Yale and he found that, "The psychiatrists—although they expressed great certainty in the accuracy of their predictions—were wrong by a factor of 500. Indeed, I have little doubt that a group of charwomen would do as well" (Blass, 2004, p. 95).

6 Milgram speculated in his notes whether the act of shocking can be described as "cooperation" with authority rather than "obedience" to authority. He says that cooperation suggests a degree of willingness to perform the action or to assist someone, while obedience suggests an action that is totally in response to a command, and the absence of motivated support from inner sources (Yale archive, Box 46) (Haslam et al., 2015b, p. 57).

7 Milgram had the highest intellectual regard for Asch and worked for him between 1959 and 1960 in Princeton. Milgram noted that his obedience experiment was in part a result of reflection on Asch's group-pressure experiment. Milgram notes that one of the provocative criticisms of Asch's experiments was "that they lack a surface significance, because after all, an experiment with people making judgments of lines has a manifestly trivial content" (Evans, 1980, p. 188). Milgram then asked himself, "How can this be made into a more humanly significant experiment?" (ibid.). Milgram called this idea of using instructions from the Experimenter and not the group "an incandescent moment" (Blass, 2004, p. 62).

8 In his *Group Psychology and the Analysis of the Ego* (1921), Freud described how the individual relinquishes his ego ideal and replaces it with the group ideal personified in the leader.

9 While psychologists have never been able to replicate Milgram's experimental procedures due to ethical guidelines, there have been creative attempts to study obedience to authority that approximate Milgram's approach. For example, Haslam and colleagues have used an Immersive Digital Realism (IDR) approach to restage and re-evaluate Milgram's original research, with findings that demonstrated "a close correspondence between the behavior observed in our IDR study and that observed in Milgram's original research" (Haslam et al., 2015b, p. 7). A virtual reality simulation of Milgram's paradigm found that obedient behavior closely corresponded with Milgram's original findings (Slater et al., 2006).

10 This is a quote from Milgram's experimental notes (Haslam et al., 2015b, p. 60).

11 As Milgram notes, "We are born with a potential for obedience, which then interacts with the influence of society to produce the obedient man." "Inborn structures" in interaction with "social influences" are what determines obedient behavior (1974, p. 125).

12 I had the privilege of having an informal chat with Milgram about thirty-five years ago thanks to his graduate doctoral student, Dr. Ronna Kabatznick. I still remember Milgram's response to my question about the difference between how a psychoanalyst and social psychologist understands human behavior, especially in terms of prediction. Milgram reached for a beautiful autumn leaf he had on his desk and held it up to us. He said something to the effect of, "you can know everything about the deep structure of this leaf, about how through its intricate parts and processes it engages in photosynthesis and transpiration. However, if you want to know where this leaf will land if I drop it, then you have to know more about the aerodynamics that the leaf is affected by." I was bedazzled by Milgram's simple but elegant metaphoric illustration of the impact that social forces can have on influencing or determining individual behavior.

13 Milgram's *Obedience to Authority* was severely criticized by analyst Steven Marcus in the *New York Times*. Marcus wrote of the "intellectual calamities that make up much of this book," and described Milgram's narrative as "moralistic," "obtrusively preachy" and "empty pious sentiments." Moreover, Milgram showed "outright contempt" toward his subjects, and overall, "this mish-mash explains virtually nothing," and "all the theoretical and explanatory parts of the book exist as an abysmal pitch of discourse" (Marcus, 1974). History has shown that Marcus's ill-conceived judgment of Milgram's studies reflected the worst of psychoanalytic arrogance and ignorance.

14 Modigliani and Rochat (1995) did a fine-grained analysis of the Yale University archive audio recordings of one of Milgram's experimental conditions and reported that the earlier the Teacher demonstrated resistance, the more inclined he was to become disobedient. Moreover, the earlier in the shock sequence the Teacher conveyed dissent, the lower the final voltage he administered, suggesting that early verbal resistance tends to diminish the pressure to rationalize, which is associated with a more docile, extended and brutal complicity (Blass, 2004, pp. 104, 105).
15 Reicher and Haslam (2017, p. 125) reported that in one replication study they reviewed, on all occasions that the Experimenter gave this prod, Teachers refused to continue administering shocks, suggesting that merely following orders, as Milgram views it, is not what was occurring psychologically; rather, Teachers are trying to generate justifications for their behavior from the Experimenter whom they trust and with whom they identify.
16 The context of Wiesel's remarks is important to appreciate, for they seem to have a somewhat rhetorical magnification to them. Wiesel made his comments a part of his improvised reply to a controversial lecture given by the "death of God" theologian Richard Rubenstein on the question of "What can be told, what can be written, where must silence be kept, what can be witnessed only by living?" (Wiesel, 1974, p. 269).
17 Bruno Bettelheim, a psychoanalyst and Holocaust survivor, regarded Milgram's research as "so vile that nothing these experiments show has any value … They are in line with the human experiments of the Nazis" (Blass, 2004, p. 123).
18 One should always be mindful that what accounts people give of their behavior, their so-called motives, may not reflect what is "really" governing them. There are many conscious and unconscious self-serving reasons why people may describe themselves a certain way. In addition, given the fact that words have no "fixed" meanings, that is, they are processive and emergent in meaning depending on the context, it is difficult to make sense of what people say and mean, let alone with the assurance that one has done so accurately and completely. Milgram seemed to be aware of some of these limitations when he wrote, "While we must take very seriously everything the subject says, we need not necessarily think that he fully understands the causes of his behavior" (1974, p. 44).

References

Akhtar, S. (2009). *Comprehensive dictionary of psychoanalysis*. London: Karnac.

Arendt, H. (1963) [1994]. *Eichmann in Jerusalem: A report on the banality of evil.* New York: Penguin.

Aristotle. (1962). *Nicomachean ethics*. M. Oswald (Trans.). New York: Macmillan.

Baron, R.A. & Byrne, D. (Eds.) (2003). *Social psychology* (10th ed.). Boston: Pearson Education.

Blass, T. (2004). *The man who shocked the world: The life and legacy of Stanley Milgram*. New York: Basic Books.

Burger, J.M. (2009). Replicating Milgram: Would people still obey today? *American Psychologist*, 64(1), 1–11.

Darwin, C. (1998). *The descent of man and selection in relation to sex*. Amherst: Prometheus Books (Original work published 1871).

Evans, R.I. (1980). *The making of social psychology: Discussions with creative contributors*. New York: Gardner Press.

Freud, S. (1921) [1955]. Group psychology and the analysis of the ego. In J. Strachey (Trans. and Ed.), *Standard edition of the complete psychological works of Sigmund Freud* (Vol. 13, pp. 65–143). London: Hogarth Press.

Fromm, E. (1973). *The anatomy of human destructiveness.* New York: Holt, Rinehart and Winston.

Gibson, S. (2014). Discourse, defiance, and rationality: "Knowledge work" in the "obedience" experiments. *Journal of Social Issues*, 70(3), 424–438.

Haidt, J. (2012). *The righteous mind: Why good people are divided by politics and religion*. New York: Vintage Books.

Haslam, S.A., Reicher, S.D. & Millard, K. (2015a). Shock treatment: Using immersive digital realism to restage and re-examine Milgram's "obedience to authority" research. *Plos One*, 10(3), 1–10.

Haslam, S.A., Reicher, D., Millard, K. & McDonald, R. (2015b). "Happy to have been of service": The Yale archive as a window into the engaged followership of participants in Milgram's "obedience" experiment. *The British Psychological Society*, 54, 55–83.

Hofling, C.K., Brotzman, E., Dalrymple, S., Graves, N. & Pierce, C.M. (1966). An experimental study in nurse-physician relationships. *Journal of Nervous and Mental Disease*, 143, 171–180.

Hollander, M.M. & Maynard, D.W. (2016). Do unto others…? Methodological advance and self- versus other-attentive resistance in Milgram's "obedience" experiments. *Social Psychology Quarterly*, 79(4), 355–375.

Jetten, J. & Mols, F. (2014). 50:50 hindsight: Appreciating anew the contributions of Milgram's obedience experiments. *Journal of Social Issues*, 70(3), 587–602.

Koltko-Rivera, M.E. (2004). The psychology of worldviews. *Review of General Psychology*, 8 (1), 3–58.

Krackow, A. & Blass, T. (1995). When nurses obey or defy inappropriate physician orders: Attributional differences. *Journal of Social Behavior and Personality*, 10, 585–594.

Marcus, S. (1974). Book review: Obedience to authority: An experimental view. By Stanley Milgram. *New York Times*, 1/13/74 (p. 1). Retrieved from www.nytimes.com/1974/01/13/archives/obedience-to-authority-an-experimental-view.html.

Milgram, S. (1963). Behavioral study of obedience. *Journal of Abnormal and Social Psychology*, 67, 371–378.

Milgram, S. (1965). Some conditions of obedience and disobedience to authority. *Human Relations*, 18, 57–76.

Milgram, S. (1974). *Obedience to authority*. New York: Harper Perennial.

Modigliani, A. & Rochat, F. (1995). The role of interaction sequences and the timing of resistance in shaping obedience and defiance to authority. *Journal of Social Issues*, 51(3), 107–123.

Phillips, B.J. (1991). Sharansky: Defying authorities as a way of life. *Tulsa World*, 05/05/91. Retrieved from www.tulsaworld.com/archives/sharansky-defying-authorities-as-a-way-of-life/article_f9278393-4af2-594f-8144-60bc26350985.html.

Reicher, S.D. & Haslam, S.A. (2011). After shock? Towards a social identity explanation of the Milgram "obedience" studies. *British Journal of Social Psychology*, 50, 163–169.

Reicher, S. & Haslam, S.A. (2017). Obedience: Revisiting Milgram's shock experiments. In J.R. Smith & S.A. Haslam (Eds.), *Social psychology: Revisiting the classic studies* (2nd ed., pp. 108–129). Thousand Oaks, CA: Sage.

Schwitzgebel, E. (2009). Do ethicists steal more books? *Philosophical Psychology*, 22(6), 711–725.

Seltzer, M. (1977). The murderous mind. *The New York Times*, 11/27/77. Retrieved from www.nytimes.com/1977/11/27/archives/the-murderous-mind-adolf-eichmanns-psychological-test-drawings-show.html.

Sharansky, N. (1988). *Fear no evil*. New York: Perseus.

Shelley, P.B. (1998). *The selected poetry and prose of Shelley*. Hertfordshire: Wordsworth Editions Ltd.

Slater, M., Antley, A., Davison, A., Swapp, D., Guger, C. & Barker, C. (2006). A virtual reprise of the Stanley Milgram obedience experiments. *PLoS ONE*, 1, e39.

Smith, J.R. & Haslam, S.A. (2017). *Social psychology: Revisiting the classic studies* (2nd ed.). Thousand Oaks, CA: Sage.

Smith, R., Mackie, D.M. & Claypool, H.M. (Eds.) (2015). *Social psychology* (4th ed.). New York: Psychology Press.

White, H.K. (Ed.) (1922). Official records of the union and confederate navies in the war of rebellion. Official Naval Records Library, US Naval War Records Office, Series II, Vol. 3.
Wiesel, E. (1974). Talking and writing and keeping silent. In F.H. Litell & H.G. Locke (Eds.), *The German church struggle and the Holocaust* (pp. 269–277). Bloomington: Wayne State University Press.

6

HELPING VERSUS INDIFFERENCE IN EMERGENCIES

Latané and Darley's bystander studies (1968)

"The opposite of love is not hate," said Elie Wiesel, "it's indifference. The opposite of beauty is not ugliness, it's indifference. The opposite of faith is not heresy, it's indifference. And the opposite of life is not death, but indifference between life and death" (Sanoff, 1986, n.p.). Indifference, defined as having no interest, concern or sympathy for someone else, is one of the most wretched and appalling qualities, for it is a spoiler of love, an anesthetic to perceiving material and spiritual beauty, and the personification of what is evil in the world. And yet, there is not a person who has not acted indifferently to someone in need, including friends and lovers. In my own life, I recall numerous instances where I have turned away from the people I love who needed me, my wife and two children, because I chose to remain self-involved, not being literally present (e.g., "I can't talk now, I am busy working on something"), or not fully present in spirit, defined as empathically inclusive of the other (e.g., appearing to be listening but thinking about something else).[1] It is the rare person who can always be ready, receptive, responsive and responsible to and for the other, let alone before oneself. This is what the great modern religious philosophers Gabriel Marcel and Emmanuel Levinas described as the ideal existential comportment. The "good news" is that by recognizing that one has been indifferent to those one cares about, there can be an upsurge of "genuine guilt" (as opposed to neurotic guilt) (Marcus, 2008, p. 60) and/or realistic shame, this being one of the psychological conditions of possibility to make reparations to the person toward which one has acted callously or insensitively. One of the greatest contemporary Jewish social philosophers, Martin Buber, recalls a personal experience of marked indifference to an acquaintance that utterly transformed Buber's outlook and behavior for the better. In *Between Man and Man*, Buber reports:

> What happened was no more than the forenoon, after a morning of "religious" enthusiasm, I had a visit from an unknown young man, without being there in spirit I certainly did not fail to let the meeting be friendly, I did not

> treat him any more remissly than all his contemporaries who were in the habit of seeking me out at this time as an oracle that is ready to listen to reason. I conversed attentively and openly with him—only I omitted to guess the questions he did not put.
>
> *(1965, pp. 13–14)*

Buber was not fully present in such a way that he did not intuit the pressing concerns of the acquaintance even before the acquaintance was mindful of what his concerns were. Buber concludes his anecdote with a searing self-accusation,

> Later, not long after, I learned from one of his friends—he himself was no longer alive [he was killed in battle or maybe suicided]—the essential content of these questions; I learned that he had come to me not causally, but borne by destiny, not for a chat but for a decision. He had come to me, he had come in this hour. What do we expect when we are in despair and yet go to a man. Surely a presence by means of which we are told that nevertheless there is meaning.
>
> *(ibid.)*

Buber notes that after this deeply troubling experience of non-presence, "I have given up being 'religious' which is nothing but the exception, extraction, exaltation, ecstasy; or it has given me up" (ibid., p. 14). Moreover, he said, "I possess nothing but the everyday out of which I am never taken" (ibid.). In other words, Buber did not simply conclude from this troubling experience that he should be a better listener to others but, more importantly, it meant that his moral focus in everyday life should be on being fully present to and for others, especially in their hour of need.

If episodically not being fully present to loved ones, a form of apathy, is fairly common, how much more so is it likely that we display such apathy toward strangers, including those in dire need of our intervention? Indeed, from the point of view of group psychology, strangers are "the others" who "have been alongside us always," and yet typically, "society includes and excludes" them, sometimes in the most horrendous of ways (Hacking, 2007, pp. 285–286). Think of Buddhist Myanmar engaging in government-sponsored ethnic cleansing and genocide against the Rohingya Muslims in 2016. However, from the point of view of moral psychology, the age-old question is how does the "ingroup" individual treat the "outgroup" stranger, especially when he is face-to-face with a stranger in harm's way?[2] What prevents ordinary people from acting more compassionately, and what can be done to promote altruistic (often called "prosocial") behavior within the context of the suffering stranger? Indeed, such apparently dehumanized and dehumanizing responses of bystanders were the focus of Latané and Darley's brilliantly choreographed bystander studies.[3]

The bystander studies

Before summarizing and discussing the main findings of Latané and Darley's studies (Latané & Nida, 1981, p. 308), and in the spirit of full disclosure and to better contextualize the bystander effect in "real life," I want to describe a personal experience when I was in graduate school in New York City about forty years ago. I still remember it with a freshness of detail. I was the "victim" to willful non-intervention in a dramatic bystander moment.

I was traveling on the fairly crowded "F" train from Kew Gardens, Queens (very close to where Kitty Genovese was murdered[4]) to 14th Street in Manhattan to go to a late afternoon class. It was still rush hour by New York City's standards. I was about twenty-five, dressed in a sports jacket, had a knapsack and was carrying a few books under my arm which I was reading while on the subway. Overall, I looked well-kempt and was obviously a college or graduate student. A few minutes before I reached my stop, I began to feel dizzy and nauseous and I felt as if I was going to pass out. I staggered out of the train and collapsed on the subway platform, still conscious but even more dizzy and nauseous. I recall the many rush hour passersby avoiding me, though I was clearly in need of some assistance. Eventually, I noticed a nurse (she was dressed in her white uniform wearing a cap and name tag), and I asked her "Are you a nurse? Please help me." Our eyes met and she walked past me, as did the other passersby whom I reached out to for about ten minutes, until someone must have called the subway personnel and two police were standing over me. Their first question to me while I was still lying on the platform feeling hot and cold flashes was "What are you on?" They assumed I was overdosed on drugs. Believe it or not, in my dire state I responded tragicomically, saying, "I am on carrot juice, I am a health nut." The cops pulled me up and an ambulance took me to a local city hospital where I waited on a gurney in the hallway for about five hours, covered in my own vomit. Apparently, I had some kind of terrible flu. When I returned home I reflected to myself that I lived in a cold-hearted "concrete jungle" where people only care for themselves.

My relatively benign story of bystander indifference is hardly novel. There are countless troubling real-life examples that anecdotally support this phenomenon being more common than one would like to believe. As Rosemary K.M. Sword and Philip Zimbardo (of the famous Stanford Prison Experiment) have indicated, "your instinct—as well as the instinct of those around you—may be to not render aid" in an emergency situation involving a victim/stranger.[5] They mentioned a tragic case that occurred in Italy when a young woman was burned alive by her ex-boyfriend on the street and people quickly drove by instead of rendering assistance (ibid.). Perhaps the worst recent example of the "bystander effect" happened on October 27, 2009, when ten men gang-raped a fifteen-year-old student outside of her homecoming dance. At least twenty witnesses did nothing to stop it or alert authorities.[6]

As Elie Wiesel noted in a *New York Times* interview regarding victims of the Darfur genocide, "Let us remember: what hurts the victim most is not the cruelty of the oppressor, but the silence of the bystander" (Kristof, 2006, n.p.)—and more so when the bystanders are sadistically enjoying sadistic victimization, even rooting it on as in the homecoming dance incident. As a result of this crime, a California state law was passed making non-intervening by a bystander illegal.

Latané and Darley's research on bystander intervention in an emergency situation provided strong support for the general claim that "the presence of other people serves to inhibit the impulse to help" (Latané & Darley, 1970, p. 38; Latané & Nida, 1981). Their assumption from the onset of their research, inspired in part by the Genovese murder, was that the failure of the bystander to helpfully respond was not due to cold-heartedness or in other ways being apathetic about the crime victim, but rather that there were other psychological considerations related to the situation that made the bystanders hesitate to intervene.

In their landmark study, Latané and Darley (1968) engaged some college students who thought they enlisted for a group discussion about what college life felt like. Allegedly making sure their anonymity was protected, each student was seated alone in a cubicle with an intercom. Each of the students were instructed that their microphone would be switched on for two minutes at a time, giving each of them an opportunity to talk while the other group members, but importantly, not the experimenter, listened to their tellings. In fact, all of this staging of the experiment was choreographed by the experimenter. Only one student at a time participated, believing two, or five other students, as represented by audio recordings, were also listening. Within this context, the staged emergency occurred. The participant heard one of the other group members, who had previously indicated his vulnerability to epilepsy, suddenly begin to have an obvious seizure. The results showed that the more other students were thought to be present, the less likely they were to help and the longer they delayed before seeking assistance. Of those who thought that four other potential helpers were present, only 62% ever came to the victim's aid. It is noteworthy, and perhaps encouraging, that the majority of group members were not apathetic per se but were stressed in their anxious ambivalence about looking inappropriate in either helping or not helping. During their debriefing, naïve subjects said such things as "I didn't know what to do," "I thought it must be some sort of fake," and "I didn't know exactly what was happening." As Latané and Darley note, their "impression" was that most naïve subjects "had few coherent thoughts during the fit" (ibid., p. 381).

Latané and Nida explained these troubling findings, the "social inhibition of helping," not in terms of personality, background or other dispositional factors, but rather in terms of three interdependent, interrelated and interactive social-psychological processes that are operative when an individual in the presence of others fails to intervene for the sake of the victim: "audience inhibition," "social influence" and "diffusion of responsibility" (1981, p. 309).

The first process that is socially inhibitive of helping, "audience inhibition" is when the bystander can feel anxious or fearful that their behavior can be viewed by others and judged negatively. The bystander may feel that if he intervenes and there is no "true" emergency he will be embarrassed; thus, the more onlookers present, the greater the risk of feeling mortified. The second process is "social influence," in which the bystander looks to other people to define the meaning of the situation that is often ambiguous and confusing. When others are present and they are not offering to help the victim, the bystander sees that they are interpreting the situation as less urgent than the bystander may have judged it to be and decides that inaction is the expected and acceptable response pattern. Finally, the third social-psychological process, "diffusion of responsibility," is a means of diminishing the psychological cost connected with not helping. When there are others present, the costs are shared and not helping becomes more probable. As Latané and Nida noted, "the knowledge that others are present and available to respond, even if the individual cannot see or be seen by them, allows the shifting of some of the responsibility to helping them."[7] It is worth mentioning that a recent meta-analysis of experimental social-psychological studies involving over 7,700 participants has confirmed the existence of the bystander effect, though it is attenuated under certain conditions (Fischer et al., 2011). For example, bystanders are more willing and able to intervene if they believe the perpetrator and victim are strangers rather than intimates (e.g., if they believe a man assaulting a woman during an argument is married to her or they are an "item," the norm of family privacy is salient), or when they share group membership with the victim (e.g., a church-going man will help a fellow church member even if they are a stranger). Likewise, if one bystander helps in an emergency, others tend to follow, the former acting as a role model for the norm of social responsibility. The point is that the original bystander effect as described by Latané and Darley (1968) is a subtle phenomenon, in that the psychological relationships between perpetrator and victim, or between bystander and victim, are important predictors of helpful intervention, rather than simply the information that bystanders have about the presence or absence of others (Levine, 2017, p. 207).[8]

Toward a psychoanalytic social psychology

There has only been one psychoanalytically oriented response to Latané and Darley's findings of which I am aware, and this was via a comment made by the late Martin Wangh, a highly respected training and supervising psychoanalyst from the New York Psychoanalytic Society, who commented on the Kitty Genovese murder in an article in an anthology on psychoanalysis and the Holocaust (Luel & Marcus, 1984). Wangh explained the inaction of the alleged thirty-eight bystanders as reflecting "self-preservative, narcissistic behavioral manifestations" (ibid., p. 198). Quoting a sociologist from a 1964 *New York Times* article, Wangh further notes "witnessing a prolonged murder under their own windows had destroyed their feeling that the world was a 'rational orderly place'…[this] deeply shook their sense of safety and sureness" (ibid., p. 197). As a result of this, says Wangh, again approvingly quoting the sociologist, there "was an 'affect denial' that caused them to withdraw psychologically from the event by ignoring it" (ibid.). In other words, in a manner that was somewhat similar to Holocaust victims who entered a Nazi death camp, bystanders did not help Kitty Genovese because they were in a state of "shock," which "was followed by apathy." Psychologically speaking, the only way that Holocaust inmates could survive their ordeal, and by analogy the bystanders to the Kitty Genovese murder, was to enter into "some form of 'denial,' of 'psychic numbing,' 'derealization,' or 'depersonalization,'" attempts to emotionally dissociate from the ordeal that "took over" their "mind and/or feeling" (ibid, p. 197).[9]

Wangh's psychoanalytic formulations are somewhat in sync with the claim made by recent social theorists, namely, that we live in a postmodern world that seriously undermines our autonomy, integration and humanity, what sociologist Zygmunt Bauman (2000) called "liquid modernity." "'Liquid modern' is a society in which the conditions under which its members act change faster than it takes the ways of acting to consolidate into habits and routines" (2000, p. 1). Liquid modernity generates a form of living called "liquid life" (Bauman, 2005), in fact they "feed and reinvigorate each other" (Bauman, 2000, p. 1). Liquidization is thus a metaphor for the fact that life and self-identity appear to be progressively fluid, fractured, flexible and frail. Furthermore, "[l]iquid life is a precarious life, lived under conditions of constant uncertainty" which fosters a widespread feeling of displacement, anxiety and insecurity which is globally operative as capitalism takes deeper hold (ibid., p. 2). Within this context of "the vexingly confusing world of flexible norms and floating values" (ibid., p. 61), with "the dense web of social bonds that tightly wrapped the totality of life's activities" having been seriously eroded (ibid., p. 20), social relations, sociality and responsibility to and for the other become less important as extreme individualism takes hold. In short, with the modern self's tendency to fold into itself for self-protection, there is not much willingness to engage in altruistic behavior, let alone to help a stranger when there is no immediate or pragmatic "pay back," except perhaps the personal satisfaction of having acted in a morally praiseworthy manner.

The main problem with Bauman's notion of liquid life characterizing "liquid modernity" and Wangh's psychoanalytic formulation is that while "self-preservative, narcissistic behavioral manifestations" may partially account for why some bystanders behaved the way they did when faced with a victim screaming for help as in the Genovese murder, these formulations lack specificity and generalizability in terms of how ordinary people act in real-life emergency bystander situations. Moreover, there is no empirical evidence that those bystanders who do not assist a stranger in an emergency situation suffer the psychopathology that Wangh describes and implies. In fact, while Latané and Darley sensed that many of the naïve subjects were highly stressed by the epileptic seizure, the idea that they were "somehow different in kind from the rest of us," such as "alienated by industrialization," "dehumanized by urbanization," "depersonalized by living in the cold society," or were "psychopaths" (1968, p. 383) was implausible, and certainly not empirically verified. Rather, they claim that to believe such explanations has a defensive purpose for the theorizer. First, they allow him to believe they know why bystanders watch others die, and second, they allow theorizers to protect themselves from realizing that they too might fail to intervene in a similar situation (ibid.). Likewise, Bauman's observations do not explain why there are so many people who feel, think and act in ways that are contrary to "liquid modernity" and "liquid living," including often doing remarkably morally praiseworthy things for others. There are many cases of bystanders intervening to help a stranger in desperate need, including putting themselves in harm's way, thus displaying great courage and selflessness. In 2009 Dominik Brunner, a CFO of a large roof tiling business, was murdered at a German railroad station by two eighteen-year-olds after he attempted to help a group of school children who were being mugged by these young criminals. Numerous bystanders witnessed the murder, but nobody physically helped Brunner (Fischer et al., 2011, p. 517).

Five-step theory

In order to prepare the way for a possible integration of psychoanalytic ideas with experimental social psychology bystander findings, I will review Latané and Darley's five-step theory that describes the conditions of possibility that make it most likely that a bystander will choose to help a stranger in an emergency. However, it needs to be stressed that each choice-point can become the context for the bystander to choose to do nothing, mainly because it is the self-serving decision.

In step one, the bystander has to recognize there is an emergency situation in play. That is, most of the time the ordinary person is involved in the flow of his everyday life, thinking about what matters to him and failing to notice with any detail what is going on in his surroundings, without expectation of witnessing a stranger's emergency. In fact, most of us work hard at shutting out the "outside" world as we attend to our "inside world," utterly preoccupied with our own concerns.

Darley and Batson's (1973) riveting study is an excellent example of this self-preoccupied phenomenon and is worth briefly describing. They examined the influence of situational variables and religiosity, as measured by numerous personality scales, on the helping behavior of forty theology students at the Princeton Theological Seminary in an emergency situation prompted by the parable of the Good Samaritan. Naïve subjects going between two buildings came upon a shabbily dressed "victim" slumped in an alleyway. Those naïve subjects in a hurry to reach their destination were more likely to pass by without stopping. Some naïve subjects were going to give a short talk on the parable of the Good Samaritan, others on a non-helping pertinent topic. In both instances, this made no significant difference in the likelihood of their giving help to the victim. (In several instances, seminary students on their way to give a talk on the Good Samaritan literally stepped over the victim!) Thus, religious personality variables did not predict whether naïve subjects would help the victim. However, if the naïve subject did stop to offer help, the nature of the helping response was connected to his type of religiosity. Moreover, what mattered most was the amount of time the naïve subjects had between classes. The more time they had, the more likely they were to help.

In step two, the bystander needs to interpret the situation as in fact being an emergency. Most of the time we go about our everyday activities with limited information and incomplete knowledge about what is going on around us. Moreover, when we do notice something out of the ordinary, we tend to interpret its meaning in a matter-of-fact, routine way. The avoidance of uncommon or improbable explanations allows us to carry on with "business as usual." Moreover, in the ambiguous situations in which many emergencies appear to occur from the bystander's point of view, there is a tendency to judge it as unimportant, thus giving oneself a less stressful "good" reason to do nothing (including the possibility of looking foolish or embarrassingly over-reactive to onlookers).

Latané and Darley (1968) conducted a famous study, "where there is smoke there is fire," that showed how "pluralistic ignorance" (when a group of strangers hesitates to do anything they believe would be "inappropriate") inhibits helping behavior. The experimenters placed the naïve subjects in a room alone or with two other naïve subjects as they completed a questionnaire. After a few minutes, the experimenters pumped smoke through a vent into the room. The results were dramatic: when naïve subjects were alone, 75% stopped completing the questionnaire and went to get help; when three people were in the room, only 38% reacted to the smoke and went for help. Most troublingly, even after the room became so smoke-filled that it became near-impossible to see, 62% did nothing. In other words, in the context of being with other strangers who do not react, there is a tendency for bystanders to act likewise, and this situational force is so powerful, in this case to not look foolish or act embarrassingly, that it would be preferable to risk serious injury or death.

Step three refers to the bystander's assumption that it is one's responsibility to help a victim stranger. After a bystander notices and judges that there is an emergency in play, he must decide whether to act responsibly by providing help. In a typical bystander emergency stranger situation when there is no obvious leader, like a firefighter, police person or doctor, bystanders tend to assume that anyone in a leadership role is the one responsible to provide help. For example, a bus driver is the one who is judged to be responsible for an emergency involving the vehicle. In other words, in a group of bystanders facing an emergency situation involving a victim/stranger in which there is no manifest leader present, bystanders assume that someone else will intervene, which allows them to do nothing. Diffusion of responsibility explains that in the context of others, responsibility is divided such that each person feels less responsible for helping than when they are alone.

Step four involves knowing what to pragmatically do in an emergency. Many emergencies are straightforward, like if a person falls in the icy street, a bystander knows how to deal with the situation, get the person out of harm's way and call the police/ambulance. However, some emergency situations demand specialized skills such as rescuing a drowning person or attending to a physical injury. Clearly, a trained lifeguard or a nurse would be more likely to offer help, that is, assume responsibility, than an ordinary person who does not have these specialized skills.

Finally, step five refers to actually making the decision to help the victim/stranger. Even if the bystander has successfully negotiated steps one to four, he still has to resolutely make the decision to provide help. This is a hugely complex issue that involves the bystander's moral outlook and inner convictions, and many other judgment and decision-making factors, in the face of what appear to be challenging situational contingencies. There are many real and imagined considerations that inhibit helping behavior, considerations that are connected to the potential negative consequences of helping. Such decision-making involves weighing the pros and cons of intervening; for example, the bystander who wants to help the person move off the icy street may reasonably be worried that he too will slip on the ice and get seriously hurt. Helping a man slumped in a doorway who appears to be sick, as in both Latané and Darley's study and my personal experience described earlier, could result in the man attacking you in some way (if he is "mentally ill"), or vomiting on you, or infecting you with a serious illness. Likewise, there are apparent victim/strangers who are actually scam artists—or worse—who will put you in harm's way. The infamous Ted Bundy, the 1970s serial killer, kidnaper and rapist, was a good-looking, well-dressed and manipulatively charming man who would play on the sympathies of young women by painfully limping and asking the women to help him get into his car, after which he would kidnap them. The point is that there are realistic considerations that a bystander has to judge as making their help worth it before deciding to intervene (Baron & Byrne, 2003, p. 398).

In general, scientifically explaining exactly how people make judgements and go about decision-making, including in these high-risk situations, is at best a "cluttered conceptual countryside" (Hacking, 2007, p. 290), and at worst, a field that is in conceptual disarray. Indeed, one behavioral decision theory authority raised two broad questions that suggest the field is in its early stages of understanding human judgements and decision-making:

> How is it that we are as competent as we evidently are? Second, what can we do about how incompetent we evidently are? Quite how it is that people perform as effectively as they do by applying non-normative mental strategies[10] to the limited information that they can process—and how we might learn to improve our decision making—remain to be explored and explained.
>
> *(Ayton, 2012, p. 362)*[11]

In my view, whether one regards feelings as most important [e.g., automatic processes, so-called moral intuitions, as "social intuitionist" Jonathan Haidt (2012) claims] in making moral judgments and decisions, or mainly strategic and conscious reasoning, it is always a mixture of these and other factors that can best account for what possibly animates moral behavior. This in keeping with my Heideggerian assumption that man is "being-in-the-world," that human existence is a unitary phenomenon of feeling/kinesthetic, thought and action enacted in the lived openness, presentness and awareness of his everyday life.

Motivations for helping

Now that we have some sense of why, social-psychologically speaking, many bystanders do not intervene in an emergency situation, the question is why some bystanders do the opposite. Social psychologists have described some of the situational factors that enhance helping, that is, that tend to generate apparently altruistic behavior. While detailing this extensive literature is beyond the scope of this chapter, a few points should be emphasized, mainly because some of these theories and findings resonate with certain psychoanalytic insights into such praiseworthy, though "deviant," behavior.

The empathy-altruism model (Batson, 2002) states that emotions associated with empathic concern generally potentiate a motivation to help someone in need, including in an emergency context, mainly for the sake of the victim/stranger. In Levinasian ethical language, this appears to be an existential mode of comportment that tends toward being for the other before oneself. In contrast, the term egoism describes a motivational state in which the main goal is to increase one's own wellbeing and best interests as an end in itself. In Levinasian ethical language, this is an existential mode of comportment that tends toward being for oneself, with little or no regard for the other. For example, bystanders experiencing high levels of empathy may feel more anguish and therefore may be more prone to help because they are largely egoistically motivated to diminish their own anguish. Another egoistically driven option is that those bystanders experiencing high levels of empathy are more inclined to help because they are more motivated to avoid feeling negatively about themselves or appearing negatively in the eyes of others should they not act helpfully. Likewise, those bystanders experiencing high levels of empathy may be more likely to help because they are more egoistically motivated to feel good about themselves or to appear good in the eyes of others.[12] Indeed, psychoanalytically speaking, all so-called altruistic acts have some kind of conscious or unconscious narcissistic "pay off," even if only the positive feeling that one has acted in accordance with one's heartfelt beliefs and values. The point is that with most intervening bystanders, the main motivation is to be other-directed, other-regarding and other-serving, even if on some conscious or unconscious level they experience an increase in self-esteem, self-coherence and self-continuity as an epiphenomenon. Indeed, Batson, one of the prominent social-psychological researchers on empathy and altruism, makes the same point in his definition of altruism: "feeling empathy for [a] person in need evokes motivation to help in which these benefits to self are not the ultimate goal of helping; they are unintended consequences" (Batson & Shaw, 1991, p. 114). In their study of the altruistic personality, the characteristics of "heroic rescuers" of Jews during the Holocaust, Oliner & Oliner (1988) have defined altruism in a useful manner: They rely on what they call "objective, measurable criteria." An altruistic act is directed toward helping another; it involves a high risk or sacrifice to the actor; it is accomplished by no external reward; it is voluntary. Heroic altruism involves greater risk to the helper, whereas conventional altruism is not life-threatening to the helper.[13] The so-called "altruistic personality" displays five personality characteristics: empathy, belief in a just world, social responsibility, internal locus of control and low egocentrism (Bierhoff et al., 1991).

Although there is substantial evidence that egoism can be a robust motivator of helping behavior, some researchers have interrogated whether all human behavior is motivated largely by self-interest. The gist of this helping model is that typically a bystander can feel two kinds of emotions when they observe a victim/stranger in an emergency situation: alarm, anxiety and fear or empathic concern such as compassion, sympathy and tenderness. Most often, I believe that a bystander will feel an ambivalent mixture of these feelings. If, however, the bystander is dominated by alarm, anxiety and fear, which are self-centric emotions, he will try to find an avenue of flight from these distressing feelings; if he is dominated by empathic concern he will offer help to the victim/stranger. It is worth mentioning that while the bystander animated by empathic concern knows he can flee the emergency situation to reduce the distress he feels, he nevertheless provides help to the victim/stranger.

In my view, he does this not only because he empathizes/identifies with him as this empathy-altruism model suggests, but because he is motivated by strongly felt, flexibly and creatively applied, transcendent beliefs and values that are firstly and mainly other-directed, other-regarding and other-serving. In other words, such a person is largely motivated by a drive to self-affirmation through the accomplishment of moral excellence in which the impulse to serve a cause greater than the self is what matters most. By residing in this atypical, "deviant" dimension of being, we sense the mystery of personal freedom and an almost unconscious openness to compassion, gloriously enacted by the bystander as he helps the suffering stranger.[14] Batson and Thompson (2001) describe a somewhat similar sounding motivation, "moral integrity," in which acting in accordance with goodness, fairness and self-sacrifice is what matters most to a bystander, but they underplay the key role of transcendent beliefs and values. They also mention "moral hypocrisy" that describes the bystander who may offer some superficial help to a victim but intentionally avoids major sacrifice or putting himself in harm's way. What matters most to him is the *appearance* of caring and helping. In a later formulation, Batson (2011) also describes what he calls "principlism," a form of moral decision-making as one of four reasons that motivate altruistic behavior (the others are egoism, altruism and collectivism), in which following moral principles is what mainly guides altruistic behavior, at least for some bystanders. While the experimental social psychology evidence for principlism is not robust as a separate motive for altruistic behavior, and not simply a form of egoism (for example, one is motivated to be observed in an emergency as acting morally),[15] the fact is that there is anecdotal evidence that some bystanders who have deeply felt, flexibly and creatively applied transcendent beliefs and values, those who are geared toward being other-directed, other-regarding and other-serving as "first principle," were most likely to act in an autonomous, integrated and humane manner toward a stranger in need. That is, moral beliefs and values that point to "something more," "something higher" and "something better" than the self that ethically animates real-life behavior in an emergency situation, a kind of "visceral ethics," may well be the lynchpin of why some bystanders help a victim/stranger, including when they put themselves at high risk for injury or death.

Clearly, what motivates altruistic behavior is a function of a number of interrelated, interdependent and interactive internal and external factors that are probably impossible to "pin down" with reasonable scientific certainty. To answer why a particular bystander behaves heroically in a particular situation and at a particular time is always multi-determined, context-dependent and setting-specific, and ultimately provisionally grasped only when one understands the idiosyncratic psychological trajectory of the hero(ine). Even then, one is only offering an informed guess as Latané and Darley imply in their five-step decision-making model. The bystander's moment of existential decision-making to help a stranger in need of intervention can never be completely predicted based on any of these factors, though it appears to have a lot to do with the psychology of courage and selflessness.[16] While courage, the ability to do something that is frightening to oneself and that demonstrates strength in the face of this fear, and selflessness, concern for the needs and wishes of others over one's own, are themselves complex phenomena that are contested both in definition and in how they are instantiated, they do appear to have a significant role in bystander intervention and other extreme rescuing/helping contexts.

It is worth describing three heroic stories of individuals whose actions during the Holocaust beautifully depict the personality and moral and emotional qualities (i.e., the beliefs and values) that are likely in play in those bystanders who acted "righteously," as Bettelheim called them (1990, p. 206). The first person mentioned by Bettelheim is the Polish priest, Father Maximilian Maria Kolbe, who, in Auschwitz, volunteered to die in the place of a political prisoner, enabling him to live and return to his wife and children (the priest had no such family). Kolbe was murdered by being starved to death, while the inmate whose life he saved lived to tell the story, as did also some other prisoners who had witnessed Kolbe's death and some of the SS guards who could not help being deeply impressed by the courage with which he suffered his terrible fate. As a result of Kolbe's extraordinary actions, he was canonized.

The second of the "righteous men" was Dr. Janusz Korczak. As is well-known, he adamantly refused many offers to be saved from extermination in the death camps. As Bettelheim describes, Korczak

> refused to desert in extremis the orphaned children to whose well-being he had devoted his life, so that even as they decided they would be able to maintain their faith in human goodness: that of the man who had saved their bodies and fed their minds; who had salvaged them from utter misery and restored their belief in themselves and the world; who had been their mentor in matters practical and spiritual.
>
> *(ibid.)*

Bettelheim, citing Pope John Paul II, agrees that Korczak was a "symbol of true religion and true morality" (ibid.).

Finally, Bettelheim describes Hermine "Miep" Gies. It is due to her,

> more than to anyone else, that Anne Frank could write her diary, since it was Miep who, at great risk to herself, provided the Frank family—and others who hid out with them—with the needed food that kept them alive, and with the human companionship they needed to be able to endure their desperate isolation.
>
> *(ibid.)*

Bettelheim further indicates "that she risked her life in efforts to rescue those in dire need not out of a feeling of obligation, but out of sheer human decency. She did what she felt was right, with disregard for her own safety, because she was the person she was." It was "her courage, her humanity, and her decency" which "give us hope for humanity" (ibid.).

In these three anecdotes, the term bystander can be defined as someone who is at an event but does not participate in it. While in these instances the bystanders were "at the event," the Holocaust, and they did not have to "take part" in it the way they did, what is common to all of these extraordinary individuals is that the responsibility to and for the other was felt as a moral imperative beyond compromise. Not to act as they did would have been too humiliating in their own judgement to allow them to continue living in a manner that they could justify. Richard Rorty starkly captures the destructive impact such humiliation has on people in terms of what they say to themselves:

> Now that I have believed or desire this, I can never be what I hoped to be, what I thought I was. The story I have been telling myself about myself—my picture of myself as honest, or loyal, or devout—no longer makes sense. I no longer have a self to make sense of. There is no world in which I can picture myself living, because there is no vocabulary in which I can tell a coherent story about myself.
>
> *(1989, p. 179)*

While there is no guarantee that the bystander will help a stranger, or for that matter predict courageous and selfless behavior in any dire situation, it should be stressed that in one of the most extreme situations imaginable, during the Holocaust, as Bauman described in another context, "The moral conscience—that ultimate prompt of moral impulse and root of moral responsibility" was not "amputated" by the Nazis (Bauman, 1993, p. 249). Moreover, "moral responsibility cannot be taken away, shared, ceded, pawned, or deposited for safe keeping. Moral responsibility is unconditional and infinite, and it manifests itself in the constant anguish of not manifesting itself enough" (ibid., p. 250). Nor was the moral conscience amputated among the many heroic bystanders who have intervened in an emergency situation involving a stranger as described earlier, often involving great personal risk (e.g., Dominik Brunner). The important point is that these bystanders are motivated by strongly felt, flexibly and creatively applied transcendent beliefs and values that are instantiated by summoning other-directed, other-regarding and other-serving behavior as they construe it. With this moral armature, they are galvanized to act righteously and heroically—call it "social deviance"—where the rest of us may do the opposite. Kolbe was motivated by his love of God and the responsibilities of self-sacrifice that emanated from his faith; Korczak by his love of the children and his intense sense of responsibility to comfort them to the end; and Giese because of her commitment to "sheer human decency," to selflessly care for those in need, another version of responsibility to and for the other. Bettelheim captures the beliefs and values of these three people by quoting the ancient rabbis who, "when asked, 'When everyone acts inhuman, what should a man do?' their answer was, 'He should act more human'" (ibid.).

Implications for treatment

For the psychoanalyst (and other psychotherapists), the most elemental, practical, clinical take home points of this discussion of the bystander effect is the need for the analyst to encourage the analysand to be a responsive bystander, to fashion his internal world in a manner that makes this morally praiseworthy way of being in the real-life world more likely. This involves, for example, the analysand cultivating greater situational awareness, being aware of one's surroundings and recognizing possible threats and dangerous situations, especially in terms of those who may be in need. Such "thin slicing" is "the ability of our unconscious to find patterns in situations and behavior based on very narrow slices of experience" (Gladwell, 2005, p. 23). Such a sensibility permits the bystander to tease out the elements that are most important from the vast number of stimuli acting on our senses. Likewise, if the analysand notices something that is out of the ordinary, it is best to generate manifold alternative accounts and seek out additional confirming/disconfirming information, rather than rely on the "usual suspects" of thought and feeling and carrying on with "business as usual." Finally, the analysand should be encouraged to be aware of what appears to be a human tendency to avoid taking responsibility, relying on "diffusion of responsibility" to rationalize not helping someone in need. Indeed, these practical tactics that are allied to the valuative attachment of social responsibility, of being for the other, are wisely worth embracing by psychoanalytic and other psychotherapists in their work with analysands and others. Ironically, engaging in socially responsible behavior, an expression of altruism, also has many documented advantages to the doer: Altruism is correlated with better marital relationships, less hopelessness, less depression, increased physical health and bolstered self-esteem. Moreover, altruistic behavior may also neutralize negative emotions that impact immune, endocrine and cardiovascular function.[17]

Indeed, Freud had a similar moral sensibility, if not aspiration, though it was severely blunted by the harsh reality of underwhelming if not deplorable individual behavior as he saw it. For example, he noted in a letter to a colleague that "the unworthiness of human beings, including the analyst, always impressed me deeply, but why should analyzed men and women in fact be better. Analysis makes for integration but does not itself make for goodness" (Hale, 1971, p. 188). He wrote in another letter "[t]hat psychoanalysis has not made the analysts themselves better, noble, or of stronger character remains a disappointment for me. Perhaps I was wrong to expect it" (ibid., pp. 163–164). Thus, Freud clearly was concerned about the moral and ethical limitations of his psychoanalytic creation as it related to clinical outcome. He also commented on altruism mainly as a masochistic manifestation, though other analysts have attempted to expand the understanding of altruism along a "normal and pathological altruism" continuum, describing proto altruism, generative altruism, conflicted altruism, pseudo altruism and psychotic altruism (Seelig & Rosof, 2001). Clearly, as Philip Rieff noted in his celebrated intellectual biography, Freud had a "mind of the moralist," in that he provided "lessons on the right conduct of life from the misery of living it" (1961, p. xix).

In contrast to Freud's reflections on clinical outcome and altruism that stressed dispositional considerations (i.e., moral beliefs and values, masochism), experimental social psychologists have shown that there are powerful contextual factors and situational forces (the "outer world") that have a significant impact on bystander behavior when a stranger is in need of intervention in an emergency situation (and other helping circumstances) And yet as the above Freud quotes suggest, from his psychoanalytic point of view, it may be one's strongly felt, flexibly and creatively applied, transcendent beliefs and values (the "inner world") that are the fertile psychological breeding ground for analysands and analysts being "better, noble, or of stronger character," and motivated by "goodness." It is such a moral armature, conceived as a meaning-giving, affect-integrating and action-guiding, ethically animated way of thinking, feeling and acting, that ultimately matters in terms of moral decision-making in many situations. This kind of existential comportment may in many instances surpass powerful contextual factors and situational forces, thus prompting altruistic bystander behavior toward the victim/stranger, and in other helping situations involving those in need. Of course, this point of view is not formulaic, absolute, or guaranteed predictive, but it does point in a direction that psychoanalysis and experimental social psychology can possibly go in, not only in terms of understanding bystander intervention, but also what child rearing could focus on in terms of educating and encouraging children to be willing and able to be for-the-other before, or at least as much as, themselves. Cultivating a willingness and ability to subjugate one's fear and anxiety, in part the basis for acting courageously, is a huge aspect of this being-for-the-other existential orientation.

The larger implications of these findings in terms of psychoanalytic clinical practice may well be controversial for some in the "postmodern camp," as it means that psychoanalysis is allying itself with a set of "virtuous" beliefs and values. While these beliefs and values are not easily, if ever, foundationally grounded, they are moral qualities that Freud has put forth explicitly, as in the above quotes from his letters, and implicitly, in his theory, that appear to be praiseworthy and worth fighting for. Lear, for example, noted "that psychoanalysis has an unavoidably ethical dimension," such as the "ethical commitment" to the "recognition and acceptance of the reality of other subjects" (2017, pp. 155, 156). Truthfulness and freedom are other valuative attachments mentioned by Lear. Even the die-hard postmodernist psychoanalyst, Barnaby B. Barratt, ends his book by saying that the deconstructive version of psychoanalysis that he puts forth is "feminist, life-affirmative, communitarian, biophilic, spiritually imbued, emancipatory and genuinely scientific" (1993, p. 223). While these terms are not elaborated in the passage quoted, they are clearly ethically provocative and morally weighty, and reflect a crypto-normativism, meaning these valuative attachments express "some of the tacit commitments that the therapeutic project subtly demands … certain hidden ethical, political, and communal commitments that the psychoanalytic ethos obliges" (Davies, 2009, p. 103). In my view, these valuative attachments are precisely the beliefs and values that constitute the moral "bedrock" of resistance to the worst aspects of modernity and postmodernity, even if these beliefs and values are difficult to define, instantiate, are not consensually grounded and involve perspective-driven personal judgments. Still they are suggestive if not summoning for how to proceed in the future both individually and societally. Richard Rorty, one of the great historicist, anti-essentialist, neopragmatic philosophers of our time, aptly made this point in an interview:

> But Dewey has a different conception of the fundamental moral fact. For him what makes us moral beings is that, for each of us, there are some acts we believe we ought to die rather than commit. Which acts these are will differ from epoch to epoch, and from person to person, but to be a moral agent is to

be unable to imagine living with oneself after committing these acts [e.g. giving in to the bystander affect].[18]

In contrast to these life-denying acts of commission and omission that constitute a lack of moral agency, there is a life-affirming way of being-in-the-world that not only points to "something more," "something higher" and "something better," but may be a redemptive counter-force to the indifference and brutality of our imperfect world: "My sense of the holy, insofar as I have one, is bound up with the hope that someday, any millennium now, my remote descendants will live in a global civilization in which love is pretty much the only law" (Rorty, in Rorty & Vattimo, 2005, p. 40).

Final remarks

I want to end this chapter by reminding the reader that Freud was concerned about "goodness" and it not being what psychoanalysis brought about in most analysands who have been in treatment. Indeed, in general, I believe that a successful analysis often makes an analysand more profound and "deeper," but not necessarily a "good" person, one who is "better, noble, or of stronger character," as Freud had hoped. Maybe it is just this quality of "goodness," a contested term that cannot be foundationally grounded, that points in the same direction which the bystander studies are also suggesting is worth striving for—namely, resisting individual apathy and indifference in whatever morally challenging setting, and intervening for a stranger in an emergency. In this sense, following Levinasian ethical reflections, but also those of Bauman and Rorty, I am suggesting that maybe psychoanalysis and experimental social psychology have to "join forces" in putting forth a theory that begins with a different assumption about what is possible for human beings to become, what they "ought" to strive for, or even what they "essentially" are, or at least appear to be in our current episteme, our socio-intellectual reality. I am suggesting a kind of Nietzschean "transvaluation of values" in which human beings are conceived differently. Call it an aspirational optic, one that recognizes that while people are prone to conformity and indifference, they are also inclined to be morally "deviant" in the positive, life-affirming sense in which people see themselves as agents of the good, the helpful; as interconnected, as each other's keepers.

As Levinas has pointed out in another context, the devout Jewish (and other spiritual aspirants) self-community and self-other relation at its best "was lived above all with the sense that belonging to humanity means belonging to an order of responsibility" (1994, p. 168). Such a notion emphasizes that the responsibility for and obligation to the other are absolute; they are greater than the individual's responsibility to satisfy them. They always demand more and are never accomplished by the fulfillment of any deed. As a moral subject, the individual is always found lacking, because ethics is not just a component of one's existence; it delimits the entire realm in which one resides (Davis, 1996). Such a conception of existence, of the subject constituted by the encounter with the other, the basis of ethical relations founded on that encounter (Bauman, 1989), suggests a reorientation for most people in contemporary society, a move from narcissism toward selflessness rooted in a commitment to an absolute responsibility to the other. In this formulation, "responsibility is the essential, primary and fundamental structure of subjectivity … the very node of the subjective is knotted in ethics understood as responsibility" (Levinas, 1985, p. 95). Levinas's main idea is beautifully captured in his often-quoted passage from Dostoyevsky, "we are all responsible for all and for all men before all, and I more than all of the others" (ibid., p. 101).

In other words, I believe that one of the best ways to protect one's personal and moral integrity from the dangerous aspects of contemporary society, whether it is distressingly called "liquid modernity" or the "mass society"—from the social control, pressures of homogeneity and conformity, normative correctness, mechanical subservience, technolatry (i.e., bedazzlement with technical competence and gadgetry that has dulled concern for human feelings), and lack of judged morality—is to embrace responsibility to the other as the existential mode of one's flourishing life. As Levinas noted, "responsibility for the other" is taken to be "incumbent on me exclusively, and what humanly, I cannot refuse" (ibid.). This way of being-in-the-world is most likely to prevent the typical person from falling under the "evil spell," as I call it, of "one of the most robust and reliable findings in social psychology" (Levine, 2017, p. 213), the bystander effect.

Notes

1 To be present, says the self-described "Christian Socratic" philosopher Gabriel Marcel, means affirming the self as a being-among-other-beings, and affirming the pertinence of other's experiences to the self, as a being. Presence thus requires being "open to openness" (www.iep.utm.edu/marcel/, retrieved 9/23/18). This being said, some have argued otherwise, raising an interesting issue. "Open-mindedness," says psychologist Gordon W. Allport, often considered a "virtue," "strictly speaking, it cannot occur." That is, "a new experience" of another person, "must be redacted into old categories. We cannot handle each event freshly in its own right. If we did so, of what use would past experience be?" Allport quotes Bertrand Russell to support his view, "a mind perpetually open will be a mind perpetually vacant" (1979, p. 20).

2 It is worth noting that in many of the ancient religious "spirituality" and "wisdom" traditions that emerged during the Axial Age (800 to 200 BCE), the socially tumultuous period when there was an explosion of spiritual creativity in four regions of the word, there was the explicit moral requirement to welcome and take care of the stranger, the foreigner and the outsider. This moral value has been embraced by most "enlightened" spiritualities and religions (Marcus, 2019).

3 The claim of the bystanders being dehumanized may sound too severe to some, since, the argument goes, the bystander was under the influence that others would do something to help the victim. However, from a Levinasian ethic of responsibility, it is precisely that relinquishment of individual responsibility that constitutes their dehumanization. Dehumanization as I am using the term means removing from a victim their unique human qualities of vulnerability and need that "ought" to summon me to help them.

4 Kitty Genovese was murdered by her probably psychotic assailant on March 13, 1964. Allegedly there were many witnesses (thirty-eight was the cited number), either seeing her stabbed, sexually assaulted or hearing her screams during the forty-five minutes of two separate attacks late at night on her way back from work. Allegedly, no one called the police or intervened in any other matter. This case became a media sensation, depicting the "homo urbanis," as Darley recollected, that is, "the city dweller who cared only for himself" and who had "personality flaws" such that he "could stand and watch while others died" (Darley, in Evans, 1980, p. 216). Later investigators have disputed the

facts of the Genovese murder, suggesting that there were not nearly as many witnesses, including those who did nothing, and the police may have been called. However, nearly all who have impartially studied this case have opined that "the behavior of the witnesses was hardly beyond reproach." In fact, one of the assistant DAs who prosecuted the case said in a 2004 interview that even if not all bystanders saw the crime, "I believe that many people heard the screams, it could have been more than 38. And anyone that heard the screams had to know there was a vicious crime taking place There's no doubt in my mind about that" (Rasenberger, 2004, n.p.). See Manning et al. (2007) for a critical discussion of the Genovese murder that claims that the received story of what happened is groundless (e.g., the number of bystanders, what they actually viewed and how they interpreted it) and has been destructively appropriated into how social psychologists researched bystander behavior and communicated it to psychology students.

5 www.psychologytoday.com/us/blog/the-time-cure/201804/heroism-vs-the-bystander-effect, retrieved 8/31/18.

6 listverse.com/2009/11/02/10-notorious-cases-of-the-bystander-effect/, retrieved 8/26/18.

7 In another study Latané and Darley (1970) discussed three very similar psychological processes that can impede bystander intervention: "Diffusion of responsibility," defined as the proclivity of a person to divide the personal responsibility to aid a victim by the number of bystanders; "evaluative apprehension," a fear of being judged by onlookers when behaving in public; and "pluralistic ignorance," the tendency to depend on the explicit behavior of others when defining an ambiguous situation.

8 As Levine summarizes the matter, the research in the bystander tradition has demonstrated that the presence of others does not necessarily lead to anti-social behavior. Rather, behavior in group settings can be prosocial or anti-social depending on what kind of identity is salient, and what the content of the identity in fact is. For example, women feel more willing and able to intervene when they have other women around them compared to having bystander men. When bystanders don't share a psychological connection, in other words, when they encounter each other as a strangers, then the bystander effect appears strong; however, when the bystanders share a salient social identity then the behavior can constrain helping, although on some occasions it can facilitate bystander intervention (2017, p. 211, 213, 214).

9 An interpersonal/relational psychoanalytic perspective focuses on the negative impact of inadequate parental caregiving and dysfunctional family life on the internalization of representations, thus psychological defects and developmental deficits, including those that are associated with adult lack of empathy and moral agency, would largely theoretically account for the bystander effect.

10 There are two kinds of decision-making theory, "normative" ones, the "ought," which is assumed to be the "ideal decision" people should make, versus "descriptive" theory, the "is," the way that people actually make decisions (Ayton, 2012, p. 335).

11 The matter is even more complicated. As Cooper points out, some neuropsychologists have claimed that decision-connected brain activity may happen up to ten seconds prior to a person actually being aware of making choices. In other words, citing researchers, "the brain evidently 'decides' to initiate or, at least, prepare to initiate the act at a time before there is any reportable subjective awareness that such a decision has taken place" (2015, p. 111). Thus, the phenomenological sense of making choices may actually be illusionary, that decisions are determined by non-conscious, a-volitional brain mechanisms. In contrast, says Cooper, perhaps human freedom is composed of the ability to say "no" to non-volitionally initiated activities. In any event, these studies raise questions about the prudence of over-valuing the authority of consciousness and the belief in self-determination. It is also worth mentioning that the psychological, adaptive unconscious of neuroscience and cognitive psychology is not what psychoanalysis means by the dynamic unconscious which for Freud was the metaphorical repository of repressed motivations, goals, desires, memories and fantasies, or the interpersonal/relational unconscious which has put forth a "dissociational" model, a kind of "motivated forgetting" of threatening experiences that serves defensive purposes (Curtis, 2009).

12 www.psychology.iresearchnet.com/social-psychology/prosocial-behavior/empathy-altruism-hypothesis/, retrieved 8/31/18. Empathy also has a down side. It can undermine rational choice. Yale professor Paul Bloom (2016), for example, describes studies that show that empathy encourages irrational moral decisions that favor one individual whose suffering is more easily metabolized compared to the masses who may be suffering more. While empathy is a contested term in that what it refers to and how it works is not agreed upon, Bloom favors rational analysis, morality and compassion as a basis for moral decision-making, though these terms' definitions and how they are instantiated are hardly agreed upon.

13 www2.humboldt.edu/altruism/definitions, retrieved 9/5/18.

14 The cultural anthropologist Ernest Becker (1975) has claimed that human beings are motivated by their wish to belong to something larger than and beyond themselves while at the same time striving to actualize themselves in a unique manner in their everyday lives.

15 Other forms of egoistic motivation include avoiding self and/or other punishment, or wanting to reduce the level of high arousal (Batson, 2011).

16 As Adam Grant noted in a recent *New York Times* book review, there has been an upsurge of books on the science of decision-making, including about choices we make in the "blink" of an eye, as Malcolm Gladwell evocatively called it, as we attempt to negotiate our everyday lives (e.g., Daniel Kahneman, *Thinking, Fast and Slow*). Most recently, Steven Johnson has written *Farsighted: How We Make the Decisions That Matter the Most*, which deals with the "big" decisions that animate our futures. However, these and other self-help books in no way provide a formula or even a credible methodology for decision-making that guarantees a successful outcome, whether as judged by the agent or an onlooker. Because you never have sufficient "information to make the best choice, all you can do is make the best of the choice you've made" (Grant, 2018, p. 16).

17 https://www.mentalhealth.org.uk/a-to-z/a/altruism-and-wellbeing, retrieved 9/24/18.

18 https://medium.com/@sean.d.norton/understanding-richard-rortys-achieving-our-country-61b7844ddd98, retrieved 9/24/18.

References

Allport, G.W. (1979). *The nature of prejudice* (25th Anniversary Ed.). Reading: Addison-Wesley Publishing Company.

Ayton, P. (2012). Judgement and decision making. In N. Braisby & A. Gellatly (Eds.), *Cognitive psychology* (2nd ed., pp. 334–365). Oxford: Oxford University Press.

Baron, R.A. & Byrne, D. (Eds.) (2003). *Social psychology* (10th ed.). Boston: Pearson Education.

Barratt, B.B. (1993). *Psychoanalysis and the postmodern impulse: Knowing and being since Freud's psychology*. London: Routledge.

Batson, C.D. (2002). Addressing the altruism question experimentally. In S.G. Post & L.G. Underwood (Eds.), *Altruism and altruistic love: Science and philosophy, & religion in dialogue* (pp. 89–105). London: Oxford University Press.

Batson, C.D. (2011). *Altruism in humans*. New York: Oxford University Press.

Batson, C.D. & Shaw, L.L. (1991). Evidence for altruism: Toward a pluralism of prosocial motives. *Psychological Inquiry*, 2(2), 107–122.

Batson, C.D. & Thompson, E.R. (2001). Why don't moral people act morally? Motivation considerations. *Current Directions in Psychological Science*, 10(2), 54–57.

Bauman, Z. (1989). *Modernity and the Holocaust*. Ithaca, NY: Cornell University Press.

Bauman, Z. (1993). *Postmodern ethics*. Oxford: Blackwell.

Bauman, Z. (2000). *Liquid modernity*. Cambridge: Polity.

Bauman, Z. (2005). *Liquid lives*. Cambridge: Polity.

Becker, E. (1975). *Escape from evil*. New York: Free Press.

Bettelheim, B. (1990). *Freud's Vienna and other essays*. New York: Knopf.

Bierhoff, H.W., Klein, R. & Kramp, P. (1991). Evidence for the altruistic personality from data on accident research. *Journal of Personality*, 59, 263–280.

Bloom, P. (2016). *Against empathy: The case for rational compassion*. New York: Ecco Press.

Buber, M. (1965). *Between man and man*. R.G. Smith (Trans.). New York: Macmillan.

Cooper, M. (2015). *Existential psychotherapy and counseling: Contributions to a pluralistic practice*. Thousand Oaks, CA: Sage.

Curtis, R.C. (2009). *Desire, self, mind, and the psychotherapies: Unifying psychological science and psychoanalysis*. Lanham: Jason Aronson.

Darley, J.M. & Batson, C.D. (1973). From Jerusalem to Jericho: A study of situational dispositional variable in helping behavior. *Journal of Personality and Social Psychology*, 27, 100–108.

Davies, J. (2009). *The making of psychotherapists: An anthropological analysis*. London: Karnac.

Davis, C. (1996). *Levinas: An introduction*. Cambridge: Polity Press.

Evans, R.I. (1980). *The making of social psychology*. New York: Gardner Press.

Fischer, P., Greitemeyer, T., Kastenmuller, A., Krueger, J.I., Vogrincic, C. & Frey, D. (2011). The bystander-effect: A meta-analytic review on bystander intervention in dangerous and non-dangerous emergencies. *Psychological Bulletin*, 137(4), 517–537.

Gladwell, M. (2005). *Blink: The power of thinking without thinking*. New York: Little, Brown.

Grant, A. (2018). Future tense: How do we make the long-term decisions that matter? *New York Times Book Review*, 10/7/18, p. 16.

Hacking, I. (2007). Kinds of people: Moving targets. *Proceedings of the British Academy*, 151, 285–318.

Haidt, J. (2012). *The righteous mind: Why good people are divided by politics and religion*. New York: Vintage Books.

Hale, N.G. (Ed.) (1971). *James Jackson Putnam and Psychoanalysis: Letters between Putnam and Sigmund Freud, Ernest Jones, William James, Sandor Ferenczi and Morton Prince. 1877–1917*. J.B. Heller (Trans.). Cambridge: Cambridge University Press.

Johnson, S. (2018). *Farsighted: How we make the decisions that matter the most*. New York: Riverhead.

Kahneman, D. (2011). *Thinking, fast and slow*. New York: Farrar, Straus and Giroux.

Kristof, N.D. (2006). The silence of bystanders. *The New York Times*, 3/19/2006. Retrieved from www.nytimes.com/2006/03/19/opinion/the-silence-of-bystanders.html.

Latané, B. & Darley, J.M. (1968). Group inhibition of bystander intervention in emergencies. *Journal of Personality and Social Psychology*, 10, 215–221.

Latané, B. & Darley, J.M. (1970). *The unresponsive bystander: Why doesn't he help?*New York: Meredith Corporation.

Latané, B. & Nida, S. (1981). Ten years of research on group size and helping. *Psychological Bulletin*, 89, 308–324.

Lear, J. (2017). *Wisdom won from illness: Essays in philosophy and psychoanalysis*. Cambridge: Harvard University Press.

Levinas, E. (1985). *Ethics and infinity*. R.A. Cohen (Trans.). Pittsburgh: Duquesne University Press.

Levinas, E. (1994). *In the time of the nations*. M.B. Smith (Trans.). Bloomington: Indiana University Press.

Levine, M. (2017). Helping in emergencies: Revisiting Latané and Darley's bystander studies. In J.R. Smith & S.A. Haslam (Eds.), *Social psychology: Revisiting the classic studies* (2nd ed., pp. 201–216). Thousand Oaks, CA: Sage.

Luel, S.A. & Marcus, P. (Eds.) (1984). *Psychoanalytic reflections on the Holocaust: Selected essays*. Brooklyn: University of Denver/KTAV Publishing.

Manning, R., Levine, M. & Collins, A. (2007). The Kitty Genovese murder and the social psychology of helping: The parable of helping. *American Psychologist*, 62(6), 555–562.

Marcus, P. (2008). *Being for the other: Emmanuel Levinas, ethical living and psychoanalysis*. Milwaukee: Marquette University Press.

Marcus, P. (2019). *The psychoanalysis of overcoming suffering: Flourishing despite pain*. London: Routledge.

Oliner, S.P. & Oliner, P.M. (1988). *The altruistic personality: Rescuers of Jews in Nazi Europe*. New York: Free Press.

Rasenberger, J. (2004). Kitty, 40 years later. *New York Times*, 2/8/2004, p. 14.

Rieff, P. (1961). *Freud: The mind of the moralist*. Garden City, NY: Anchor Books.

Rorty, R. (1989). *Contingency, irony, and solidarity*. Cambridge: Cambridge University Press.

Rorty, R. & Vattimo, G. (2005). *The future of religion*. E. Sambalo (Ed.). New York: Columbia University Press.

Sanoff, A. P. (1986). "One must not forget," Interview of Elie Wiesel. *US News & World Report*, 10/27/86.

Seelig, B. & Rosof, L.S. (2001). Normal and pathological altruism. *Journal of the American Psychoanalytic Association*, 49, 933–959.

Internet sources

https://medium.com/@sean.d.norton/understanding-richard-rortys-achieving-our-country-61b7844ddd98, retrieved 9/24/18.

https://psychology.iresearchnet.com/social-psychology/prosocial-behavior/empathy-altruism-hypothesis/, retrieved 8/31/18.

www.iep.utm.edu/marcel/, retrieved 9/23/18.

www.mentalhealth.org.uk/a-to-z/a/altruism-and-wellbeing, retrieved 9/24/18.

www.psychologytoday.com/us/blog/the-time-cure/201804/heroism-vs-the-bystander-effect, retrieved 8/31/18.

listverse.com/2009/11/02/10-notorious-cases-of-the-bystander-effect/, retrieved 8/26/18.

www2.humboldt.edu/altruism/definitions, retrieved 9/5/18.

7

SELF-CONTROL VERSUS LACK OF SELF-CONTROL

The Marshmallow Experiment of Mischel (1970)

As Ben Zoma, the great interpreter of the Hebrew Bible, famously said in the Talmud, "Who is Mighty? He who subdues his passions. As it is written" (Proverbs 16:32) and "He that is slow to anger is better than the mighty, and he that rules over his own spirit than he that conquers a city" (Bokser, 1982, p. 242). Indeed, this moral/psychological ideal is expressed in most ancient religious wisdom and spirituality traditions and their modern variants, for the person who has a high degree of self-control is viewed as more willing and able to enact a holy way of being-in-the-world. Indeed, most thoughtful people would agree that without a robust capacity for self-control it is nearly impossible to effectively engage in the business of everyday living, let alone artfully fashion a morally praiseworthy, flourishing existence.

Self-control is one of those words that nearly everyone bandies about, but it is difficult to define. For example, in positive psychology the term "self-regulation" is often used synonymously with self-control. It has been defined as "how a person exerts control over his or her own responses so as to pursue goals and live up to standards" (Peterson & Seligman, 2004, p. 500). Self-regulation "means different things to different people" (Carver & Scheier, 2016, p. 3), while Berkman notes, "the dominant models lack specificity regarding exactly how self-regulation actually works" (2016, p. 451).[1] "Self-discipline" is another synonym for self-control and it refers "to making oneself do things that one does not want to do and restraining temptation" (Peterson & Seligman, 2004, p. 500). Others use self-control to specifically refer "to controlling one's impulses so as to behave in a moral fashion" (ibid.). In his final book before his death, Mischel defined self-control as "the ability to delay immediate gratification for the sake of future consequences" (2014, p. 3). Overall, "research has yet to resolve how self-control should be best conceptualized and measured empirically" (Rocque et al., 2016, p. 522).

Four points about defining self-control are worth noting. First, all of the aforementioned definitions resonate with the ancient virtue of "patience" (in the Judeo-Christian tradition it is equated with forbearance or endurance), what spiritual aspirants regard as a vital lifelong practice that potentiates emotional freedom among other manifestations of autonomy, integration and humanity. Second, in five highly respected psychoanalytic dictionaries that I consulted, there was no entry for self-control, and only the most recent one had a short entry defining self-regulation: "the tendency and capacity for maintaining or restoring the baseline functional integrity during environmental perturbations" (Akhtar, 2009, p. 260). To further emphasize the lack of cross-fertilization between academic/experimental social psychology and psychoanalysis, in Vohs and Baumeister's (2016) *Handbook of Self-Regulation: Research, Theory, and Applications*, which codifies the cutting-edge knowledge of this burgeoning field, there are no index entries for psychoanalysis, and only three each for Freud and John Bowlby in a 640-page book. The three Freud citations only total about ten lines of text. Third, self-regulation, whether defined by a positive psychologist or a psychoanalyst, often happens in an automatic (Fitzsimmons & Bargh, 2004) or unconscious manner (Emde, 1988). Fourth, given the near conceptual disarray among researchers and scholars about exactly what self-control refers to, it is reasonable to agree with Watts et al. (2018), who did an important replication of the Marshmallow Experiment (with some important contrary findings). Watts noted that self-control is best understood an "an umbrella construct that includes gratification delay but also impulsivity, conscientiousness, self-regulation, and executive function" (2018, p. 1160). Impulsivity, a term "that has been conceived in many different and often inconsistent ways" (DeYoung & Rueter, 2016, p. 357),[2] is roughly the incapability of delaying gratification and engaging in split-second decisions without taking time to reflect (Rocque et al., 2016, p. 226). Conscientiousness refers to a cluster of traits that characterize people who regularly demonstrate self-control, work diligently and follow rules (Laurin & Kay, 2016, p. 307). Executive function roughly describes a collection of higher-order processes like planning, task switching and inhibition of thought and behavior (Hipple & Henry, 2016, p. 479). Indeed, self-control is one of those rather "slippery" concepts that change markedly depending on your perspective.

Notwithstanding the above, whatever definition of self-control one uses, there are valuative attachments that animate the definition and how a particular instance of self-control is instantiated. While self-control is conceived as involving a person's thoughts, emotions, impulses and performances, its standards consist of ideals, moral prohibitions, social norms, performance targets and the expectations of others (Peterson & Seligman, 2004, p. 500). As Mischel noted, "we can fail to develop our self-control skills, and even if we have them in abundance, we may lack the goals, values, and social support needed to use them constructively" (2014, p. 230). Indeed, the valuative character of self-control is starkly illustrated when we consider that it takes robust self-control to disregard one's personal survival when a mother throws herself in front of a careening car to save her child as it does for a terrorist patiently waiting to blow himself up to maximize human carnage. Thus, self-control, or what I prefer to call, following Nietzsche, "self-mastery"—an ethic of self-rule over one's emotions and passions and a striving for excellence—is best viewed as an important aspect of moral psychology, in part because one's freedom is truncated to the extent that one is not master of himself. Such a valuative attachment is entirely in sync with a psychoanalytic outlook, for as Freud noted, "Analysis does not set out to make pathological reactions impossible, but to give patients the freedom to decide one way or another" (1923, p. 50).

In this chapter I will first briefly summarize Mischel's original Marshmallow Experiment with preschoolers, followed by what he claimed were the "real-life" consequences of early self-control for adolescence and adulthood. Next, I will discuss how Mischel (and other researchers) and psychoanalysts have understood the development of self-control, what enables and constrains it, and briefly what can be done to promote this important potential, however ambiguously defined, that needs to be developed to create a praiseworthy moral existence and a flourishing life.[3]

The Marshmallow Experiment and follow-ups

In the original Marshmallow Experiment (Mischel & Ebbesen, 1970), the investigators were interested in studying "voluntary postponement of immediate gratification for the sake of more distant long-term gains" (p. 329). Their way of doing this was brilliantly simple and elegant.

Sixteen boys and girls from ages three years and six months to five years and eight months who were attending the Bing Nursery School at Stanford University were the subjects of the experiment. Four boys and girls were randomly assigned to each of the four experimental conditions. In each condition, one of the two experimenters ran two boys and girls so as to reduce any biasing effects from the gender of the children or of the experimenters.

The four conditions of the experiment were: (1) Both the immediate (less favored) and the delayed (more favored) reward (marshmallows, pretzels, cookies—henceforth, marshmallows) were put in front of the child and accessible; (2) Neither reward was available for the child's notice, both rewards having been eliminated from the field of vision; (3) Only the delayed reward was left in front of the child and accessible for notice while the child waited; (4) Only the immediate reward was left in front of the child and accessible for notice while the child waited.

On the table in the small chamber where the experiment was implemented there were five one-third of an inch-long pieces of pretzels and an opaque cake tin (Mischel & Ebbesen, 1970, pp. 32–33). Underneath the cake tin were five pretzels and two animal cookies. There were two chairs in front of the table, on one chair there was an empty cardboard box. There were four battery-operated toys on the floor close to the chair with the cardboard box. The experimenter made notice of the four toys, but before the child could play with the toys, the experimenter requested that the child sit in the chair and then demonstrated each toy briefly and in a cordial manner, saying that they would play with the toys later. Then the experimenter placed each toy in the cardboard box and out of the child's field of vision. The experimenter explained to the child that the experimenter occasionally has to go out of the room but if the child consumes a pretzel the experimenter will return to the room. These instructions were repeated until the child appeared to comprehend them totally. The experimenter departed the room and waited for the child to consume a pretzel, which was repeated four times. Next, the experimenter opened the cake tin to disclose two sets of rewards to the child: five pretzels and two animal crackers. The experimenter inquired which of the two the child favored more, and after the child chose, the experimenter explained that the child could either continue waiting for the more favored reward until the experimenter returned, or the child could desist waiting by bringing the experimenter back using a signal bell. If the child desisted waiting, then the child would receive the less favored reward and relinquish the more favored one. Depending on the condition the child was in, and the child's choice of favored reward, the experimenter lifted up the cake tin and along with it, either nothing, one of the rewards, or both. The experimenter came back into the experimental chamber either the moment the child alerted him via the signal bell or after fifteen minutes had elapsed.

The results were as follows: "Unexpectedly," Mischel and Ebbesen noted, "voluntary waiting was substantially increased when subjects could not attend to rewards during the waiting period" (1970, p. 329). That is, in more than 600 children who participated in the experiment, a minority consumed the marshmallow straightaway. Of those children who made efforts to delay, one-third delayed gratification long enough to obtain the second marshmallow. The age of the child was a significant factor in determining which child delayed gratification, as common parenting experience would predict, the younger the child (typically under age four years), the less likely s/he could delay immediate gratification. The ability to delay allegedly indicated superior determination that would pay the child later dividends at school and in the adult workplace.

From this and his subsequent research (Mischel et al., 1988, 1989; Shoda et al., 1990), Mischel concluded that self-control was "an acquired cognitive skill," more or less synonymous with "will power,"[4] and it "is the 'master aptitude' underlying emotional intelligence, essential for constructing a fulfilling life" (Mischel, 2014, pp. 3, 6).[5] Few thoughtful people would argue with Mischel's emphasis on the importance of delay of gratification in early childhood and its likely usefulness as a cognitive/affective/behavioral skill in adulthood; however, what has been challenged is whether learning a delay of gratification in early childhood actually predicts greater competence and success in adulthood, or whether there are other interrelated, interdependent and interactive individual and social factors at play. Given the fact that self-control is reasonably described as an "umbrella construct" (Watts et al., 2018, p. 1160), the latter perspective is more plausible.

In their first follow-up study twelve years later, questionnaires were sent to parents and teachers who were requested to "think about your child in comparison to his or her peers, such as classmates and other same-age friends. We would like to get your impression of how your son or daughter compares to those peers" (Mischel, 2014, p. 23). They rated their child on a scale from one to nine ("Not at all" to "Extremely"), and teachers were asked to rate the children on cognitive and social skills during school. Mischel summarizes his findings:

> Preschoolers who delayed longer on the Marshmallow Test were rated a dozen years later as adolescents who exhibited more self-control in frustrating situations; yielded less to temptation; were less distractive when trying to concentrate; were more intelligent, self-reliant, and confident, and trusted their own judgment. When under stress they did not go to pieces as much as low delayers did, and they were less likely to become rattled and disorganized or revert to immediate behavior. Likewise, they thought ahead and planned more, and when motivated they were more able to pursue their goals. They were also more attentive and able to use and respond to reason, and they were less likely to be sidetracked by setbacks.
> *(ibid., pp. 23–24)*

Mischel also notes that the adolescents' actual academic achievement as measured by SAT verbal and quantitative scores for those preschoolers who "delayed longer," were "on the whole … much better" (ibid., p. 24). He further claims that similar findings were self-reported into adulthood. That is, longer delayers in preschool were more capable of pursuing and achieving long-term goals, used dangerous drugs less often, achieved higher education levels and had significantly less body mass. In addition, they were more resilient and adaptive in coping with relationship difficulties and better at sustaining close relationships. Likewise, brain scan images suggested that the preschoolers who delayed longer, and who continued this behavior into adolescence and adulthood, had more active prefrontal cortexes, the part of the brain that gets activated for effective problem-solving, creative thinking and control of impulsive behavior (ibid., p. 26).

It is worth mentioning that Mischel and his colleagues' research on self-control (Shoda et al., 1990) has not been adequately replicated by an often-cited study (Watts et al., 2018). These researchers focused on children whose mothers had not completed college, and they found that the majority of the variation in adolescent achievement emanated from being able to wait at least 20 seconds. Moreover, associations between delay time and measure of behavioral outcomes at age fifteen were much smaller and rarely statistically significant (ibid., p. 1159). Notwithstanding Watts et al.'s findings, Mischel's studies have been characterized as "the most influential roots of contemporary research on self-regulation" (Peterson & Seligman, 2004, p. 500). In fact, "Mischel and Shoda's longitudinal studies still stand as the foundational examinations of the long-run correlates of the ability to delay gratification in early childhood" (Watts et al., 2018, p. 1160).

Development of self-control

Mischel et al. (1988, 1989) described some of the delay of gratification tactics used by preschool children. Most of these tactics are fairly obvious to anyone who has observed children, especially at home, in school or the clinical context. Moreover, with some recasting and retrofitting, these tactics are used by adolescents and adults who show good self-control. Conversely, these psychic capacities appear to be underdeveloped and/or underfunctioning in those people who have difficulties in controlling emotions and desires or the enactment of them in their behavior, particularly in stressful circumstances.

As Mischel notes, those children who successfully delayed immediate gratification were willing and able to distract themselves, and in so doing, they reduced the conflict and stress that the experimenters put the children in. They did this by drawing on their imaginative faculty, creating enjoyable distractions that diminished the great subjective effort of deploying their willpower. In other words, the children made the waiting period easier to tolerate by changing the meaning of the aversive waiting circumstances. The children made up songs, such as "This is such a pretty day, hooray;" they engaged in making amusing and misshapen or ugly faces; they picked their noses and cleaned their ear canals and played with what they extracted; and they made up games with their hands and feet, such as playing their toes as if they were piano keys.[6] When these distractions became ineffective, some of the children tried to go to sleep. Mischel poignantly mentions "one little girl who finally dropped her head into her folded arms on the table and fell into a deep slumber, her face inches from the signal bell" (Mischel, 2014, p. 31). Finally, it should be mentioned that when the children's self-created distracting thoughts were not primed by the experimenter, they were willing and able to wait only about a minute for their reward. Moreover, when they were cued to reflect on the reward while they were waiting, they would usually ring the bell once the experimenter left the chamber (ibid., p. 32).

The distraction tactics used by preschool children in Mischel's experiments are very much in sync with research on the beneficial impact of distraction on adults, at least in certain contexts. We know, for example, that distraction can reduce physical and psychological pain and other types of aversive experiences. One important experiment will suffice to illustrate this well-known point as reported by Jane McGonigal (2016). The study tested whether playing a cancer-themed video game known as "Re-mission" would facilitate cancer patients to comply with their treatment plan and regularly and properly take their medication. In this context, the game didn't fight pain directly, but enhanced patients' capabilities (in part because it sophisticatedly distracted them from their pain). Patients who played the game were more inclined to take their medications, increase their sense of self-efficacy and manifest more knowledge regarding how to fight their cancer diagnosis. From McGonigal's perspective, digital games are awesome tools to build inner strength, self-control and self-confidence because "… Constantly escalating challenge requires a willingness from [patients] to keep trying, even when they fail. It instills a belief that if they keep practicing and learning, if they put in the hard work, they will eventually be able to achieve more difficult goals" (2016, p. 81). By surmounting challenges within a game, the cancer patients fortified their determination to press on, to keep fighting their life-threatening diagnosis. Such distraction is "self-expansive," including increasing self-control, rather than "self-suppressive," (ibid., p. 106), including decreasing self-control.

This and other research on distraction suggests that personal technology distractions like video games and puzzles can, in certain contexts, give us strength and the self-control to bear difficult and distressing experiences and fortify our willingness and ability to take on new challenges. Thus, for many people, personal technology can be a "healthy" if not life-affirming distraction, one that requires good self-control. However, it can be subverting when it is used as an avenue of flight from a distressing problem (i.e., from facing reality), as with some adolescent or young adults who are obsessive/compulsive "gamers."

"Abstraction" is another tactic that the children used to exert self-control in Mischel's experiments. Abstraction is a higher order mode of thinking in which common elements are identified (or abstracted). This cognitive process of isolating common characteristics between different things is vital for many high-level kinds of thinking such as learning from experience, inference and making judgments. When something is abstracted it turns into an abstraction or an abstract idea, and abstract concepts are to be distinguished from concrete or literal ones.

In this context, Mischel and his colleagues showed the children pictures of the marshmallows rather than the rewards themselves. The results of this study were the total reverse of the previous finding. When the children were exposed to the real marshmallows, most of them found delay of gratification impossible; however, exposure to the realistic pictures of the marshmallows made their willingness and ability to wait much more likely. Those children who were exposed to pictures of the marshmallows waited twice as long as those who viewed irrelevant or no pictures or those who were exposed to the real marshmallows. Importantly, says Mischel, the pictures had to be of the goodies for which the child was waiting, not of similar goodies that were not pertinent to what the child had chosen. In other words, "an image of the object of desire, not the tempting object itself, makes it easiest to wait" (Mischel, 2014, p. 33).

Mischel's conclusion agrees with Freud's "hallucinatory wish fulfillment" notion (1950). Freud theorized that an infant makes efforts to gratify his unfulfilled instinctual needs and wishes, say, for food, by generating mental pictures of them and their gratification (similar to what happens in dreams). Rather ironically, however, such hallucinatory wish fulfillment does not actually gratify the instinctual need and desire, and thus facilitates in the child the beginning of reality-testing (i.e., the ability to differentiate mental images and external percepts, fantasy and reality, and modify subjective notions by considering external facts). This being said, Mischel's findings point to the necessity of having a robust imagination to enhance our self-control. For example, role playing has been shown to promote self-control in children. In one experiment, children were given a red cape and told to "pretend to be Superman," and they performed better on the delay of gratification task compared to their peers (Eskreis-Winkler et al., 2016, p. 389). Perhaps even more important is the role of the imagination to help artfully fashion a flourishing life. As Ralph Waldo Emerson said, "the revelation of thought [i.e., the imagination] takes man out of servitude into freedom. We rightly say of ourselves, we were born and afterwards we were born again, and many times" (Geldard, 2001, p. 114).[7]

A third tactic for enhancing self-control mentioned by Mischel focuses on how the child conceptualized the stimulus, the marshmallow. That is, "the power is not the stimulus ... but in how it is mentally appraised: if you change how you think about it, its impact on what you feel and do changes" (2014, p. 36). What the marshmallow experiments "convinced" Mischel of was "that if people can change how they mentally represent a stimulus, they can exert self-control and escape from being victims of the hot stimuli [that which activates an impulsive reaction, the automatic, reflexive, unconscious limbic system] that have come to control their behavior" (ibid.). Mischel is reaffirming an ancient Stoic principle famously articulated by Epictetus, "People are not disturbed by things, but by the view they take of them."

Likewise, Mischel's research suggested that the children's moods impacted how quickly they rang the signal bell. For example, if the experimenters suggested prior to leaving the children by themselves with the marshmallows that during their waiting they might want to think of some events that made them sad (e.g., crying and no one coming to assist them), they stopped waiting as quickly as if the experimenter had suggested thinking about the marshmallows. If, however, the children were primed to think about fun happenings, they waited almost three times longer. As Mischel notes, if you give a nine-year-old child compliments about their drawn pictures, they will choose delayed rather than immediate marshmallows much more frequently than when given criticism of their work (Mischel, 2014, p. 33). That mood affects decision-making, judgement and consequential thinking is obvious, though Mischel showed that it is a correlation that begins early in child development. For example, anxiety, anger, depression and other expressions of emotional dysregulation can influence how a person appraises situations in ways that impact his choices in both work and love contexts. Research has shown that under stress, a person's ability to thoughtfully control their actions is significantly diminished (Wood, 2016, p. 100). If how a child or adult thinks about temptation really matters, as seems to be true based on the research of Mischel and others, then these strategies can possibly be taught and become a habituated way of behaving.

Psychoanalytic views on the development of self-control

As I have earlier noted, the term self-control was not listed as an entry in the prominent psychoanalytic dictionaries I consulted, and from what I can tell, it is generally regarded as an aspect of self-regulation which itself is composed of a number of inter-reliant and interacting elements. That is, self-control can be usefully psychoanalytically conceived as a conscious and unconscious self-regulating strategy, though one that is an amalgamation of a number of related constructs rather than a single undifferentiated capacity (Hoyle & Davisson, 2016, pp. 396, 397, 399). The capacities associated with the basic infant motivation of self-regulation are "arousal, attentiveness, and sleep-wakefulness cycles, and in the long-term sense, for growth and vital developmental functions" (Emde, 1988, p. 29). Issues related to self-control are part and parcel of any psychoanalytic rendering of a wide range of psychological conditions, such as addictions, risky behavior and criminality, but also in terms of having the will and ability to flourish in work and love. Though the matter is not simply a self-control issue, to the extent that one can exert self-control one is less susceptible to feeling as wounded or rejected by others and obsessively dwelling on hurtful or anger-inducing experiences. Indeed, Freud famously affirmed his civilized dislike of the primitive id when he claimed what the goal of analysis was: "where id was, there ego shall be" (1932, p. 80).

For Freud, self-control, the ability to inhibit or modulate undesirable impulses, was the foundation of civilization.

In light of the fact that self-control per se is not a category that is typically written about in psychoanalysis, I will discuss a few related notions to give some "thick" description to the possible origins and later meanings of self-control in everyday life, especially as it relates to fashioning a morally praiseworthy, flourishing life.

Superego functioning

When an analyst thinks about self-control, he will probably first consider the analysand's superego functioning (roughly, the conscience). For Freud, the superego is the psychic structure that is the consequence of the resolution of the Oedipus complex. Most importantly, the superego is composed of "dos and don'ts," what a child should and should not say or do that is consciously and unconsciously learned and internalized during his upbringing. When the child does not comply with these rules, customs and prohibitions, or even thinks of such wrongdoings, he experiences an upsurge of guilt. During development, especially in adolescence, the child later abstracts these dos and don'ts as well as the guilt response, the latter often experienced as deserved punishment. In fact, how parents engage their child in terms of attention (e.g., neglectful versus empathic attunement) and discipline (e.g., harsh versus reasonable) will to some extent impact this internalization process. Likewise, permissive parenting and an inordinate focus on increasing children's self-regard may be damaging to self-control in that it could create a character that is feeble, self-occupied and self-indulgent. This being said, psychologists have recently reported that "issues related to the source of self-control and the effect of parenting remain in question" (Rocque et al., 2016, p. 520). It is common knowledge that once a child reaches adolescence, and maybe earlier (some researchers claim self-control is "set" at about eight or nine years of age), the influence of parental instructions and prohibitions (and schools and other influences) have much less impact, if any, on the development of self-control (ibid., pp. 519, 525).

Put simply, psychoanalytically speaking, a child learns self-control in early childhood, learns to behave in accordance with the norms of society and feels guilty when these norms are violated. However, as part of his upbringing he develops unconscious defenses against his instinctual impulses; for instance, his infantile wishes and desires, say for sexual gratification with an inappropriate person like one's mother or father (as the individual/society judges this). Sometimes these are reasonable defenses and sometimes they are neurotic in character in adulthood. So-called superego analysis is focused on helping the person to modulate or resolve earlier internalizations, both before and after the Oedipus complex, that in adult life have become self-defeating and possibly distressing. A person will activate ego defenses against instinctual impulses and it is through analysis that he can acquire conscious control of his previously repressed instinctual impulses. For example, a man may not be able to exert self-control during intercourse, and prematurely ejaculates because he unconsciously experiences the woman as having a "vagina dentata," a male fantasy that the vagina encloses sharp teeth and can bite off the penis that is put into it. During analytic exploration, what may be animating his sexual performance failure is that the debilitating vagina dentata fantasy is a displacement of castration fear from his father to his mother. In a sense, then, the man's lack of self-control during sex is an effort at self-control of an unconscious anxiety about punishment for his incestuous wishes toward his mother.

Ego weaknesses

Ego weaknesses is a term that describes limitations a person has in his ability to navigate between both the requirements of external reality and instinctual desires and superego directives. For example, a person with a severely "weak ego," such as someone with borderline personality disorder, is not capable of generating clear boundaries between "inside" and "outside," such as whether a feeling is emanating from within oneself or from the other person. Such a perceptual difficulty contributes to questionable reality-testing. Most importantly for this chapter, while a severely weak ego can be characterized with a wide range of primitive defenses (e.g., splitting and denial), a less severely weakened ego, like of a neurotic person, uses defenses that call to mind self-control problems, such as poor impulse control, impaired tolerance for anxiety and limited ability to sublimate. For example, poor impulse control can be said to be manifest by focal, repetitive and ego-syntonic acts such as in a child or adolescent with attention-deficit hyperactivity disorder (ADHD), or as a more generalized lack of control over one's desires such as with borderline personality disorder. Impaired tolerance for anxiety in stressful circumstances can lead to regression, the development of discrete symptoms or a tendency to enact the anxiety in ill-conceived and often ill-fated behavior. Poor sublimation capacities, such as not being able to direct one's unconscious desires into intellectual and artistic activities are said to reflect inadequate ego-strength (Akhtar, 2009, p. 92). The point is that, for most people in the neurotic range (which in psychoanalysis pertains to just about everyone), psychoanalysis views a lack of self-control as a reflection of a lack of ego-strength, that is, the inability for adequate impulse control, anxiety tolerance and sublimation, the roots of which reside in ineffective parenting and negative environmental influences.

Too much self-control

Rather simplistic is the fact that in an important positive psychology research review article on self-control, it was claimed that there is hardly a "downside" to too much self-control: "we are unaware of any undesirable consequence or correlates of high self-control," including "over-control," and while the authors acknowledge that self-control can be used for anti-social purposes, "by and large it appears to produce mainly positive effects" (Peterson & Seligman, 2004, p. 508). In contrast, to the psychoanalyst, self-control is often a case of "too much of a good thing." For example, in the classic Freudian description of the obsessive character, the personality is typified by the qualities of orderliness, parsimony and obstinacy. Lack of tolerance of grime and untidiness, exacting record keeping, promptness, a proclivity toward perfectionism and a generalized need and desire for control are frequently observed characteristics of the obsessive character. While these aforementioned characteristics can have their positive side to them in certain social contexts, they can also make one's life, and the lives of those one interacts with, hard-going if not miserable. Put simply, the obsessive character maintains a high degree of self-control in his way of being-in-the-world; however, in many instances it can be self-defeating. Indeed, a person with a diagnosed obsessive-compulsive disorder can have routines that can become all-encompassing and all-consuming, seriously undermining their relationships with their significant other, children and colleagues. Likewise, treatment for a neurotic woman who is so overcontrolled that she cannot let herself have an orgasm would focus on learning to let go. Her capacity to be more sexually free, flowing and unrestrained may emerge only when she perceives that the psychic pain connected with not relinquishing control is more than the pain connected with relinquishing control.

As Lynch (2018) reports, researchers have found that too much self-control is linked with social isolation, reduced interpersonal effectiveness and serious mental health problems that are hard to treat and negatively impact artful living, such as chronic depression, obsessive-compulsive personality disorder and anorexia nervosa. Ill-conceived and ill-fated self-control often involves four types of core deficits, or personal limitations that have been described as maladaptive: (1) "Low receptivity and openness," which involves a lack of receptivity to novel, unanticipated, or disconfirming feedback; evasion of uncertainty or unintended risks; suspiciousness; hyper-vigilance for possible threat; and the proclivity to ignore or dismiss critical feedback; (2) "Low flexible-control," which involves compulsive demands for structure and order; extreme perfectionism; high social obligation and dutifulness; compulsive rehearsal, premeditation and planning; compulsive fixing and approach coping; rigid rule-governed behavior; and high moral certitude, such as believing their way is the only right way of doing something; (3) "Pervasive inhibited emotional expression and low emotional awareness," which involves context/setting inappropriate inhibition of emotional expression; for example, not reacting when complimented, and/or inauthentic or incongruent expressions of emotion, such as smiling when upset, displaying concern when not actually feeling it, frequent under-stating of upset like anxiety/depression, and reduced awareness of body sensations; (4) "Low social connectedness and intimacy with others," which involves aloof and remote relationships, feeling estranged from other people, recurrent social comparisons, pronounced envy and bitterness, and truncated empathy (ibid.).

More generally, research on self-control has approached the subject of having too much or too little self-control by suggesting an interesting distinction between two types of self-control, by "inhibition" or by "initiation" (Hoyle & Davisson, 2016, p. 399). Self-control by inhibition is necessary when personal forces (e.g., desires, impulses and habits) or situational forces (e.g., norms, requests/demands of others) pull for thoughts, feelings or behaviors that are inconsistent with one or more active goals, and thus consciously override a pull toward goal-inconsistent behavior. For example, self-control by inhibition is necessary to constrain checking an e-mail while at work on the computer. In contrast, self-control by initiation is necessary when those aforementioned personal or situational forces pull for inaction when the pursuit of an active goal demands action. An example of this is someone who finishes an exercise workout that started as an act of self-control by initiation yet demands that she stay the course when she feels tired, achy or bored. Finally, Hoyle and Davisson mention "self-control by continuation," that is, acts that involve the conscious decision to persevere at inhibition or to carry on following initiation, notwithstanding the pull to desist when a challenging self-control situation is continuing (ibid.).

Self-control can be short- or long-term in its enactment, and one can have self-control in one domain and not in another; hence, to describe self-control as a "trait" is problematic. For example, an obsessive-compulsive personality who in general is averse to dirt and untidiness usually has one domain, like a bedroom or a closet, that is a filthy mess.

To be or not to be in control of life

The issue of control is one of the most common in psychoanalytic treatment. Analysands and psychotherapy patients are frequently complaining about feeling out of control, of being controlled by others or of wanting to control others. This is especially the case in contexts that are stressful, painful and require endurance such as while coping with extended suffering. While Western-based psychoanalysis aims to assist people with gaining control of their lives (e.g., by increasing self-control), certain kinds of so-called religious/spiritual outlooks, like those lodged in the Axial tradition (Marcus, 2019),[8] assist people with coming to terms with the limits of their control. When it comes to every major aspect of living—birth, who your parents are, who you fall in love with,[9] your children's lives, illness and death—one realizes the more deep and decisive issue than trying to control one's life and world is learning to come to terms with how little control we actually have regarding things that matter. Chance, accident and other contingencies are hugely operative. Anxiety masks a powerful wish, and as Freud noted, the wish for control is rooted in the desire to reclaim one's lost childhood narcissism, the time when he existed as his own ideal. A religious/spiritual outlook can help a person internalize this rather harsh truth about reality while at the same time offers some hope, especially through a sacred/spiritual language that is embedded in a "sacred canopy." For example, by living in the present, moment by moment, even amid intense pain as the Buddha taught, as opposed to getting stuck in the past and dwelling on the future, the analysand can better endure his suffering. Suffering, says the Buddha, follows the same pattern, one that requires patience and a transcendent perspective. Suffering arises, dwells, changes and ultimately fades away. As the Taoist-sounding, motivational saying goes, the anxious person is lodged in the future, the depressed person in the past and the peaceful person in the present.

Where self-control fits into the aforementioned discussion is that it requires the person's will and ability to give up control of control, to have the discernment, if not the wisdom, to begin with the opposite of what is sought. Indeed, there is vast literature that has shown that perceived personal control (which is a belief about the self) improves personal adaptation, including emotional stability and the capacity to skillfully manage life. For example, Thompson (2009) cites studies that show that perceived personal control, defined as "the judgment that one has the means to obtain desired outcomes and to avoid undesirable ones" (p. 271), can be strengthened by a person who concentrates on reachable goals, generates new opportunities for control and accepts unmodifiable situations. All of these techniques to enhance perceived personal control assume a robust capacity for self-control by engaging in reasonable judgment and sensible decision-making, including about what can and cannot be controlled. Perceived personal control needs to be realistic to be psychologically beneficial, but in some contexts, such as with serious loss or trauma, illusory control can be helpful through increasing self-regard (though this can morph into narcissistic self-absorption). Laboratory studies have suggested that sometimes those who overestimate their personal control are inclined to be better at coping and more persistent with tasks (ibid., p. 273). To some extent, this last finding is a reaffirmation of Freud's observation, "We welcome illusions because they spare us unpleasurable feelings, and enable us to enjoy satisfactions instead. We must not complain, then, if now and again they come into collision with some portion of reality and are shattered against it" (1975, p. 280).

Enabling and constraining factors in self-control

The aforementioned discussion suggests that adequate self-control involves a number of interconnected and interactive factors that are synergistically at play. For example, Baumeister and colleagues (Baumeister et al., 1998; Maranges & Baumeister, 2016) have put forth the ego depletion theory, known as the strength or resource model of self-control.[10] The gist of the theory is that self-control, which is defined as "the ability to alter one's thoughts, emotions and behavior, or to override impulses and habits, allows people to monitor and regulate themselves to meet expectations," (Maranges & Baumeister, 2016, p. 55) uses a limited repository of psychological resources that are available. When the energy for psychological activity is low, self-control is usually reduced, which is what is meant by ego depletion ("ego" here means psychological, it is not a reference to psychoanalysis). Ego depletion describes "a state of diminished self-control resources, when one cannot or does not successfully implement further control" (ibid.). In other words, a subjectively felt instance of ego depletion truncates self-control in the future: a depleting task that demands self-control can have a thwarting impact on a later self-control task, even if the tasks are apparently disconnected. Chronic dieting can bring about ego depletion in a person as a function of having to engage in so much self-control in circumstances that would otherwise not be experienced as depleting, such as in the presence of ice cream. Dieters spend so much mental energy attempting to curtail their food intake (i.e., a form of resource depletion), that paradoxically, these efforts are likely to be subverted when faced with irresistible temptation. In this theory, self-control operates analogously to the self-regulatory abilities of a muscle (perhaps an emotional muscle), that is, similar to a muscle it can become depleted with intense or protracted use, though it can also be enhanced with practice and exercise (ibid., p. 50). In some sense, this model calls to mind Freud's emphasis on psychic energy, in his case as it related to controlling the instincts.

While the ego depletion theory has been seriously criticized, with even the main claims questioned (Engber, 2016), what the theory highlights is that to live a flourishing life requires one to be mindful that one's capacity for self-control is not an ever-flowing, gushing resource, and that depending on the context, sensible self-control can give way to insensible gratification (especially if there is extended temptation). For example, a businessman analysand of mine who did a lot of airline traveling was a devoted and faithful husband for years, until one day his flight home was cancelled for a few days due to a terrible snow-storm. Feeling a bit lonely and disoriented, he went to the hotel bar to hang out, something he never did while traveling (he usually watched a movie in his room and went to sleep). By the end of evening, he found himself in bed with an attractive woman who was lodged by the airlines in the same hotel. While there are many psychodynamic considerations to his infidelity and guilty aftermath, what he did not realize at the time was that by situating himself in the bar, drinking and talking to this attractive single woman he was depleting his self-control. That is, put succinctly in psychoanalytic language, the superego is soluble in alcohol and travel! Indeed, it is for this reason that ego completion theory puts forth the pragmatic claim that one should live one's everyday life animated by habit, routine and other automatic processes, so that when one has to make conscious decisions, one has not depleted one's self-control resources (Peterson & Seligman, 2004, p. 510). This being said, those cognitive behavior therapists who draw from the mindfulness tradition believe just the opposite, that living on "automatic pilot" instead of with awareness of the present and conscious choice more or less dooms you to experience psychological distress or worse. Automatic cognitive habits, for example, are regarded as an aversion (avoiding/escaping from unpleasant internal experience) or desire (attaching/clinging to pleasant internal experience) and awareness and acceptance of these habits is the way to break their destructive hold on one's outlook and behavior (Segal et al., 2018, pp. 89, 92). To further complicate an already ambiguous matter, some positive psychologists disagree with the tenor of the mindfulness-based claim, "People who live only in the present moment are unlikely to exhibit good self-control, whereas future-mindedness will facilitate self-regulation" (Peterson & Seligman, 2004, p. 511).

Self-control can be enhanced with self-monitoring (such as tracking how many drinks one consumes at a party), and when the psychological distance[11] between the current state and the goal state (to leave the party able to drive and function) is relatively clear (ibid., p. 510). As this example suggests, in general, self-control focuses on behavior and not merely thoughts and feelings. The aforementioned businessman who cheated on his wife in the hotel had a breakdown in his control over his behavior, and if he had simply fantasized about sleeping with the woman while drinking and talking with her, or masturbated alone to her in his room, the psychological consequences of his lack of behavioral self-control would have had a much more favorable outcome in a variety of ways.

Other factors that appear to have an enabling or constraining impact on effective self-control include how one is raised and the environment that one is in. If parents and teachers encouraged a child to delay gratification and generated clear standards, expectations and consequences, a child is more likely to learn reasonable self-control. This is especially the case if the child has had a fairly good upbringing by parents who were loving and supportive, discipline and punishment were fair and moderate, and the child was not in other ways traumatized or had to contend with long-standing stress (the latter of which can generate significant diminution of prefrontal cognitive capacities). Similarly, in the workplace, if an employee is faced with multiple, discrete goals that appear to be in conflict, they tend to obsessively dwell about what to do, and rarely effectively mobilize themselves and reach any of the goals. In another variation, if a person is ensconced in a situation with competing desires, say finishing some important paperwork that has a deadline, and watching over his young children, the competing goals will likely immobilize him, or if not immobilize him, he will do neither task effectively, a manifestation of poor self-control among other factors. Indeed, multi-tasking has been shown to increase distractibility, and decrease efficiency and productivity, the opposite consequences of effective self-control.

Implications for treatment

There are hundreds of professional and lay books and articles on how to improve a child and adult's self-control, however it is defined and instantiated, and many of them are worth reading. Some of these evidence-based metacognitive strategies are useful in some social contexts, and cognitive behavioral therapists formally apply them while psychoanalysts informally use them in terms of giving "ego support" meant to enhance ego-strength (e.g., to help the analysand avoid unwise immediate instinctual gratification, to engage in consequential thinking and to avoid regression in the face of anxiety).

For example, academic psychologists have claimed that behavior modification takes place only when individuals implement "mental contrasting," first imagining the desired future (e.g., sorting out a difficulty with one's significant other), then trying to identify and imagine the impediments of reality (e.g., anger, anxiety). This is due to the fact that in mental contrasting, the future fantasies provide the direction in which to proceed, and the impediments of reality potentiate the energy to transcend the difficulties on the way to wish-fulfillment. In other words, when the impediments are manageable (i.e., expectations of success are high), people are highly committed and determinedly pursue the desired future; when the impediments are perceived as insuperable (i.e., when expectation of successes are low), people tend to delegate, postpone or relinquish the satisfaction of their wishes, or otherwise adjust to a more achievable wish. Thus, mental contrasting assists people in making wise and skillful distinctions between possible and impossible wishes (Oettingen & Cachia, 2016, pp. 555–556).

Likewise, "If–Then implementation plans" is a self-control strategy that can facilitate improved goal accomplishment, as well as bring about habit and behavior change (Gollweitzer & Oettingen, 2016). It is secondary to goal intentions as it delineates the when, where and how aspects of behavior that are goal-directed. The focus is on modifying a person's time perspective from "now" to "later" (Mischel, 2014, p. 135). Briefly, the If–Then implementation plans involve four steps: (1) Choose a goal; (2) Identify the one action (the "Then") that you'll concentrate on to achieve your goal.

The action should be uncomplicated, one that you can implement immediately; (3) Identify a particular cue for the action (the "If"), something that will remind and motivate you to implement your action. This cue must be simple to identify; (4) Rehearse your plan, the more often the better. The notion underlying implementation intentions is that when the decisive time arrives and your If presents itself, you implement your self-control action automatically. For this to occur, you must encrypt your If–Then Plans into your brain, for instance, writing them down and re-reading them a few times a week, even out loud. As Mischel notes, if the If–Then plans are well-rehearsed and established, the self-control response will become automatically triggered by the stimulus that it is linked to: "If I approach the fridge, then I will not open the door" (ibid., p. 258).

While there are other such metacognitive strategies and behavioral interventions that are available to enhance self-control in children and adults in discrete contexts (Vohs & Baumeister, 2016), I want to conclude this chapter by suggesting one somewhat underappreciated aspect of self-control that can contribute to artful fashioning of the morally praiseworthy flourishing life: the cultivation and enactment in behavior of strongly felt, flexibly and creatively applied, transcendent-pointing moral beliefs and values that tend to be other-directed, other-regarding and other-serving. At the deepest level of the self, this exemplary "other" can be an intimate presence called God, an Idea and/or a Person, one that is perceived as a cherished objective reality that is meaning-giving, affect-integrating and action-guiding. As sociologist W.I. Thomas famously said, "If men define situations as real, they are real in their consequences" (Thomas & Thomas, 1928, pp. 571–572). Indeed, Mischel noted that

> to be able to delay gratification and exert self-control is an ability, a set of cognitive skills, that, like any ability, can be used or not used depending primarily on the motivation to use. Delay ability can help preschoolers resist one marshmallow now to get two later, but they have to want to do that.
>
> *(2014, p. 189)*

Mischel specifically emphasizes, but does not elaborate on, the fact that self-control is not just cognitive skill but involves "internalizing goals and values" (ibid., p. 9). Such goals and values "direct the journey" and provide the "motivation that is strong enough to overcome the setbacks along the route" (ibid., p. 9). Indeed, researchers lodged in self-affirmation theory have found that "affirming core values," those values that are most significant to oneself, can increase self-regulation or related constructs (such as self-control), including by counteracting ego depletion effects (Berkman, 2016, p. 448).

While space limitations do not allow me to detail how the aforementioned moral beliefs and values can enhance self-control and potentiate morally praiseworthy, artful fashioning of a flourishing life, I want to say something about this topic that is underappreciated and undertheorized in mainstream psychoanalytic thought, though less so in experimental social psychology. Indeed, as sociologists and criminologists have pointed out, "the incorporation of morality and self-control into a larger theoretical framework remain in its infancy, with empirical research slowly emerging but with mixed results" (Rocque et al., 2016, p. 521).

For example, the role of how one "frames" one's frustrating situation, as with Mischel's children, or more generally and profoundly, how one conceptualizes one's extreme suffering, has bearing on to what extent one can exert patient self-control and persevere. Indeed, this capacity is lodged in deeply internalized transcendent-pointing beliefs and values that is both an expression and affirmation of one's autonomy, integration and humanity. Drawing from an extreme example of the human condition, Primo Levi described "the saving force" of the religious (e.g., devout Jews and Catholics, Jehovah's Witnesses) and secular (e.g., devout Marxists) believers' faith in the Nazi concentration camps, in contrast to the secular intellectual lodged in a skeptic-humanistic category:

> Their universe was vaster than ours, more expanded in space and time, above all more comprehensible, they had a key and point of leverage, a millennial tomorrow so that there might be a sense to sacrificing themselves, a place in heaven or earth where justice and compassion had won, or would win in a perhaps remote but certain future: Moscow or the celestial or terrestrial Jerusalem. Their hunger was different from ours. It was a Divine punishment or expiation, or votive offering, or the fruit of capitalist putrefaction. Sorrow, in them or around them, was decipherable and therefore did not overflow into despair.
>
> *(Levi, 1988, p. 146)*

What Levi is getting at is that it was through the believers' strongly felt, flexibly and creatively applied, transcendent-pointing moral beliefs and values, specifically as they related to pressing on amidst the horror of the immediate future, that the devout religious and political camp inmate was able to transform their dehumanizing reality into something "more." It is a gross understatement to say that this required self-control and other qualities associated with self-mastery. For it is documented that many camp inmates threw themselves into the electrified barbed wire, or allowed themselves to become a *muselmann*, slang for one of the "walking dead." As Auschwitz survivor Jean Améry put it, the believer was to some extent shielded from the worst of Nazi dehumanization in that he was paradoxically both more distant and closer to his horrifying reality:

> Further from reality because in his Finalistic attitude he ignores the given contents of material phenomenon and fixes his sight on nearer or more distant future; but he is also closer to reality because for just this reason he does not allow himself to be overwhelmed by the conditions around him and thus can strongly influence them.
>
> *(Améry, 1980, p. 14)*

The aforementioned observations of Levi and Améry have been supported by research-based psychologists of religion. They "have shown that religion as experienced and practiced by many people in the 21st century is associated with higher self-control and specific elements of self-regulation" (McCullough & Carter, 2013, p. 127). That is, "research suggests that religion and self-control are indeed related at the level of personality" (ibid., p. 128). In other words, at its best, religion can be a fertile breeding ground for the development and implementation of self-control, which can have positive outcomes in a wide range of behavioral and psychological domains. For example, many of the unruly impulses, emotions and desires that get people into trouble, making their existence and the existences of those they care about miserable, are reinforced by the highly valued self-control-oriented features of the world religions, such as moralizing gods, a belief in an afterlife and the self-monitoring/policing aspects of the sanctification of everyday life (ibid., pp. 124, 126, 129). Of course, this is not to say that religion at its worst can't promote self-control failures, like when religious fanatics have apocalyptic notions or engage in murder of innocents for the "sake of god." Religion can also facilitate over-control that inhibits and self-alienates a person, that, to quote one of my Catholic analysands, made them "feel twisted up like a pretzel."

My point is that when self-control is understood within the context of self-mastery as a manifestation of a broad set of strongly felt, flexibly and creatively applied, transcendent-pointing moral beliefs and values that tend to be other-directed, instead of being understood in the short-term (e.g., resisting ice cream while dieting), chances are that one will be willing and able to exert reasonable self-control, especially in important matters and exceptional accomplishments. Such self-mastery resonates with what has been called "grit," which has been "defined as passion and perseverance for long-term goals despite setbacks, failures and competing pursuits" (Eskreis-Winkler et al., 2016, p. 380). Grit requires having a superordinate goal that, along with sound judgment and empathy, motivates a person to struggle toward a culminating point of actualization, sometimes for a lifetime (ibid., p. 390). Such self-mastery includes resisting foolish or dangerous temptation and summoning the courage to act in the face of challenge or assault. In both of these contexts, one's behavior is perceived as an affirmation of one's autonomy, integration and humanity that is rooted in one's identity-congruent, life-promoting moral beliefs and values. Indeed, "one of the recent shifts in self-regulation theory has been to propose that effective self-regulation operates through habits or habitual avoidance of conflict" (Maranges & Baumeister, 2016, p. 103). That is, "People with good self-control do not necessarily resist temptation and desires, more often or more effectively than others. Rather they seem to set up their lives to be less exposed to temptations" (ibid.). This shift in self-regulation and self-control theory clearly suggests that certain moral beliefs and values and their associated other-directed, other-regarding and other-serving enactments in "real life," such as those of aforementioned religious/political believers, potentiate high levels of habitual self-control that can be a significant factor in living a morally praiseworthy, flourishing life.

Notes

1 Berkman (2016) reviews the three major models for understanding the development of self-regulation: the strength model, that alleges that by practicing self-regulation a person will enhance his general self-regulatory capacity or strength; the motivational model, that alleges that self-regulation can be enhanced by increasing goal-directed motivation; and the cognitive model, that alleges that cognitive manipulation such as If–Then implementation strategies can increase self-regulation. Some additional discussion of these models is provided throughout this chapter.

2 DeYoung and Reuter claim that there are "at least four different types of impulsivity" (2016, p. 351). Also worth mentioning is that sometimes impulsivity, conceived as "undercontrol," is not harmful because it permits spontaneous exploration and utilization of unexpected opportunities. For example, there are contexts where acting, talking and implementing rapid decisions with little or no reflection, such as in fast-paced discussions, sport or in the presence of transient opportunity, can be highly functional (ibid., p. 346).

3 Mischel seems to be talking about a similar overarching goal, "constructing a good life" (2014, p. 101).

4 See Baumeister and Tierney (2011) for a useful book on the psychology of willpower written by a social psychologist and journalist.

5 Mischel appears to be an essentialist in his outlook, even writing a chapter in his book on "Human Nature" (2014), strongly suggesting that he believes that humans have goals and needs that are fixed by nature. For example, he writes, "That leaves us with a view of human nature in which we potentially have more choice, and more responsibility, than in the purely deterministic scientific views of the past century" (ibid., p. 278). Playing off Descartes's *cogito, ergo sum*, "I think, therefore I am," he declares his view of human nature, "I think, therefore I can *change* what I am" (ibid.). While the take home message is uplifting and in certain ways a useable truth, the fact that Mischel believes it is human nature, and not a historically contingent formulation, is troubling to this postmodernist.

6 Engaging in distracting activities isn't merely a way of deferring or not thinking about what you're not getting. It carries its own reward, before the "ultimate reward" for deferring gratification. This is, every time you engage in this substitute behavior it's a reward in of itself because it means you've successfully deferred.

7 For a detailed discussion of the role of imagination in the context of surmounting suffering, and of how to fashion a flourishing life, see Marcus (2019).

8 The Axial Age was a pivotal time from 800 to 200 BCE when the spiritual foundations of our current society were established. Confucius, Lao Tse, Zarathustra, Buddha, Isaiah, Jeremiah, Homer, Plato, et cetera, all lived during this period (Marcus, 2019).

9 See Marcus (2017) for an explication of Freud's suggestion as it relates to the psychology of work.

10 Baumeister did an often-cited "Radish Experiment" as part of his study of ego-depletion. University students came to the laboratory hungry, as they were asked to fast before arriving. Once they were in the laboratory, some were asked to compel themselves to relinquish the tempting chocolate chip cookies and chocolate-flavored confections and instead consume radishes, while others were permitted to eat the cookies. Immediately afterwards, both groups were requested to work on challenging geometry problems that were, in fact, unsolvable. The study demonstrated that the radish students gave up on their problem-solving efforts much sooner than the students who had been permitted to consume the cookies and candy. As Mischel noted, "in more than a hundred other experiments, there were similar results: Engaging in self-control at Time 1 reduced self-control at Time 2, which immediately followed Time 1. This was true no matter which act of self-control the students were instructed to perform" (2014, pp. 217–218). See Baumeister et al. (1998) to read the details of the classic study.

11 Psychological distance is a construct that has been studied as a discrete phenomenon. Distance can be a temporal dimension, such as the present in contrast to the future or the past; a spatial one, such as near in contrast to far; a social one, such as the self in

contrast to strangers; and one of certainty, such as definite in contrast to hypothetical. The more the psychological distance, the more the individual uses the "cool" system, his high-level information processing capacities that are thoughtful, rational and problem-solving. The goal is to live one's life mainly by the "cool" system (the "ego," an analyst might say) where self-control is lodged, rather than the "hot" system, the automatic, reflexive, unconscious limbic system (the "id") (Mischel, 2014, p. 132).

References

Akhtar, S. (2009). *Comprehensive dictionary of psychoanalysis.* London: Karnac.

Améry, J. (1980). *At the mind's limits: Contemplations by a survivor on Auschwitz and its realities.* A. Rosenfeld & S.P. Rosenfeld (Trans.). Bloomington: Indiana University Press.

Baumeister, R.F., Bratslavsky, E., Muraven, M. & Tice, D.M. (1998). Ego depletion: Is the active self a limited resource. *Journal of Personality and Social Psychology*, 74, 1252–1265.

Baumeister, R.F. & Tierney, J. (2011). *Willpower: Rediscovering the greatest human strength.* New York: Penguin.

Berkman, E.T. (2016). Self-regulation training. In K.D. Vohs & R.F. Baumeister (Eds.), *Handbook of self-regulation: Research, theory, and applications* (3rd ed., pp. 440–457). New York: Guilford.

Bokser, B.Z. (1982). *The prayer book: Weekday, Sabbath and festival.* B. Z. Bokser (Ed. & Trans.). New York: Behrman House Publishers.

Carver, C.S. & Scheier, M.F. (2016). Self-regulation of action and affect. In K.D. Vohs & R.F. Baumeister (Eds.), *Handbook of self-regulation: Research, theory, and applications* (3rd ed., pp. 3–23). New York: Guilford.

DeYoung, C.G. & Rueter, A.R. (2016). Impulsivity as a personality trait. In K.D. Vohs & R.F. Baumeister (Eds.), *Handbook of self-regulation: Research, theory, and applications* (3rd ed., pp. 345–363). New York: Guilford.

Emde, R. (1988). Development terminable and interminable: Innate, motivational factors. *International Journal of Psychoanalysis*, 69, 23–42.

Engber, D. (2016). Everything is crumbling. *Slate*, 3/6/16. Retrieved from www.slate.com/.../ego_depletion_an_influential_theory_in_psychology_may_have_j.

Eskreis-Winkler, L., Gross, J.J. & Duckworth, A.I. (2016). Grit: Sustained self-regulation in the service of superordinate goals. In K.D. Vohs & R.F. Baumeister (Eds.), *Handbook of self-regulation: Research, theory, and applications* (3rd ed., pp. 380–395). New York: Guilford.

Fitzsimmons, G. M. & Bargh, J.A. (2004). Automatic self-regulation. In K.D. Vohs & R.F. Baumeister (Eds.), *Handbook of self-regulation: Research, theory, and applications* (3rd ed., pp. 151–170). New York: Guilford.

Freud, S. (1923). The ego and the id. In J. Strachey (Ed. & Trans.), *The standard edition of the complete psychological works of Sigmund Freud* (Vol. 19, pp. 3–66). London: Hogarth Press.

Freud, S. (1932). New introductory lectures on psychoanalysis. In J. Strachey (Ed. & Trans.), *The standard edition of the complete psychological works of Sigmund Freud* (Vol. 22, pp. 3–182). London: Hogarth Press.

Freud, S. (1950). Project for a scientific psychology. In J. Strachey (Ed. & Trans.), *The standard edition of the complete psychological works of Sigmund Freud* (Vol. 1, pp. 295–343). London: Hogarth Press. (Original work published 1895).

Freud, S. (1975). Thoughts for the times on war and death. In J. Strachey (Ed. & Trans.), *The standard edition of the complete psychological works of Sigmund Freud* (Vol. XIV, pp. 273–288). London: Hogarth Press. (Original work published 1915).

Geldard, R. (2001). *The spiritual teachings of Ralph Waldo Emerson* (2nd ed.). Herndon, VA: Lindisfarne.

Gollweitzer, P.M. & Oettingen, G. (2016). Planning promotes goal striving. In K.D. Vohs & R.F. Baumeister (Eds.), *Handbook of self-regulation: Research, theory, and applications* (3rd ed., pp. 223–246). New York: Guilford.

Hipple, W.V. & Henry, J.D. (2016). Aging and self-regulation. In K.D. Vohs & R.F. Baumeister (Eds.), *Handbook of self-regulation: Research, theory, and applications* (3rd ed., pp. 479–494). New York: Guilford.

Hoyle, R.H. & Davisson, E.K. (2016). Varieties of self-control and their personality correlates. In K.D. Vohs & R.F. Baumeister (Eds.), *Handbook of self-regulation: Research, theory, and applications* (3rd ed., pp. 396–413). New York: Guilford.

Laurin, K. & Kay, A.C. (2016). Religion and self-regulation: Integrating skills-based and motivation-based accounts. In K.D. Vohs & R.F. Baumeister (Eds.), *Handbook of self-regulation: Research, theory, and applications* (3rd ed., pp. 305–322). New York: Guilford.

Levi, P. (1988). *The drowned and the saved.* New York: Summit Books.

Lynch, T.R. (2018). *The skills training manual for radically open dialectical behavior therapy: A clinician's guide for treating disorders of overcontrol.* Oakland, CA: New Harbinger Publications.

McCullough, M.F. & Carter, E.C. (2013). Religion, self-control, and self-regulation: How and why are they related. In K.I. Pargament (Ed.), *APA handbook of psychology, religion, and spirituality: Vol. 1, Context, theory, and research* (pp. 123–138). Washington, DC: American Psychological Association.

McGonigal, J. (2016). *SuperBetter: The power of living gamefully.* New York: Penguin.

Maranges, H.M. & Baumeister, R.F. (2016). Self-control and ego depletion. In K.D. Vohs & R.F. Baumeister (Eds.), *Handbook of self-regulation: Research, theory, and applications* (3rd ed., pp. 42–61). New York: Guilford.

Marcus, P. (2017). *The psychoanalysis of career choice, job performance, and satisfaction: How to flourish in the workplace.* London: Routledge.

Marcus, P. (2019). *The psychoanalysis of overcoming suffering: Flourishing despite pain.* London: Routledge.

Mischel, W. (2014). *The Marshmallow Test: Mastering self-control.* New York: Little, Brown and Company.

Mischel, W. & Ebbesen, E.B. (1970). Attention in delay of gratification. *Journal of Personality and Social Psychology*, 16(2), 329–337. doi:10.1037/h0029815.

Mischel, W., Shoda, Y. & Peake, P.K. (1988). The nature of adolescent competencies predicted delay of gratification. *Journal of Personality and Social Psychology*, 54, 687–696.

Mischel, W., Shoda, Y. & Rodriguez, M. L. (1989). Delay of gratification in children. *Science*, 244, 933–938.

Oettingen, G. & Cachia, J.Y.A. (2016). Problems in positive thinking and how to overcome them. In K.D. Vohs & R.F. Baumeister (Eds.), *Handbook of self-regulation: Research, theory, and applications* (3rd ed., pp. 547–570). New York: Guilford.

Peterson, C. & Seligman, M.E.P. (2004). *Character strengths and virtues: A handbook and classification.* Oxford: Oxford University Press.

Rocque, M., Posick, C. & Piquero, A.R. (2016). Self-control and crime: Theory, research, and remaining puzzles. In K.D. Vohs & R.F. Baumeister (Eds.), *Handbook of self-regulation: Research, theory, and applications* (3rd ed., pp. 514–532). New York: Guilford.

Segal, Z., Williams, M. & Teasdale, J. (2018) *Mindfulness-based cognitive therapy for depression* (2nd ed.). New York: Guilford.

Shoda, Y., Mischel, W. & Peake, P.K. (1990). Predicting adolescent cognitive and self-regulatory competencies from preschool delay of gratification: Identifying diagnostic conditions. *Developmental Psychology*, 26, 978–986.

Thomas, W.I. & Thomas, D.S. (1928). *The child in America: Behavior problems and programs.* New York: Knopf.

Thompson, S.C. (2009). The role of personal control in adaptive functioning. In S.J. Lopez & C.R. Snyder (Eds.), *Oxford handbook of positive psychology* (2nd ed., pp. 271–278). Oxford: Oxford University Press.

Vohs, K.D. & Baumeister, R.F. (Eds.) (2016). *Handbook of self-regulation: Research, theory, and applications* (3rd ed.). New York: Guilford.

Watts, T.W., Duncan, G.J. & Quan, H. (2018). Revisiting the Marshmallow Test: A conceptual replication investigating links between early delay of gratification and later outcomes. *Psychological Science*, 29(7), 1159–1177.

Wood, W. (2016). The role of habits in self-control. In K.D. Vohs & R.F. Baumeister (Eds.), *Handbook of self-regulation: Research, theory, and applications* (3rd ed., pp. 95–108). New York: Guilford.

8

TYRANNY VERSUS AUTONOMY

Zimbardo's Stanford Prison Experiment (1971)

What are the psychological conditions of possibility for "normal," "good" people to engage in deeply morally troubling actions? While in previous chapters I discussed the dramatically stressful moral conflict situations that two "classic" experimenters creatively put naïve subjects in to find answers to this question—Asch's 1951 study of conformity versus independence, and Milgram's 1961 study of obedience versus resistance—in this chapter I focus on the last of the triumvirate, Philip Zimbardo's 1971 Stanford Prison Experiment of tyranny versus freedom. All of these investigators were focused on understanding what and how social influences can foster behavior that is judged by most "reasonable" and "decent" people as not only ill-conceived and ill-fated but most importantly, "immoral" (i.e., deliberately harmful to innocent others). While Asch and Milgram's studies were done in an experimental laboratory, Zimbardo created a prison simulation using "normal average" (Haney et al., 1973, p. 3) male college students playing either "guards" or "prisoners" in a mock prison he built in the basement of the psychology department at Stanford University. The results were surprisingly disturbing. Some of the guards became sadistic while most of the prisoners became mentally unhinged. Moral feelings like guilt or shame, moral thinking like ethically animated strategic reasoning and moral behavior like not doing harm to innocent people, gave way to powerful situational forces that produced "demonic" (Zimbardo, 2007, p. 208) guard behavior. As Zimbardo notes, the Stanford Prison Experiment "serves as cautionary tale of what might happen to any of us if we underestimate the extent to which the power of social roles and external pressures can influence our actions."[1] Such actions can be a loss of moral agency and moral autonomy instead of doing "good" things and desisting from "bad" ones (Bandura, 2016, p. 2).

The Stanford Prison Experiment (SPE)

Like Asch and Milgram who were deeply influenced by their childhood backgrounds, Asch by his Jewish religious life in Poland, and Milgram by the Holocaust, Zimbardo, an Italian American, was impacted by his early childhood experience of poverty and prejudice. It was these childhood experiences that he claims led him to become a social psychologist:

> I grew up in a South Bronx ghetto in a very poor family. From Sicilian origin, I was the first person in my family to complete high school, let alone go to college.
>
> Prejudice and discrimination have always been a big part of my life. When I was 6, I got beat up and called "dirty Jew boy" because they thought I looked Jewish, even though I wasn't. Then I almost didn't get accepted into Yale University graduate school because many on the psychology faculty thought I was black. And when I was teaching at NYU, I was carrying furniture in from a rented moving van, wearing a bandanna on my head, and some neighbors passed and said to each other, "Oh my God, the Puerto Ricans are moving everywhere."
>
> So I was discriminated against because I was Jewish, Italian, black and Puerto Rican. But maybe the worst prejudice I experienced was against the poor. I grew up on welfare and often had to move in the middle of the night because we couldn't pay the rent.
>
> *(Maslach, 2000, n.p.)*

Given Zimbardo's childhood of poverty and prejudice it is not surprising that he ended up researching the "psychology of evil" for much of his professional life (2007, p. xi), for as Mahatma Gandhi argued, "poverty is the worst form of violence" (Martin, 2014, p. 41). Researchers have found that being poor can contribute to short- and long-term depression and anxiety, and a downward psychological spiral of fearfulness, self-hatred and failure (Foster, 2015, n.p.)

Zimbardo and two research assistants did a brilliant study of prison life in which they showed that when ordinary people are enmeshed in a group, the group norms become the governing force in terms of individual feeling, thinking and action, sometimes to the extent that the individual does not even view himself as an individual anymore, or at least not as the person he usually saw himself as before the group immersion (Haney et al., 1973; Zimbardo, 2007). This process, called deindividuation (or "anonymity") by social psychologists, is the psychological condition in which a group or social identity utterly controls personal or individual identity such that the group norms become maximally available. Needless to say, the meaning of deindividuation is context-dependent and setting-specific and involves valuative judgments—that is, when deindividuation occurs it does not necessarily lead to sadistic behavior as it did among the guards in Zimbardo's study. For as researchers have shown, the character of deindividuation is that it maximally increases the proclivity of individuals in a group to participate in whatever behavior the group is doing, which could be, for example, rescuing tsunami victims. Deindividuation can lead to prosocial group behavior that is perceived as normative because it increases the saliency of whatever behavior is characteristic of the group. In other words, deindividuation can be "bad" as in Zimbardo's study, or "good" in other contexts (Smith et al., 2015, p. 357).

In the SPE, the researchers randomly assigned twenty-four psychologically and physically fit men to be either mock guards or mock prisoners (they were given a background questionnaire, interviewed and psychologically tested before being accepted into the study). The research spared almost nothing to make the prison look and feel real to the participants. For example, prisoners were surprise arrested by real police on a Sunday at their home, handcuffed, put through the "booking" process, driven hooded to the prison, stripped searched, deloused and they were given identical baggy uniforms with a number that replaced their name by which they were subsequently identified. The guards wore the same military style uniforms and reflective glasses that concealed their eyes and carried billy clubs. The power and control that the guards had over the prisoners was reinforced by the prison "Superintendent" (i.e., Zimbardo), while the two researchers kept notes and audio and visually recorded some of the behavior of both groups. Though the study was supposed to last fourteen days (the participants were contracted and paid in advance), due to the negative effects it had on both groups and Zimbardo, it was ended in six days. The guards, particularly after a rebellion by the prisoners, became abusive and degrading, denying the prisoners food, humiliating them and putting them in solitary confinement. The prisoners were at first oppositional and defiant, but soon became passive, docile and in many instances, so emotionally compromised that they had to leave the study early. Zimbardo called this the Lucifer Effect, "the process of transformation at work when good or ordinary people do bad or evil things." This process was evoked in the infamous Abu Ghraib Prison and in other diabolical contexts. Zimbardo, putting forth his strict situationalism (i.e., the environment made me do it) and anti-dispositionalism (i.e., it wasn't "me" who decided to do it), unsuccessfully testified for the defense of one soldier from Abu Ghraib Prison who received a stiff sentence (Zimbardo, 2007, p. 5).

Zimbardo describes the great care he put into creating a mock prison environment geared to bring out the most extreme behavior in the participants: (1) The prisoners were there twenty-four hours a day while the guards worked eight-hour shifts, which over time promoted situational norms to emerge and induced the corresponding behavior of each group; (2) All participants were as "normal as possible initially, healthy both physically and mentally" (ibid., p. 40); for example, they did not have any prior history of drug involvement, crime or violence, which was important in order for Zimbardo to be able to sort out the role of dispositional and situational factors in understanding guard and prisoner behavior; (3) Neither the guards nor prisoners had any training or real-life experience in how to play their randomly assigned roles, and as such they were left to their own improvisational abilities rooted in their previous knowledge and beliefs; (4) Zimbardo created an experimental context that came as close to a "functional simulation of the psychology of imprisonment" (ibid.) as was doable. The aforementioned was accomplished by the use of depersonalizing uniforms; realistic, menacing props like handcuffs, police clubs, whistles, signs on doors and halls; substituting corridor hall doors with prison bars to generate prison cells;

using cells without windows or clocks so there was no indication of the time of day; a make-shift solitary confinement cell; and implementation of the institutional rule that removed/substituted individual names with numbers for prisoners or titles for staff (Mr. Correction Officer who was an ex-convict, Warden, an undergraduate research assistant, Superintendent, the principal investigator). All of this allowed guards to have near absolute power and control over prisoners.

As Haslam and Reicher (2017, pp. 135–136) note, the guards and prisoners appeared to go through three phases prior to the simulation being stopped. Phase one was "settling in," which involved the participants gearing themselves up for their new roles, albeit with some hesitation and awkwardness. For instance, some prisoners did not take their inferior position earnestly during roll call and the guards were not sure how to authoritatively respond to this oppositional behavior. Likewise, some guards felt tinges of guilt and anxiety, sometimes feeling they were too courteous to prisoners and they should be tougher about discipline. Zimbardo mentions one night-time guard nicknamed "John Wayne" (in general night shift guards were more comfortable with their role) who enjoyed punishing prisoners if they erred during roll call by ordering them to do press-ups. In one instance when one of the prisoners defied the night guards, he was ordered into "the Hole," a small windowless closet Zimbardo created that was used for solitary confinement. This and a few similar incidents tended to create group solidarity against the guards rather than the prisoners simply viewing themselves as "lone wolves" trying to survive their ordeal.

Phase two was "rebellion" wherein the prisoners as a group were frustrated and angered by their maltreatment by the guards and began to plan for a rebellion, beginning with small acts of insubordination, such as protesting the conditions of their imprisonment, cursing at the guards and refusing to obey orders. The culminating point of this defiance was when the prisoners in two cells removed their caps and prisoner numbers and barricaded themselves in their cell, one of them crying out, "Fight them! Resist violently! The time has come for violent revolution" (Zimbardo, 2007, p. 61).

Phase three involved an increased empowerment of the prisoners along with a more troubling "tyranny" that guards implemented. They requested reinforcements and forcefully put down the rebellion. They crashed through the barricaded cells, disrobed all of the prisoners, removed the ringleader and put him into "the Hole." Along with intensifying their harassment and intimidation of the prisoners, the guards aggressively used a "divide and conquer" tactic that included pulling out the prisoners in the cell who had not willingly participated in the rebellion for special privileges and reconfiguring the cells so that those prisoners who had rebelled were combined with those who had not done so.

Zimbardo, acting as "Superintendent," was not an impartial experimenter but was swept into his role similar to how the other participants were, only stopping the experiment when a woman he was dating (and subsequently married) who just got her Ph.D. pointed out to him the inhumanity of the course of the experiment, including his participation (Haslam & Reicher, 2017). For example, Zimbardo recruited one of the rebelling prisoners to act as a "snitch," bribing him with privileges. Another prisoner who Zimbardo coerced began to believe that there was no exit out of the prison, even screaming to his fellow prisoners that "I couldn't get out! They wouldn't let me out! You can't get out of here" (Zimbardo, 2007, p. 70), an affirmation that had a powerful, decisive impact on other prisoners. As Haslam and Reicher point out, "with the prisoners' collective will now crushed, and that of guards consolidated, the scene was set for the guards to progressively dominate, oppress, and brutalize the prisoners" (2017, p. 136).

Zimbardo indicated that about eight of the twenty-four guards became "tyrannical" in their capricious use of their power, often using considerable sadistic inventiveness to destroy the prisoners' self-respect. The guard John Wayne, for example, was gradually more degrading of the prisoners. He ordered the roll calls to last hours, and disobedient or new prisoners who went on a hunger strike were targeted for especially mean-spirited abuse. Other tyrannical guards ordered prisoners to do push-ups with a guard forcefully holding his foot on the prisoner's back, wash out toilets without gloves and play homoerotic games of leapfrog. Another group of guards became "tough but fair" while others were "good guards," being cordial and doing an occasional favor for a prisoner like giving him an apple.

Not only did Superintendent Zimbardo get swept into the destructive social dynamics of the mock prison, so did the other experimenters. For example, once when there was a rumor in the prison that there was an escape to be initiated, Zimbardo inserted a new prisoner/informant to undermine the escape. When this tactic did not work, Zimbardo used a second tactic in which the guards were ordered "to chain the prisoners' legs together, put bags over their heads" and relocate them to another part of the building (Zimbardo, 2007, pp. 97–99). The other experimenters showed great vigor in attempting to convince the visiting relatives that the prison was non-injurious while simultaneously conducting mock parole boards which verbally disparaged and abused the prisoners. By day number six of the planned fourteen-day experiment, Zimbardo traumatically realized that not only could he have quite easily behaved the same way the most brutal guards did, but he had become "blinded … to the reality of the destructive impact of the System that I was sustaining … I was the 'Iceman' in that house of inhumanity" (ibid., p. 179). Hence the experiment was ended.

Social-psychological explanations of the SPE

There have been two social-psychological accounts to explain Zimbardo's findings, one vigorously given by Zimbardo that puts forth a strict situationalist-based behavioral perspective, while the other by Reicher and Haslam (2006), puts forth an interactionist one. I will discuss them in kind and then offer some psychoanalytic reflections that help integrate the two perspectives.

The situationalist explanation

Zimbardo views his study as following in the grand situationalist tradition of Asch, Milgram and Bandura:

> In Solomon Asch's classic research … the power of the group majority distorted the perceptual judgments of individual college students. In Stanley

> Milgram's obedience research … the power of an authority figure induced actions that went against the moral conscience of adult male participants to harm a stranger. In experimental research on moral disengagement [when a person actively disengages their self-regulating efficacy for moral conduct] Albert Bandura ([et al.,] 1975) showed that college student participants shocked the "errors" of other student with highest intensity when they had been labeled "animals," compared to other [neutral or humanized] conditions. In the SPE, we witnessed the creation over time of two mentalities, that of dominating guards and of helpless, hopeless prisoners in a setting that validated these alternative personas. I believe that these four psychological studies … illustrate the extent to which the power of a social situation can come to dominate and distort individual perceptions judgements, values and behavior.
>
> *(Zimbardo, 2018, n.p.)*

As a strict situationalist, Zimbardo believes that external determinants of behavior should be in the foreground of any attempt to understand why people act as they do, which is well beyond viewing them as merely mitigating background circumstances (Zimbardo, 2007, p. 21). In particular, he claims that with "relative ease, ordinary, 'good' men and women can be induced into behaving in 'evil' ways by turning on or off one or another social situational variable" (ibid., p. 22). Evil, says Zimbardo, is "defined as intentionally behaving, or causing others to act, in ways that demean, dehumanize, harm, destroy, or kill innocent people" (ibid.). Zimbardo quotes a respected colleague, saying, "Evil is knowing better but doing worse," (ibid.) implying that the guards had a choice in their behavioral orientation.

It is important to note that Zimbardo is an essentialist.[2] For example, he refers to his study being concerned with "profound questions about human existence and human nature;" "We are not born with tendencies toward good or evil but with mental *templates* to do either … we all share the human condition" (ibid., p. 23). He also described guard behavior as a "'natural' consequence" of their role playing (Haney et al., 1973, p. 12) and uses the phrase "what is best in human nature" (Zimbardo, 2018, n.p.). Zimbardo's claims are questionable because he makes these assertions as if what constitutes "human nature," "the human condition," and is "natural" and "best in human nature," has a fixed and absolute meaning, rather than being historically contingent (i.e., context-dependent and setting-specific circumstances of the present historical mode of being and way of dealing with reality). Similar to the historical Freud, who puts forth a notion of the subject that was allegedly natural, essential, ahistorical and universal, a subject constituted by sexual desire, Zimbardo claims that the subject is hardwired or at least prewired (i.e., he has "mental templates" and "natural" inclinations) to be largely governed by external determinants and situational variables. All human beings, according to Zimbardo, have "vulnerability to situational forces" (2007, p. 26). This being said, he also makes the questionable assertion, "We can assume that most people, most of the time, are moral creatures" (ibid., p. 17). In fact, ironically, Zimbardo accuses those who apply internal dispositional analysis to understanding observed behavior, such as personality/character, free will, responsibility and conscience (including to the SPE), and who ignore or underplay the impact of situational variables, as being guilty of committing the fundamental attribution error (FAE) (ibid., p. 24). The FAE alleges that people have a proclivity to exaggerate the role of personal qualities and ignore situational forces in judging others' behavior. Because of the FAE, we are inclined to believe that others do "bad" things because they are "bad" people. That is, we are prone to ignore situational forces that might have played a decisive role. While there appears to be some truth to the FAE, Zimbardo commits a reverse FAE by overutilizing situational explanations while underutilizing dispositional ones. Clearly, the most robust analysis of observed behavior such as in the SPE, looks at both the individual and situation in dynamic interaction,[3] and this, I believe, includes using psychoanalytic insights to expand and deepen our understanding of the behavior of the guards and prisoners.

In Zimbardo's view, "anything that makes a person feel anonymous [i.e., deindividuated], as if no one knows who he or she is, creates the potential for that person to act in evil ways—if the situation gives permission for violence" (2007, p. 29). Drawing from Milgram and Bandura's studies, Zimbardo notes that the latter showed how individuals can become willing and able to morally disengage from destructive behavior through applying an array of "cognitive mechanisms" (or what I would call forms of strategic reasoning that are probably mainly unconscious), that change one's perception of the morally objectionable behavior. This includes, for example, engaging in moral rationalizations, like making soothing comparisons and using euphemistic labeling for one's objectionable behavior. The morally disengaged agent also changes his sense of the destructive impact of his behavior by minimizing, ignoring or misinterpreting the consequences. A third cognitive mechanism used involves relinquishing his sense of personal responsibility for the connection between his immoral behavior and its destructive impact, for example by displacing or diffusing personal responsibility. Finally, says Zimbardo, the morally disengaged actor changes his perception of the victim by dehumanizing him, assigning the blame for the destructive outcome onto the victim (ibid., p. 31). According to Zimbardo, what his study adds to Milgram and Bandura's theorizing to account for "evil deeds" is his emphasis "on the role of cognitive controls" that usually animate behavior in socially and personally acceptable ways:

> The shift from good to evil behavior can be accomplished by knocking out these control processes, blocking them, minimizing them, or reorienting them. Doing so suspends conscience, self-awareness, sense of personal responsibility, obligation, commitment, liability, morality, and analysis in terms of costs-benefits of given actions.
>
> *(ibid., p. 32)*

Finally, Zimbardo notes that there are two strategies to accomplish the aforementioned goal. First, the actor diminishes the cues of social accountability by saying, for example, "No one knows who I am, nor cares to know." Such a strategy bypasses anxiety about social evaluation and approval by assuming a sense of anonymity and diffusing personal responsibility onto others in the situation. The second strategy diminishes the actor's anxieties about self-evaluation. It halts self and consistency monitoring by using tactics that change forms of consciousness by, for example, using drugs, arousing powerful emotions or hyperintense actions, generating a highly focused present-time existential orientation such that there is no concern for past or future, and by projecting personal responsibility onto others (ibid.). As Zimbardo notes, unlike Milgram's studies in which an authority figure was present, coaxing the naïve subject to obey, Zimbardo is emphasizing the role of the totality of circumstances that constitute the situation, such that subjects behave in conformance to paths made available to them, without critically reflecting on the meaning or consequences of their behavior. Their behavior is not cognitively guided in the way it usually is. Rather, it is guided by the behavior of others in proximity to them, or by their powerfully generated emotional states and situationally accessible cues, such as the existence of weapons, like the billy clubs in Zimbardo's study (ibid., p. 33).

What these factors did according to Zimbardo was to demonstrate how ordinary men can be radically transformed by the circumstances in which they find themselves and engage in evil behavior, more or less irrespective of their pre-situational (i.e., pre-imprisonment) personality/character and other dispositional factors. In other words, individuals descend into evil behavior because they unreflectively conform to the "toxic roles" that have been assigned to them without needing specific orders, this being a "natural" result of being a uniformed guard and enforcing the power that the role entails (Haslam & Reicher, 2012a, p. 1). To be fair to Zimbardo, in his 2007 book, *The Lucifer Effect*, he somewhat softens his strict situationalism of his 1973 paper, claiming that he is against those researchers who "focus on the actor as the sole causal agent," while they "minimize or disregard the impact of situation variable and systemic determinants that shape behavioral outcomes and transform actors" (Zimbardo, 2007, p. 445). In other words, Zimbardo is acknowledging that the "actor" is one important "causal agent," though not the only or most important one.

The interactionist perspective

Zimbardo's essentialist, situationalist perspective has been challenged by social psychologists who believe that while situational forces have a significant role in the actions of the guards, as Zimbardo undeniably demonstrated, other interdependent, interrelated and interactive dispositional factors of equal or greater importance were also at play.

The interactionist explanation of the SPE is lodged in social identity theory developed by Henri Tajfel and John Turner in the 1970s. The gist of the theory is succinctly summarized by Haslam and Reicher:

> People do not automatically take on roles associated with group membership, but do so only when they come to *identify* with the group in question … This suggests that the roles will only be accepted when they are seen as an expression of a person's sense of self (i.e., the social identity of "us"). Moreover, the theory suggests that when members of a low status group (e.g., prisoners) came

> to develop a sense of shared social identity this can be a basis for them to collectively *resist* oppression rather than just succumb to it.
>
> *(2017, p. 141)*

The point that Haslam and Reicher are making is that to comprehend tyranny we need to go beyond Zimbardo's claim that there is a "natural" inclination, the Lucifer Effect, in which guards are bound to enact without critical reflection or power to do otherwise, and therefore cannot be reasonably held responsible for their actions (Haslam & Reicher, 2012a, p. 3). Indeed, while Zimbardo puts forth a strict situationalist explanation for the guards' behavior in his original study, he nonetheless illogically also affirms, without a reasoned argument, that his situationally based behavioral explanations are never forms of "excusiology" (Zimbardo, 2018, n.p.). In other words, Zimbardo wants it both ways: He claims that humans are governed by external determinants and situational forces but they should still be held personally accountable for the atrocities they commit. In fact, in *The Lucifer Effect*, he correctly (in my view) advocates for behavioral resistance to unwanted, if not evil, influences by drawing from the beliefs and values of "heroes and heroism," what amounts to a dispositional analysis that affirms human freedom (2007, p. 460). He says, "I also endorse the power of people to act mindfully and critically as informed agents directing their behavior in purposeful ways" (ibid., p. 21).

Like the SPE, in the British Broadcasting Study (henceforth, BBC Prison Study), Reicher and Haslam (2006), also randomly assigned men to groups as guards and prisoners and investigated their behavior within a specially designed prison.[4] The difference between their study and Zimbardo's is that they took no leadership role in the study and thus put into sharp focus the question of whether participants would conform to a hierarchical script or resist it. For example, Zimbardo gave the guards specific instructions during their orientation,

> You can create in the prisoners feelings of boredom, a sense of fear to some degree, you can create a notion of arbitrariness that their life is totally controlled by us, by the system, you, me … We're going to take away their individuality in various ways. In general, what all of this leads to is a sense of powerlessness.
>
> *(2007, p. 55)*

While Zimbardo has claimed that it was the "behavioral scripts associated with the oppositional roles of prisoner and guard [that were] the sole source of guidance" (Zimbardo, 2004, p. 39), these instructions given raise questions about whether it was the role-related scripts that most motivated the abusiveness of the guards or some other factors related to leader/follower (Reicher & Haslam, 2006, p. 2). As Haslam and Reicher note, without the guidance of the experimenters in the SPE and giving the guards "a script of terror," as Philip Banyard called it, it is unlikely that the guards would have behaved as brutally as they did. Other studies done on guard behavior in a prison have indicated that guard brutality is hardly "natural or inevitable" as Zimbardo argues. Lovibond et al. (1979) found that if guards were urged to act more respectfully of prisoners' humanity and encouraged their decision-making participation, the resulting prison regime was considerably more modulated and benevolent (Haslam & Reicher, 2017, p. 130).[5]

Drawing from the critique of Zimbardo's experiment by Banuazizi and Movahedi (1975), Haslam and Reicher (2017) point out that it was not so much that in the SPE the guards on their own creatively abused the prisoners. Rather, it was the demand characteristics of the situation they were in that mattered most. In cognitive psychology, demand characteristics refers to the situation where the results of an experiment are biased because the experimenters' expectancies regarding the performance of the participants on a particular task create an implicit demand for the participants to perform as expected. Thus, the guards behaved as brutally as they did because they were merely exploiting the props and procedures that the experimenters made available, such as chains, bags over the prisoners' heads and forced nudity. Likewise, in some contexts, the guards were directed to apply these tools against the prisoners, and in other contexts, neither Superintendent Zimbardo nor the Warden attempted to halt any prisoner abuse, in effect endorsing it by their non-intervention. In other words, it was the demand characteristics of the overall prison environment, Zimbardo's experimental design, that most influenced guard brutality, rather than the individual's sadistic inventiveness in his role playing (ibid., p. 139).

Erich Fromm (1973), coming from a psychoanalytic angle of vision, also points out that the demand characteristics of Zimbardo's experiment may have influenced prisoner behavior. For example, he mentions that the prisoners could not have possibly expected to find themselves in the degrading and humiliating situation they found themselves in when they agreed to participate in the experiment. That is, there was considerable confusion from the start. Prisoners did not know if the police arrest was "real" or part of the experimental role playing because their questions to the police were not answered and they had no lawyer to advocate for their rights. Likewise, throughout the experiment, there was confusion about what was reality and fantasy, as the prison experiment was just that, an experiment, and not a "real" prison. Such a context almost inevitably produced a high degree of feeling puzzled, tricked and helpless, leading to corroborating behavior. It was not completely clear to the prisoners that they could leave the experiment whenever they wanted, that they did not need permission from the parole board or other staff ("we could not detain our subjects for extended or indefinite periods of time"; Haney et al., 1973, p. 4),[6] though some prisoners were released earlier for mental health reasons. As a result of not knowing whether they had the "right" to leave, this condition became other demand characteristics that negatively influenced them, such as their confused thoughts, anxious feelings and compliant behavior. The upshot of this is that it is not clear whether the prisoners' hopeless and helpless behavior was due to a lack of clarity about whether they had the power to intervene in their situation to leave the experiment (unlike a real prison), or were simply doing what any person would do who was role playing as part of a contractual agreement (ibid., pp. 58, 59, 60).

Finally, there is some evidence that the so-called "normal average" participants in Zimbardo's study may not have been as psychologically healthy as Zimbardo believed. Carnahan and McFarland (2007) researched whether students who selectively volunteer for a study of prison life have dispositions linked with abusive behavior. Two sets of college students were recruited for a study of prison life using a nearly identical newspaper ad as used in the SPE, or for a psychological study, which was an identical ad without the words "prison life." Volunteers for the prison study scored statistically significantly higher on a measure of the abuse-related dispositions of aggressiveness, authoritarianism, Machiavellianism, narcissism and social dominance, and lower on empathy and altruism. These findings contradict Zimbardo's claim that the participants were not distinguishable on authoritarianism before the experiment and they are in sync with Zimbardo's reporting that only one-third of the guards engaged in tyrannical behavior.[7] According to Carnahan and McFarland, these findings suggest that a person–situation interactionism account may be more plausible in understanding guards' abusive behavior than Zimbardo's strict situationalism, or an account that views the individual and environment in isolation (Haslam & Reicher, 2017, p. 140).

The BBC Prison Study produced three important findings that challenge Zimbardo's explanatory framework. First, the participants did not mechanically conform to their designated role. Second, the participants acted in terms of group membership to the degree that they actively identified with the group and made it part of their self-system. And third, group identity did not mean that participants merely embraced their assigned role. Rather, it emboldened them to resist it. As Reicher and Haslam (2006) note, early in the study, the prisoners' identification as a group permitted them to effectively challenge the authority of the guards and generate a more egalitarian system. Later on, however, a highly dedicated group developed out of displeasure with the system and they collaborated to create a new hierarchy that was excessively harsh and severe (ibid., pp. 2–3).

The significance of these three findings is that it was not passive conformity to roles that mattered most, as in Zimbardo's explanation of guard and prisoner behavior. Rather, it was the internalized roles and rules that were constituent elements of a system that the guards and prisoners used as an animating guide for their behavior. In other words, it was not conformity to roles that was the guarantee of the tyrannical regime as Zimbardo theorized, but rather, it was the shared identification, creative leadership and engaged followership within a group of sadistically inclined believers (ibid., p. 3).[8]

Psychoanalytic reflections on the SPE

The only response to the SPE done by a psychoanalyst was by Fromm in *The Anatomy of Human Destructiveness* (1973). Fromm critically evaluated Milgram's and Zimbardo's findings and conclusions and found them to be highly questionable. While some of what Fromm commented on appears to be dated, he makes a few thoughtful points that will lead into the heart of my psychoanalytically inspired reflections.

Fromm indicates that despite the fact that the methods used in the prison were those of severe and systematic humiliation and degradation, two-thirds of the guards did not engage in sadistic behavior toward the prisoners. This finding suggests the opposite of what Zimbardo concluded, namely, that the situation itself in a few days can transform "normal average" people into ruthless sadists and abject, submissive prisoners. Rather, says Fromm, the experiment appears "to prove that one can *not* transform people so easily into sadists by providing them with the proper situation" (ibid., p. 58). Indeed, as I will suggest shortly, there were forms of resistance among the guards and prisoners from the onset of the study, though to be fair to Zimbardo, this was the minority of participants and it tended to peter out.

A second Fromm criticism of Zimbardo's study was the difference between fantasy and reality, a mock prison versus a real one (e.g., one could leave the mock prison but couldn't simply walk out of a real prison because of mental instability), that pervaded the experimental environment (both consciously and unconsciously), as the guards were less inclined to call forth their usual superego considerations in terms of their behavior. That is, since they were never sure if the mock prison was real, and probably knew it was only role/game playing, what may have been the guard's usual conscience (i.e., their moral feeling, reasoning and consequential thinking) in the service of doing the "right" thing, was not in play. As Fromm notes, due to the confusion between fantasy and reality of the SPE, guards' (and prisoners') critical judgements and moral inhibitions were greatly diminished. Therefore, the ruler over the fictitious reality (aka, the experimenter) becomes "the reality" for the guards and prisoners, somewhat akin to a hypnotist/hypnotee relationship: "The experimenter relieves the subject, to some extent, of his responsibility and of his own will, and hence makes him much more prone to obey the rules than the subject would be in a nonhypnoid situation" (ibid., p. 65). Discerning exactly what reactions of the prisoners were due to character structure and the social structure of the experiment becomes nearly impossible (ibid., p. 66).

Fromm also criticizes Zimbardo's claim that the battery of unspecified psychological tests given to the participants the day prior to the experiment (but kept confidential to avoid experimental bias) had demonstrated that there was no proclivity toward sadistic or masochistic behavior, or put in psychoanalytic terms, that they had no such "character traits" (Haney et al., 1973; Fromm, 1973, p. 58). The tests administered, we learned many years later, were the F-Scale, The Machiavellian Scale, the Comrey Personality Scales and during and after the experiment the Mood Adjective Self-Reports. For the most part, "there were no prior dispositional tendencies that could distinguish those individuals who role played the guards from those who enacted the prisoner role" (Zimbardo, 2007, pp. 198–199).

As Fromm noted, while such psychological tests may relate to observable behavior, and therefore Zimbardo's conclusion is plausible from a psychoanalytic perspective, characterologically based sadism and masochism are not easily discernible via psychological testing, let alone the "objective" self-reporting types that Zimbardo administered. For example, there were no projective tests given, which are better at assessing unconscious processes. Even then, accessing the unconscious material which allegedly animates sadistic and masochistic characters ("unconscious sadists," ibid., p. 5) is not straightforward to identify and interpret, and some believe projective testing has questionable reliability and validity even if done by an experienced clinician. It is noteworthy, however, that Zimbardo gives some credence to unconscious processes in his understanding of guard and prisoner behavior, when, for example, he says that the systemic and situational forces that can operate to influence individual behavior in negative or positive directions is "often without our personal awareness" (2018, n.p.). Also worth mentioning is Carnahan and McFarland's (2007) findings that suggest that those who took part in a study of prison life were inclined to be more authoritarian, Machiavellian, narcissistic and socially dominating, suggesting that Zimbardo's participants may not have been as "normal and average" as he thought, and that their pathology was more so characterological than manifest behavior accessed via "objective" self-reporting psychological testing.

While Fromm believed that the one-third of guards who acted most sadistically probably had unconscious sadistic characters, and the prisoners who became quickly compliant were masochistic characters, the fact is that there have been many subsequent studies to Zimbardo's that detail the range of psychological processes that can take hold of ordinary people, let alone those with sadistic or masochistic characters, and transform them into abusers or abusees. Lifton's psychoanalytically animated work on medicalized killing in Auschwitz (1986) showed the relationship of SS doctors who were respectable doctors pre-Holocaust to the killing process in the transformation from healer to killer via such mechanisms as psychic numbing and splitting. As Haslam and Reicher noted, studies that have revisited the SPE have intimated that "dispositions play a role in drawing people into particular contexts and also in orienting them towards particular group activities once there" (2017, p. 143). Bruno Bettelheim's study of inmate behavior in the "extreme" situation of the concentration camp has shown how inmates regressed, embraced destructive camp values, and lost their autonomy, integration and humanity amidst the Nazi assault (1960). Whether the perpetrator or the victim, processes of psychic fragmentation were paramount, somewhat similar to Zimbardo's observations in his comparatively limited study. By way of concluding this chapter, I want to explore in more detail a theme that Zimbardo takes up in *The Lucifer Effect* in which he recaps his 1973 research and augments it with other data both from the original experiment and other sources, namely, how prisoners and others in extreme situations, as well as those who feel social influences of various kinds to be bearing down on them, can resist such assaults on their autonomy, integration and humanity.

Toward a psychoanalytic social psychology of freedom/resistance

In his conclusory chapter, Zimbardo noted of the prisoners in his study that

> Experiencing a loss of personal identity and subjected to arbitrary continual control of their behavior, as well as being deprived of privacy and sleep, generated in them a syndrome of passivity, dependency, and depression that resembled "learned helplessness" … Most of them who remained for the duration generally became mindlessly obedient to the guards' demands and seemed "zombie-like" in their listless movements while yielding to the whims of the ever-escalating guard power.
>
> *(2007, p. 196)*

Zimbardo explained this outcome as mainly due to the clear-cut results of the assignment of participants to the prisoner group with its distinct role, that is, the prisoners conformed to the role that their group assignment induced via arbitrary control by the guards (Haslam & Reicher, 2012b, pp. 155, 156). In fact, Zimbardo compares the prisoners to "Method actors who continue to play their roles when offstage and off camera, and their role has come to consume their identity" (2007, p. 143).[9] Zimbardo says more generally that those situational forces that were operative to produce prisoner and guard behavior were "roles, rules, norms, anonymity of person and place, dehumanizing processes, conformity pressures, group identity" (ibid., p. 197).

This being said, Zimbardo does mention in passing that some of the prisoners displayed resistant behavior, mainly early in the experiment. For example, one prisoner, the "most evenly balanced" one, mainly survived his affliction by "turning inward" as the prisoner later reflected, with little interest in assisting others, though he behaved heroically by refusing an order to verbally abuse a fellow prisoner (ibid., p. 196). The early "settling in" and "rebellion" phases, expressions of resistance, were effectively put down by the guards, and after the rebellion the prisoners assumed an intensified "prisoner mentality" (ibid., p. 205) in which they were automaton-like, utterly self-centric and self-serving. In fact, "the two most *infrequent* behaviors we observed over the six days of our study were individuating others and helping others. Only one such incident of helping was recorded—a solitary sign of human concern for a fellow human being occurred between two prisoners" (ibid., p. 213).

The above rendering of how prisoners lost their pre-incarceration autonomy, integration[10] and humanity is entirely in sync with studies of inmates in perhaps the most extreme prison circumstances that both Zimbardo (2007) and Haslam and Reicher (2012a) liberally draw from, namely the Nazi concentration camps, but also in similar persecutory contexts (Bettelheim, 1960; Marcus, 1999). The literature of survival has affirmed many of the observations that Zimbardo and his colleagues have made; namely, that most ordinary people who find themselves in an extreme situation of long-term imprisonment or other types of total institutions[11] lose most of their pre-incarceration moral compass and personal integrity as they try to endure their ordeal of suffering by embracing a "survival at any price," self-centric, self-serving way of being (Marcus, 1999; Sofsky, 1997).

Zimbardo, the strict situationalist, seems to have expanded and deepened his analysis of resistance toward a decidedly dispositional analysis in his 1973 paper. Such a perspective affirms what I have described in previous chapters as being vital to maintaining one's autonomy, integration and humanity both inside and outside the morally challenging situations that Asch, Milgram and Zimbardo have designed; namely, an ethic of freedom and care. Such an existential orientation is rooted in a person having strongly felt, flexibly and creatively applied, transcendent-pointing moral beliefs and values that are primarily other-directed, other-regarding and other-serving. Resistance is possible against "influences that we neither want nor need but that rain upon us daily. We are not slaves to the power of situational forces. But we must learn methods of resisting and opposing them" (Zimbardo, 2007, p. 446). This is the weakest section in *The Lucifer Effect*, for he describes his "ten-step program" in which "the key to resistance" resides in developing "the three Ss: self-awareness, situational sensitivity, and street smarts" (ibid., p. 452). "We are best able to avoid, prevent, challenge, and change such negative situational forces only by recognizing their potential power to 'infect us,'" including the all-important "framing provided by the System" which imposes "pervasive top-down dominance"[12] (ibid., pp. 211, 227). While these factors are surely important as I have mentioned in other chapters [and Bettelheim (1960) has described in detail in the concentration camps and beyond], they hardly constitute the "whole story," and they do not adequately indicate "how" the three Ss and other pertinent factors actually help one maintain one's autonomy, integration and humanity. While detailing all of this is beyond the scope of this chapter, a few points are worth making in the service of developing the rudiments of a psychoanalytically animated "social psychology of resistance" that goes beyond Zimbardo's cognitive and environmental determinism (Haslam & Reicher, 2012b, p. 154).

To understand resistance in a prison, and by extension in similar situations, it is important to consider not only the individual dispositions, like beliefs and values (which they underplay in my view), but contextual, group factors. That there is a collective basis to resistance, including a strong link between physical and psychological survival and a feeling of group identity (ibid., p. 167), is a familiar observation from the Nazi concentration camp and other such survivalist literatures. However, these collectivities are held together by an existential commitment of individuals to particular beliefs, values and practices that function prophylactically in terms of maintaining autonomy, integration and humanity, at least to some degree. As Auschwitz survivor Jean Améry noted, those inmates with strong beliefs/values or ideology had a "firm foothold in the world from which they spiritually unhinged the SS state ... They survived better or died with more dignity than their irreligious or unpolitical intellectual comrades" (1980, p. 13).[13]

What Zimbardo underplays in his analysis of resistance to the extreme situation is that resistance is not only recognizing that there are cognitive alternatives, "the three Ss," to how one responds to oppressiveness of long-term imprisonment and the like. Rather, resistance both expresses and affirms a cluster of interrelated, interdependent and interactive, meaning-giving, affect-integrating and action-guiding processes that are enacted in the person's way of being in the world. That is, following Heidegger, a person is best understood as an integrated unit of thoughts, feelings/kinesthetics and overt behavior. For example, Albert Bandura, a social cognitive theorist, has a similar point of view when he comments that the unidirectional dispositional and situational perspectives, and the debate about which matters more, is a fruitless one. Rather, he puts forth a "triadic codeterminism" in which human functioning, including in terms of maintaining moral agency, is best understood as a result of the interaction of personal influences (e.g., intrapsychic and biological factors), the behavior in which individuals engage (e.g., physical, social and emotional forms), and the environmental forces that impinge on them (the selected lived environments) (Bandura, 2016, pp. 6–7). I briefly describe below how resistance, conceived as reflecting the totality of a person's way of being-in-the-world, is instantiated in a real-life extreme prison situation, the Nazi concentration camps (Haslam & Reicher, 2012b; Zimbardo, 2007).

The German sociologist Wolfgang Sofsky has aptly summarized how having strongly felt, flexibly and creatively applied, transcendent-pointing moral beliefs and values that are primarily other-directed, other-regarding and other-serving helped inmates resist the Nazi dehumanization:

> As different as the specific content of their belief was, religious Jews and Christians and staunch communists had the benefit of a critical resource for survival not available to their nonreligious, nonideological fellow prisoners; the belief and trust in the future. They considered themselves to be part of a spiritual-intellectual continuum that could not be called into question. In this way, they passed beyond their concrete, momentary existence, gaining distance from the presence of terror. Their conviction served to secure the experimental, project-oriented character of human existence and the ability to act. Although the future was a fiction, its consequences were practical and real. It reduced powerlessness, integrated the individual into a group, and bolstered the power to resist. It counterposed a higher temporal plane to the all-powerful time of the camp, salvaging in this way the prisoner's personal time, which had been threatened to its very foundation.
>
> *(1997, p. 93)*

What Sofsky and others have described is that those inmates with such aforementioned beliefs, values and practices, in part expressed and fortified through communal solidarity and social bonding, tended to be most willing and able to maintain their autonomy, integration and humanity in the camps. For example, religious faith and moral convictions operated to some extent as a "sacred canopy" (Berger, 1990). That is, it provided a system of meaning and metaphor by which inmates organized and interpreted their suffering and thus gave it, relative to most other inmates, manageable emotional form and moral coherence, rendering it endurable. Put differently, where suffering become sufferable is an expression of the living truth of resistance. Religious beliefs and values permitted an inmate to integrate his suffering into a theoretical-practical framework of expectation and interpretation in terms of an imagined, longed-for, glorious future. The belief in deliverance such as through divine grace, the transforming and comforting power of religious practices, rituals and communal prayers, the expectation of an afterlife—all of this provided the inmates with resources for giving their suffering meaning, and made their pain more endurable. Religious faith, like any symbolic world, whether political or in other ways secular, generated order out of chaos. However, its special characteristics allowed the inmate to interpret luck and contingency as part of a cosmic plan of divine providence, strengthening moral beliefs and values in a morally ambiguous, contradictory, capricious context where good and evil were knotted together in ethical paradox. As is well-known, Judaism and Christianity assume the existence of evil in the world, juxtaposing it with the potential antidotes of messianic hope, the belief in divinely inspired mercy, compassion and selflessness. Through these beliefs and values the inmate's determination to survive in the camps was strengthened, and perhaps most importantly, they helped maintain the moral structure of the inmate's existence. That is, the inmate's religious beliefs and values enlarged the horizon of expectation and hope beyond the immediate situation to a transcending plane of comforting cosmic meaning, thus giving the inmate a moral, cognitive, affective basis for making his suffering sufferable. Many inmates "owed their unshakeable steadfastness to the strength of the dissociative wedge of terror, and that was true not only of the Jehovah's Witnesses and the isolated clerics in Dachau; groups of Jews, Polish, French and Dutch Christians also formed a haven of solidarity and resistance" (ibid., p. 92).

Strongly held political beliefs, values and practices, especially of the Marxist variety, acted in a similar manner as religious orientation. As Sofsky summarized the matter, communist ideologies situated the camp experience within a more comprehensive, all-embracing world-historical process, so that it was possible to interpret the horrible present as a transitional phase that could be endured and ultimately triumphed over. Past experiences in political organizations and party membership provided the basis for internal group solidarity within the camp. Political beliefs and values also provided a clear delineation of who and what was the enemy, providing resistance with a clear focus, direction and rationale. Political ideology, says Sofsky, also generated the basis for social organization. It gave the death of the individual inmate a world-historical, transcending meaning. No matter how many might die as martyrs, the just cause would eventually be victorious. Compared to religious beliefs and values, continues Sofsky, political ideology had the advantage that it was more directly linked with concrete reality. It defined a secular future whose form was also dependent on the position generated in the camp, and the struggle for gains of fellow communists beyond the camp gates. While religious beliefs and values provided the standards and norms for morally correct action in the camp, by contrast, political beliefs and values offered a standard for strategically effective action (ibid., p. 93).

These observations are in sync with research using a social identity model of resistance dynamics. In this model it is assumed that members of low-status groups (e.g., camp inmates) are tied together by a feeling of shared social identity (e.g., religious and political beliefs/values), which becomes a foundation for effective leadership and organization that permits them to offset stress (at least to some degree), obtain support, contest authority and foster social change in even the most extreme situations of social inequality such as the concentration camp society of Nazi Germany, and the carceral regimes of Northern Ireland and South Africa (Haslam & Reicher, 2012b). Haslam and Reicher reject the assumptions of SPE, including as they relate to resistance, that people automatically accept the social roles and social group memberships that they are assigned by others, and that any acceptance of roles or group membership automatically means acceptance of the ways in which they are positioned in society (ibid., p. 173). In fact, as I have suggested, the opposite is sometimes true, that prisoners and camp inmates do not always identify as such. They may adapt alternative identities as did the religious or political inmates, or refuse collective identification of themselves as an expression of self/group autonomy, integration and humanity. Even when prisoners and inmates accept in a nominal sense that they are prisoners or camp inmates, it does not necessarily mean that they accept their role as subordinated, subjugated or victimized (ibid.). In fact, sometimes in the camps, inmates opted for strategic anonymity (deindividuation as Zimbardo calls it)[14] in order to avoid standing out during a Nazi roll call/selection. In other words, deindividuation had a positive function. As Terrence Des Pres noted, "the survivor must be in the world but not of it" (1977, p. 116). Inmates with strong beliefs and values were more inclined to recognize that there was a "duality of behavior" (ibid., p. 136) in the camps, that they were forced to cooperate with Nazi demands and adapt to the system. At the same time, they resisted the system and found ways to stand apart from the role and self that was taken for granted by the Nazis. Goffman refers to these two modes of behaving in the camps as "primary and secondary adjustments" (1961, pp. 188–189) and suggests that these secondary adjustments, the unauthorized modes of resisting the Nazi system, comprise what can be called the "underlife" of the camp life (and other total institutions). What Zimbardo under-theorizes is the fact that it is largely in this realm that the inmate with strong beliefs and values waged his resistance against Nazi dehumanization. Moreover, my hunch is that if the SPE had continued for many weeks, so would some of the "zombie-like" prisoners who moved through the initial phase of being overwhelmed by their imprisonment begin to fight back against their dehumanization as the survivor literature suggests was the case with inmates who held strong beliefs and values.

Implications for treatment

I am not simply suggesting that the key to resistance in a total institution is to somehow become a die-hard homo-religious or homo-politicus, despite the seeming personal advantages in terms of maintaining autonomy, integration and humanity in such contexts. By way of concluding this chapter, extrapolating from the SPE and Haslam and Reicher (2012b), the two-part question I want to briefly focus on is this: What practical wisdom can we derive from those prisoners incarcerated in an "extreme prison" for resisting the total institutions that characterize the worst aspects of modernity? How can such practical wisdom help the ordinary person struggling to live a flourishing life in the less extreme but challenging social contexts that constitute our at times dehumanizing and depersonalizing world? Of course, detailing all of this is beyond the scope of this chapter. Three points emanating from Zimbardo's experiment and the subsequent literature that it generated may be helpful to analysands and the psychotherapists working with them.

First, in the concentration camps those inmates with strong beliefs and values maintained their autonomy, integration and humanity by accessing their capacity to re-create their community in fragmented and limited but life-affirming and self-fortifying ways. Whether it was religious Jews, Catholics or Jehovah's Witnesses collectively practicing their religion, or Marxists planning and strategizing together against their Nazi rulers, these inmates were better able to maintain and express their deeply internalized beliefs and values through their re-creation of community. This gave the inmates the feeling that their pre-incarceration narrative of self-identity (i.e., the story they told themselves about who they were) and the basis of their sense of personal dignity was not completely destroyed. Without such self-respect, they become vulnerable to perhaps the most personally devastating self-relation, that of self-hatred

(Bandura, 2016, p. 29). Thus, reconstituting their "home world" (i.e., the stable, real and symbolic world they resided in prior to incarceration), however fragmented and limited, had personally sustaining consequences that tended to help inmates reinforce their ontological security (following Anthony Giddens, the stable mental condition emanating from a feeling of continuity in relation to the events in one's life), strengthen their sense of autonomy and integration, and defend against Nazi attempts to dehumanize and depersonalize them. As Auschwitz survivor and self-psychologist Anna Ornstein has pointed out in another context,

> the creation of small groups provided an opportunity to experience and express aspects of the nuclear self [i.e., an individual's most cherished ambitions and ideals], specifically related to the pole of ideas, and it provided the all-important empathic selfobject matrix [i.e., relationships that support the cohesion and vitality of the self] that reinforced a modicum of self-esteem.
>
> *(1985, p. 115)*

Moreover, it is a well-known fact that those inmates who were part of a community or group were more likely to physically survive and stay relatively psychologically intact: the community was a crucial source of emotional sustenance, morale-building, protection, information, advice and practical help to its members.

The aforementioned observations are in agreement with social identity theory of resistance in at least two ways. First, they emphasize that in most circumstances shared social identity is a source of social power. The sense of "us-ness" and "them/us" fosters a marshalling of resources by a group of like-minded people to proactively resist tyranny. Second, shared social identity, the sense of "us-ness" and "them-us" on its own is not enough to mobilize people to generate agreement on what and when effective action should be taken to achieve particular goals. Rather, social identity generates the expectation and motivation to affirm that a course of defiant action is necessary, wherein leaders and organization are necessary. Only then can social identity be the basis for transforming expectation into reality (Haslam & Reicher, 2012b, p. 174).

The take home point for resisting the extreme situation (e.g., total institutions) that also applies to less dehumanizing and depersonalizing contexts is that membership in a group that generates communal loyalty and devotion and is guided by "higher" moral beliefs and values as construed by members is an important way to help maintain one's autonomy, integration and humanity. Such group affiliation tends to counteract dehumanization, the stripping away of human qualities or assignment of demonic ones, and depersonalization, the negative effects of being treated with emotional detachment and little regard for one's personhood (Bandura, 2016, p. 89). Recall in the SPE that there was a rebellion early on that involved a few prisoners, suggesting a degree of group solidarity. By group affiliation I am not thinking of the group membership that takes place in the work context, like an entrepreneurial or work group, that gives its members and employees enhanced knowledge, connections, resources, and ideally inspiration and support (Marcus, 2017). Rather, I am imagining the kind of spiritual fellowship that one sees in firefighters or the military, in which integrity, community/team playing, flexibility/adaptability, tolerance, self-sacrifice and perhaps above all, altruism, are what matter most. As one believing Catholic fireman, quoting St. Francis of Assisi, told me in treatment, "For it is in giving that we receive."

Second, while thankfully most of us don't find ourselves in a total institution, we do have to contend with institutions and social systems that are at times dehumanizing and depersonalizing. Whether our current age is described as The Age of Anxiety (Auden, 2011), The Age of Virtuality (Van Deurzen, 2009) or The Age of Violence (Bernstein, 2013), many people living in Western society feel themselves "under siege," as if one's "world," the once comfortably self-sustaining, meaning-giving, affect-integrating, action-guiding ways of being, of thinking, feeling and acting, no longer "make sense." As we saw in the SPE, both the initially "normal average" guards and prisoners were dehumanized, the guards became abusive and sadistic while the prisoners became "zombie-like" (calling to mind the grotesque imagery of the "*muselmann*," the "walking dead" of the concentration camp) and utterly self-absorbed.[15] As Bandura pointed out, "dehumanization weakens moral self-restraints by undermining prosocialness [e.g., cooperativeness, helpfulness and sharing], blunting empathy for other's suffering, and excluding devalued individuals from the concept of common humanity" (2016, p. 36). Most of these aspects of moral disengagement were to some degree observed in the guard behavior in the SPE, while most of the prisoners became almost completely self-centric and self-serving. In contrast, says Bandura, "Perceived self-efficacy [a person's beliefs about his capabilities to produce effects] for empathy not only curtails inhumane behavior but fosters prosocial humane behavior as well" (ibid.). In other words, to become less prone to engaging in dehumanizing and cruel behavior like the SPE guards, and to be more willing and able to maintain autonomy, integration and humanity, unlike most of the SPE prisoners, an existential orientation of "empathy-induced altruism," is probably your best bet (Batson, 2018). In fact, Zimbardo quotes one prisoner who displayed "considerable principle" rather than being "blindly obedient" to the orders of the guards that affirms Batson's point: "When I entered the prison I determined to be myself as closely as I know myself. My philosophy of prison was not to cause or add to the deterioration of character on the part of fellow prisoners or myself, and to avoid causing anyone punishments because of my actions" (2007, pp. 124–125).

Very briefly, the "empathy-altruism hypothesis" defines "empathic concern" as the "other-oriented emotion elicited by and congruent with the perceived welfare of someone in need," while altruism "is the motivational state with the ultimate goal [that which is pursued for its own sake] of increasing another's welfare" (ibid., pp. 29, 22). The opposite of altruism is egoism in which the ultimate motivational goal is increasing one's welfare, though this too can be the basis for prosocial behavior like cooperativeness, helpfulness and sharing in certain contexts. "Principlism," where the ultimate goal is maintaining a moral principle, standard or ideal (i.e., "core" belief and values), and "collectivism," the ultimate goal of increasing the welfare of a group or collective (ibid., pp. 261, 260), are other general motivations of human behavior. In particular, they help maintain autonomy, integration and humanity in the face of a wide range of subverting if not destructive social influences and contexts. As Batson summarizes it, research has supported the benefits of empathy-induced altruism. For example,

> More and better help for those in need; less aggression towards them; less derogation and blaming of victims of injustice; increased cooperation in conflict situations (business negotiations, political conflicts, and tensions between students in school); less negative attitudes toward stigmatized groups; increased willingness to help those groups; more sensitive and responsive care in close relationships; increased happiness and self-esteem; less aggression; more meaning in life; even longer life.
>
> *(ibid., p. 229)*

What is important about all of this is that by enacting empathy-induced altruism in one's way of being in the world, one can draw from "a powerful force for good" (ibid.) that is potentially humanizing and in other ways beneficial to the individual, group and society.

Finally, Zimbardo's experiment emphasizes the need to resist coercive, remunerative and normative modes of power that are meant to induce obedience and conformity, as it did to the abusive guards and submissive prisoners in the SPE, or in other situations where one is vulnerable to destructive social control as a powerless outsider. Power, as Foucault has shown, is not only manifest in overt attempts to coerce, dominate and threaten the vulnerable and weak such as in the SPE, concentration camps, and other lesser but potentially destructive institutional crystallizations of power. Power is also enabling, "it produces reality; it produces domains of objects and rituals of truth," such as the expert-driven, binary labeling vocabularies of "healthy"/"adaptive," "unhealthy"/"maladaptive" and "normal"/"pathological" that can be dangerous to individual freedom and expressiveness. They deny the uniqueness, originality and specificity of the person (Foucault, 1979, p. 194). That is, power and knowledge are two elements of the "comportment-conditioning environment" (the sum of influences on actions) within which individuals act, and thus within which subjects are shaped and enact their being (Prado, 1995, pp. 71, 72), including through norm-driven, prescriptive versions of psychoanalysis and psychotherapy. The point is that power conceived as "multiplicity of force relations," as a "set of actions upon other actions" (ibid., p. 72) is enabling and inhibiting, and it is the job of the analysand and analyst to discern how these context-dependent, setting-specific force relations can be resisted in the service of one's autonomy, integration and humanity as they construe it. What Foucault said about the inventive philosopher at his best is also true for the analysand and analyst. The task is "to question over and over again what is postulated as self-evident, to disturb people's mental habits, the way they do and think things, to dissipate what is familiar and accepted, to reexamine rules and institutions" (Foucault, 1988, p. 265). By doing this, by critiquing accepted truths, institutions and practices that constitute the totality of circumstances of one's life, the analysand is better situated to be willing and able to "think differently" about his way of being-in-the-world (Foucault, 1986, p. 9). This is the key psychological condition of possibility for fashioning a credible identity and flourishing way of life that one judges as reflecting and affirming of one's moral agency and moral autonomy.

Notes

1 www.prisonexp.org/response/, retrieved 11/1/18.
2 Prominent social psychologist Albert Bandura (2016, p. 16), and C. Daniel Batson (2018, p. 252) also appear to be essentialists in their maintaining there is a non-historical "human nature."
3 Zimbardo, a strict situationalist, makes this point when he says that "[p]eople and situations are usually in a state of dynamic interaction" (2007, p. 8).
4 Similar to Milgram's study, the SPE could not be fully replicated due to ethical considerations governing social psychology research.
5 Zimbardo cites Lovibond et al. (1979) as supporting his central conclusion: "Our results thus support the major conclusion of Zimbardo et al. that hostile, confrontive relations in prison result primarily from the nature of the prison regime, rather than the personal characteristics of inmates and officers" (2007, p. 251).
6 In his book, Zimbardo says that "the student volunteers could have elected to quit at any time. No guns or legal statues bound them to their imprisonment, only a subject selection form on which they promised to do their best to last the full two weeks" (2007, p. 222).
7 The only difference between the randomly assigned participants in terms of personality variables, says Zimbardo, was that the higher the F-scale authoritarianism score, the more days the prisoner survived in this authoritarian environment (Zimbardo, 2007, p. 40). Reicher and Haslam (2006, p. 32) suggest that authoritarianism is best conceptualized as a variable outcome of social structure rather than a stable individual difference variable.
8 As Haslam and Reicher point out (2012b), the resistant prisoners gained the upper hand because: (1) modifications to the social structure allowed them to define themselves in terms of a shared identity; (2) their condition of defiance was empowered through group-based interaction; and (3) an emergent leadership served to encourage and justify acts that opposed the guard's regime that ultimately led to its defeat (p. 159).
9 Lee Strasberg, the founder of "Method" acting, noted that his Method "was the use of the soul of the actor as the material for his work—the necessity for the study of the emotions and the analysis of simple and complicated feelings." Strasberg's main way of evoking the actor's emotions, imagination and inspiration were through concentration and affective memory. The prisoners in the SPE did not engage in such deliberate conscious processes in the service of fashioning a great theatrical performance (Marcus with Marcus, 2011, p. 38).
10 Following Bruno Bettelheim, autonomy "has to do with man's inner ability to govern himself, and with a conscientious search for meaning despite the realization, that as far as we know, there is not purpose in one's life. It is a concept that does not imply a revolt against authority qua authority, but rather a quiet acting out of conviction, not out of convenience or resentment, or because of external persuasion or controls" (Bettelheim, 1960, p. 72). By integration Bettelheim means having attained an internal harmony between one's evolving personal strivings, one's values and the changing demands of the environment, such as the state, without submitting to either one at the expense of the other (Marcus, 1999, p. 17)
11 Total institution is Erving Goffman's (1961) term for a continuum of institutions in which clusters of people are bureaucratically processed while being physically removed from the normal round of activities. They are compelled to sleep, work and play within the boundaries of the same institution. Prisons and mental hospitals are Goffman's main illustrations, but he discusses other such socially controlling environments including concentration camps, boarding schools, barracks and monasteries. Exactly how "total" a total institution is depends on the degree of bureaucratization, openness versus closedness, the official intention/function of the institution and the modes used to compel compliance (Davies, 1989, p. 94). Goffman stresses that in such institutions the bureaucratic regimentation and manipulation of residents is always governed by the best interests of the staff as opposed to the residents; however, the latter group develops a wide

range of resistances to the assaults on their autonomy, integration and humanity, the "underlife."

12 "The System," says Zimbardo, is composed "of the agents and agencies whose ideology, values and power create situations and dictate the roles and expectations for approved behaviors of actors within its spheres of influence" (2007, p. 446).

13 Likewise, Primo Levi noted, "The believers in any belief whatsoever, better resisted the seduction of power … they also endured the trial of the Lager and survived in proportionately higher number … Not only during the crucial moments of selection or the aerial bombings but also in the grind of everyday life, the believers lived better" (1986, pp. 145–146).

14 Zimbardo quotes one prisoner saying after the experiment, "A good prisoner is one who knows how to strategically unify himself with other prisoners without getting put out of action himself" (2007, p. 186).

15 As one guard put it, "I realized that I was just as much a prisoner as they were … We were both crushed by the oppressiveness, but we, the guards had an illusion of freedom" (Zimbardo, 2007, pp. 187–188).

References

Améry, J. (1980). *At the mind's limits: Contemplations by a survivor of Auschwitz and its realities.* S. Rosenfeld & S.P. Rosenfeld (Trans.). Bloomington: Indiana University Press (Original work published 1964).

Auden, W.H. (2011). *The age of anxiety: Baroque Eclogue.* Princeton: Princeton University Press (Original work published 1947).

Bandura, A. (2016). *Moral disengagement: How people do harm and live with themselves.* New York: Worth Publishers.

Bandura, A., Underwood, B. & Fromson, M.E. (1975). Disinhibition of aggression through diffusion of responsibility and dehumanization of victims. *Journal of Research in Personality*, 9, 253–269.

Banuazizi, A. & Movahedi, S. (1975). Interpersonal dynamics in a simulated prison: A methodological analysis. *American Psychologist*, 30, 152–160.

Batson, C.D. (2018). *A scientific search for altruism: Do we care only about ourselves?*Oxford: Oxford University Press.

Berger, P. (1990). *The sacred canopy: Elements of a sociological theory of religion.* New York: Anchor.

Bernstein, R.J. (2013). *Violence: Thinking without banisters.* Cambridge, UK: Polity.

Bettelheim, B. (1960). *The informed heart: Autonomy in a mass age.* Glencoe: Basic Books.

Carnahan, T. & McFarland, S. (2007). Revisiting the Stanford prison experiment: Could participant self-selection have led to the cruelty? *Personality and Social Psychology Bulletin*, 33(5), 603–614.

Davies, C. (1989). Goffman's concept of the total institution: Criticisms and revisions. *Human Studies*, 22(1/2), 77–95.

Des Pres, T. (1977). *The survivor: An anatomy of life in the death camps.* New York: Pocket Books.

Foster, D. (2015). How being poor can lead to a negative spiral of fear and self-loathing. *The Guardian*, 6/30/15. Retrieved from www.theguardian.com/society/2015/jun/30/poverty-negative-spiral-fear-self-loathing.

Foucault, M. (1979). *Discipline and punishment.* A. Sheridan (Trans.). New York: Pantheon.

Foucault, M. (1986). *The use of pleasure.* R. Hurley (Trans.). New York: Vintage.

Foucault, M. (1988). *Michel Foucault: Politics, philosophy, culture: Interviews and other writings 1977–1984.* L.D. Kritzman (Ed.). Oxford: Blackwell.

Fromm, E. (1973). *The anatomy of human destructiveness.* New York: Holt, Rinehart and Winston.

Goffman, E. (1961). *Asylums.* New York: Anchor Books.

Haney, C., Banks, C. & Zimbardo, P. (1973). A study of prisoners and guards in a simulated prison. *Naval Research Reviews* (September), 1–17. Washington, DC: Office of Naval Research.
Haslam, S.A. & Reicher, S.D. (2012a). Contesting the "nature" of conformity: What Milgram and Zimbardo's studies really show. *PLOS Biology*, 10(11), 1–4.
Haslam, S.A. & Reicher, S.D. (2012b). When prisoners take over the prison: A social psychology of resistance. *Personality and Social Psychology Review*, 16(2), 154–179.
Haslam, S.A. & Reicher, S.D. (Eds.) (2017). *Social psychology: Revisiting the classic studies* (2nd ed.). Los Angeles: Sage.
Levi, P. (1986). *The drowned and the saved.* New York: Summit.
Lifton, R.J. (1986). *The Nazi doctors: Medical killing and the psychology of genocide.* New York: Basic Books.
Lovibond, S.H., Mithiran, X. & Adams, W.G. (1979). The effects of three experimental prison environments on the behavior of non-convict volunteer subjects. *Australian Psychologist*, 14, 273–287.
Marcus, P. (1999). *Autonomy in the extreme situation: Bruno Bettelheim, the Nazi concentration camps and the mass society.* Westport: Praeger.
Marcus, P. (2017). *The psychoanalysis of career choice, job performance, and satisfaction: How to flourish in the workplace.* London: Routledge.
Marcus, P. with Marcus, G. (2011). *Theatre as life: Practical wisdom drawn from great acting teachers, actors and actresses.* Milwaukee: Marquette University Press.
Martin, C. (2014). *Moral decision making: How to approach everyday ethics. Course guidebook. The great courses.* Chantilly: The Teaching Company.
Maslach, C. (2000). Emperor of the edge. *Psychology Today.* Retrieved from www.psychologytoday.com/us/articles/200009/emperor-the-edge.
Ornstein, A. (1985). Survival and recovery. *Psychoanalytic Inquiry*, 5(1), 99–130.
Prado, C.G. (1995). *Starting with Foucault: An introduction to genealogy.* Boulder: Westview.
Reicher, S.D. & Haslam, S.A. (2006). Rethinking the psychology of tyranny: The BBC Prison Experiment. *British Journal of Social Psychology*, 45, 1–40.
Smith, R., Mackie, D.M. & Claypool, H.M. (Eds.) (2015). *Social psychology* (4th ed.). New York: Psychology Press.
Sofsky, W. (1997). *The ordeal of terror: The concentration camps.* W. Templer (Trans.). Princeton: Princeton University Press.
Van Deurzen, E. (2009). *Psychotherapy and the quest for happiness.* Los Angeles: Sage.
Zimbardo, P. (2007). *The Lucifer Effect: Understanding how good people turn evil.* New York: Random House.
Zimbardo, P. (2004). A situationalist perspective on the psychology of evil. Understanding how good people are transformed into perpetrators. In A. Miller (Ed.), *The Social psychology of good and evil* (pp. 21–50). New York: Guilford.
Zimbardo, P. (2018). Philip Zimbardo's response to recent criticisms of the Stanford Prison Experiment. *Stanford Prison Experiment.* Retrieved from www.prisonexp.org/response/.

9

STEREOTYPES AND UNDERPERFORMANCE

Steele and Aronson's stereotype threat studies (1995)

It was the great interactionist sociologist Erving Goffman who famously used the term "stigma" to denote the labels that society applies to devalue members of particular social groups (1963). These moral "blemishes" or "abominations" of physical identity (facial disfigurement or blindness), individual character (imprisonment or mental disorder) or group identity (being from a specific race, nation or religion), discredit a person's claim to "normal" identity (p. 4). The person is viewed as having an "undesired differentness from what we had anticipated … the person with a stigma is not quite human" (ibid., p. 5). In our episteme, our sociocultural reality, people are typically stigmatized on their physical or behavioral characteristics. Indeed, there probably isn't a person in Western society who has not felt stigmatized in some way during their lifetime through real or imagined exclusion, marginalization or discrimination. Shame and guilt, anxiety and fear, and anger and hostility are some of the troubling emotions that are evoked when one has to live with a "spoiled identity," as Goffman calls it. This being said, as Erçetin et al. (2016)[1] point out, if stigma is defined as a notion that makes reference to socially ostracized individuals and/or groups that have objectionable characteristics as judged by society (lodged in prejudices, stereotypic thoughts and labeling), then individuals who have lives that transcend societal standards and characteristics that entice public attention that is societally inconsistent also experience stigmatization. By this definition, they suffer from positive stigma (Goffman, 1963, p. 141)[2], such as "beautifulness stigma, success stigma, intelligence stigma, wealth stigma, sexiness stigma, independence stigma, happiness stigma, power stigma, and prophet-hood stigma and so on" (ibid.). While I believe that positive stigma has its deleterious psychological features, some which have a "family resemblance" to "negative stigma," in this chapter I focus on the adverse impact of negative stigma on an ordinary person's way of being-in-the-world,[3] in particular the stigma pressure associated with work (i.e., performance on tasks), as this is the domain of Steele and Aronson's research and the thousands of studies that followed.

In their "now-classic series of studies" (Shapiro & Neuberg, 2007, p. 108), Steele and Aronson (1995) described how the salience of stigmatized status negatively impacted African American academic performance and aspiration in terms of what they called "stereotype threat." Stereotype threat

> can be thought of as the discomfort targets feel when they are at risk of fulfilling a negative stereotype about their group; the apprehension that they could behave in such a way as to confirm the stereotype—in the eyes of others, in their own eyes, or both at the same time.
>
> *(Aronson et al., 1998, pp. 85–86)*

Stereotype threat does not only involve academic underperformance of stigmatized groups like African Americans who have been discriminated against as being unintelligent and academically inept. In addition, it has been found in a variety of groups with alternative stereotypes regarding performance, such as women who are thought to be less competent in math compared to men,[4] elderly folks who display diminished cognitive/memory performance, Latinxs whose performance spirals down on tests labeled as predictive of intelligence, negotiations and financial decision-making (Shapiro & Neuberg, 2007; Spencer et al., 2016). Even so-called high-status and non-stigmatized groups such as white males, in such areas as "natural athletic ability" (i.e., in golf putting) where negative stereotypes are operative about them (i.e., that whites have less natural ability than blacks), have shown stereotype threat (Stone, 2002). In fact, when modifying the definition of the putting task from "natural athletic ability" to being an assessment of "sports strategic intelligence," the performance ranking of white and black players were totally reversed (Steele, 2010, p. 215). As Spencer et al. noted in their review of the vast literature on stereotype threat, "Every individual is potentially vulnerable to stereotype threat, because every individual has at least one social identity that is targeted by a negative stereotype in some given situation" (2016, p. 417). And Claude M. Steele, the senior co-originator of the concept of stereotype threat, puts this point even stronger: "Stereotype threat … is a general phenomenon. It happens to all of us, all the time" (2010, p. 209). This being said, as sociologist William B. Helmreich notes, diverse research suggests that among Americans, "it turns out that approximately one third of the stereotypes can be said to have a good deal of truth to them" (2009, p. 244). However, while some of the negative stereotypes tend to be true, "most of the stereotypes for which support can be found are positive and flattering to the group involved, whereas those that seem highly inaccurate tend, by and large, to be negative" (ibid.).

In this chapter I will first summarize Steele and Aronson's "ground-breaking set of studies" (Schmader & Forbes, 2017, p. 245) on stereotype threat, which is the dread of confirming others' negative stereotyping of one's group, and how this threat affects individual performance. Next, I will provide some psychoanalytically animated remarks on the personal impact on the stigmatized person when in a situation in which there is a negative stereotype about their group (Spencer et al., 2016, p. 416). Finally, I will describe strategies of people who feel stereotype threat but are good at self-mastery over its negative personal consequences. For as Goffman has noted, while the experience of being stigmatized can powerfully negatively impact individual self-esteem, self-concept, academic attainment and motivation,[5] there are those stigmatized people who have high self-esteem and a good self-concept, who academically and in other ways perform at impressive levels, and describe themselves as fairly resistant to their negative social experiences associated with stigma pressure (Heatherton et al., 2000). Indeed, Steele's memoir (2010) of his intellectual odyssey as an African American social psychologist appears to be an example of this phenomenon: "When barriers arise, we're supposed to march through the storm, picking ourselves up by our bootstraps. I have to count myself a subscriber to this creed" (Steele, 2010, p. 4). While Steele acknowledges "the psychic damage of self-doubt and low expectations" (ibid., p. 57) associated with stereotype threat that can negatively influence one's ability to effectively work and love, and notes that "internal characteristics are hard to change" (ibid., p. 216),[6] he emphasizes from his own experience that "situational identity contingencies [roughly the totality of circumstances you have to cope with], the cues that signal them, and the narratives that interpret them are easier to change" (ibid.).

Steele and Aronson's stereotype threat studies

Steele and Aronson (1995) administered a challenging verbal test derived from the Advanced Graduate Record Examination to African American and white students at Stanford University. The investigator led half of the students from each race to believe that he was measuring their intellectual ability ("this is a genuine test of your true ability") and they had to mark their race, the diagnostic condition[7] that was intentionally meant to stimulate stereotype pressure among the African American students [i.e., that they were intellectually inferior; books like *The Bell Curve* (Herrnstein & Murray, 1994) allegedly supported this stereotype].[8] The white group was made to believe that the investigator was simply attempting to further develop the validity and reliability of a new test, and therefore their performance was irrelevant to their actual intellectual ability. The results were astonishing: white students performed equally well whether they believed the test was a measure of their intellectual ability or not, while African American students who believed they were taking a test of intellectual ability performed significantly worse compared to whites (i.e., 4.4 test items correct out of 20 compared to 10.2 for whites). However, African American students who believed the test was not measuring their intellectual ability performed as well as whites. Thus, the manner in which people explain to themselves their academic performance can have significant effects on how well they perform.

In explaining their findings, Steele and Aronson were not sure of the precise mechanisms at play, but they focused on "how social context and group identity come together to mediate an important behavior" (ibid., p. 810). Specifically, stigma pressure on intellectual performance for African Americans reflected "pressure [that] was a contingency of these group's identities," one that had a "serious toll—impaired performance on the kind of test on which one's opportunities can depend" (Steele, 2010, p. 52). "Identity contingencies" are "the things you have to deal with in a situation because you have a given social identity" (ibid., p. 3). Social identity refers to those elements of the self-concept that emanate from a person's knowledge and feelings about his group affiliations that he has in common with others. Thus, identity contingencies are the "circumstances you have to deal with in order to get what you want or need in a situation," such as being African American, a white man, elderly, young, gay, a woman, Latinx, politically conservative or liberal, diagnosed with mental illness, a cancer or an AIDS patient, et cetera (ibid.). Steele and Aronson (1995) mentioned such performance-interfering/worsening factors among their African American naïve subjects as "inefficiency of processing" and "impaired efficiency" similar to that generated by other kinds of evaluative pressures (ibid., p. 809) and "lower expectations" that "can play a role in mediating stereotype threat" (ibid.).

As Aronson et al. (1998) noted, more precisely explaining their stereotype threat finding regarding African Americans was hardly straightforward, and they urged fellow social psychologists to tease out the potentially different threats that may be operative in the general phenomenon of stereotype threat (Shapiro & Neuberg, 2007, p. 112).

> Is stereotype threat self-threatening because it arouses a fear of being a bad ambassador of one's group to mainstream society? Or is it more simply the apprehension about appearing incompetent—for the sake of one's reputation? Or, alternatively, is it merely the result of worrying that one might lack ability? Or is it some combination of these concerns? These are important questions that will have to await the results of future research for answers.
>
> *(Aronson et al., 1998, p. 43)*

Steele more recently summarized the "chief discovery of our research," suggesting possible explanations for the negative impact of stereotype threat:

> The protective side of the human character can be aroused by the mere prospect of being negatively stereotyped, and that, once aroused, it steps in and takes over the capacities of the person—to such an extent that little capacity is left over for the work at hand. It shows that this side of the human character, aroused this way, affects our thoughts, emotions, actions and performances in ways that have nothing to do with our internal traits, capacities, motivations, and so on. And that these effects contribute importantly to group differences in behavior, ranging from math performance to the interest when in interracial conversations to playing golf.
>
> *(2010, p. 214)*

Steele more precisely elaborates why he believes stereotype threat can have such a negative impact on the person, saying, "Even the mild short-lived doses of stereotype threat that can be implemented in these experiments are enough to raise your blood pressure, dramatically increase ruminative thinking, interfere with working memory, and deteriorate performance on challenging tasks" (ibid., p. 132). And even worse, if you carry on for an extended period of time to care and labor in a domain "where your group is negatively stereotyped, disadvantaged, and discriminated against," the likelihood of having serious health problems like hypertension greatly increases (ibid.). Aspects of stereotype threat and performance are hotly contested, and it "continues to be an intensely debated and researched topic in educational, social and organizational psychology" (Spencer et al., 2016, p. 415). Thus, a more in-depth understanding of some of the mediating and moderating factors animating this harsh situational predicament is warranted.

The bases of stereotype threat

Steele et al. (2002) have emphasized that an important source of stereotype threat is related to the social cues that put the threat into sharp emotional focus, a fertile breeding ground for later psychological problems that contribute to impaired performance. While the psychoanalyst would be inclined to look for dispositional factors, such as lack of self-confidence, an over-reactivity to potential discrimination or poor frustration tolerance, Steele and his colleagues looked at other contextual factors to explain what governs how much an individual is impacted by stereotype threat (Steele, 2010, p. 138).[9]

Social cues are the social symbols manifested through body language, tone or words that are meant to convey a positive or negative message between people. They are a form of "hint-based" communication that assists us in navigating our relationships and interactions with other people. Stereotype threat pertains to any cue that suggests a cultural stereotype that is potentially negatively judged and therefore makes the target feel vulnerable. When this feeling of vulnerability, of worrying, escalates, a sense of identity threat is prone to arise. In short, it is not individual traits that matter most in terms of one of the identities of a person, but "contingency-signaling cues in a setting" (Steele, 2010, p. 139). Examples of such social cues that call to mind identity contingencies are numerical under-representation, like being the only African American in a board meeting or the only woman in a university math department, or prejudicial attitudes that are expressed by high-status individuals during interactions in the workplace. In fact, anything in the ongoing environment, whether human or object and explicit or ambiguous, can put into question a person's sense of being welcomed and belonging. They feel "identity unsafe." "Identity safe" classrooms, for example, are those in which teachers attempt to guarantee that students feel that their social identities are an advantage as opposed to an impediment or barrier to flourishing in the classroom. Thus, for Steele, identity threat is not "rooted in an internal psychological trait, or vulnerability of some sort," but context-dependent, setting-specific "cues and contingencies" (ibid., p. 151). It is important to note that in Steele's view, stereotype threat need not be blatant and harsh; in fact, it is typically "cues—often innocent-appearing cues that seemed to be natural, unavoidable ingredients of the situation," that "regulate how much identity threat a person feels" (ibid., p. 139). In other words, stereotype threats are omnipresent, "in the air" (ibid., p. 5).

Stereotype mediators

Given the fact that stereotype is such a diffuse phenomenon that operates among a wide range of populations and settings, it is not surprising that it is mediated by many factors. Such contributions to underperformance like additional pressure to succeed, threats to self-integrity and priming of stereotypes have been researched and found to have a role in stereotype threat (Spencer et al., 2016, p. 419).

Additional pressures to succeed

Researchers have found that additional pressure can subvert performance, by the negative effects of exerting greater effort, working memory diminution and conscious attention to automatic processes. Exerting greater effort simply means that individuals experiencing stereotype threat are driven to perform well on tasks that matter to them so they can disconfirm the stereotype. This effort potentiates the dominant response on a particular task, specifically on tough tasks that challenge a skill set, such as academic examinations, and can lead to underperformance (stereotype threat often leads to better performance on easy tasks, probably the consequence of increased effort).

Working memory (or short-term memory) is a system for temporarily storing and managing the information necessary to do complex cognitive tasks such as learning, reasoning and comprehension. Working memory is operative in the selection, initiation, and termination of information-processing functions like encoding, storing and retrieving data. Working memory is not only operative in test-taking contexts, but also in conversations and discussions with others, or, say, with the white student reading homework assignments for an African American political science class by himself in a dorm room (even more so if he were the only white student in the class) (Steele, 2010, p. 123). When stereotype threat is in play, the negative stereotype becomes disturbingly pertinent to one's task performance. It can bring about a full-blown stress response (i.e., one that is psychophysical) and a hyper-vigilant monitoring process to discern information pertinent to self-identity and indications of failure. Efforts to suppress troubling thoughts and uncomfortable feelings are also at play, and thus diminish working memory, which impairs successful performance (Spencer et al., 2016, p. 421). Thus, it is not hard to imagine the detrimental influence of stereotype threat on working memory that serves to undermine performance with so much "performance-worsening rumination"—racing thoughts, hyper-vigilance to those things pertinent to the threat and generating tactics to avoid them, self-distrust about what is reality-based or imagined, anxious scanning of the totality of circumstances of how one is faring, and efforts to stay task focused (Schmader et al., 2008; Steele, 2010, p. 123). The psychological lynchpin of this ruminative dwelling is what has been called a "discrepancy monitor." This is an anxiety-driven process that repeatedly monitors and assesses the self and the present circumstances against a model, standard or norm, such as a notion of what is wished for, required, expected or feared. Once this discrepancy monitor is activated, it will locate mismatches between how things are and how we believe they should be. Noting these mismatches stimulates additional efforts to diminish these discrepancies in a seemingly endless, unproductive "single loop" that feels to the person like he is on "a runaway train" (Segal et al., 2013, p. 66).

Likewise, when one is self-monitoring perceived threats, activated by stereotype threat, there can be a subversion of the automaticity of behavior, of well-learned skill sets that do not depend on working memory that one usually does without conscious attention. For example, highly skilled, seasoned golfers have been found to have diminished putting skills under stereotype threat, seemingly because anxious attention is utilized on procedure-oriented processes that ordinarily operate outside of working memory. When these golfers are given a secondary task to use up working memory, their performance under threat is reinstated to its previous level (Beilock et al., 2007; Spencer et al., 2016, p. 421).

Threats to self-integrity

Though enigmatic, the virtue term self-integrity is one of the most frequently used terms by psychologists and philosophers.[10]

Its meaning and how it is instantiated is radically philosophical, yet its definition is "up for grabs." In stereotype threat literature, it is roughly equivalent to "self-worth," that is, "the sense of oneself as a coherent and valued entity" (Spencer et al., 2016, pp. 421, 420). Thus, it is alleged that the underperformance that one observes in a stereotype threat situation is rooted in the defensive tactics that targets implement to shield and sustain self-worth or self-esteem. Such self-sabotaging behavior may be manifest in not adequately practicing, as was the case in the golf-putting example, in reporting full-blown stress reactions that self-justify impaired performance, or by trying to answer fewer questions on a test (ibid., p. 421). Ultimately, the self-sabotaging person is implementing avenues of flight from reckoning with what he imagines are the "real" reasons for his lack of optimal performance, namely his lack of objective competence and ability. Thus, he generates responsibility-dodging rationalizations like lack of effort and lower expectations to account for his poor performance. As Steele notes, citing Cohen et al.'s (2006) research on minority student classroom behavior in K through 12, identity threat is similar to self-image or self-worth threats, namely, a threat to a student's sense of himself as being "morally and adaptively adequate" (Steele, 2010, p. 173). In a classroom there can be a number of continuous social cues that threaten a minority student's perceived self-integrity, such as being a member of a devalued if not debased minority group, having a negative stereotype about your group being repeatedly pertinent to significant classroom activities, and confronting a group-based social organization that intimates your marginal status. In the classroom setting, identity threat can profoundly undermine a minority student's sense of competence and belonging (ibid.).

Priming the stereotype

Priming is an unconscious process which happens as a consequence of learning. A famous example of priming was Pavlov's dog experiment, wherein the dog learned to expect food at the sound of a bell and salivated upon hearing the sound. Salivation was not consciously controlled by the dog, but rather it was an unconscious response to the bell. Likewise, if an individual consistently responds in a particular way to a stimulus, his future response will be implemented in an unconscious automatic manner. Such behavior is not produced by a person's idiosyncratic perceptions or judgments. Thus, when a stereotype becomes mobilized, stereotype-consistent behavior automatically follows from the mobilization. For example, if a person dresses in softer, mild colors and talks and walks slower, he will prime his targets to be calmer and more accepting, or young adults primed with an elderly stereotype usually walk more slowly (Spencer et al., 2016).[11]

Thus, in this ideomotor model, where involuntary motor activity is viewed as caused by an idea, all persons mindful of the primed stereotypes are equally vulnerable to their effects. In other words, the actual pertinence of the stereotype is irrelevant. This is decidedly not the case in most stereotype threat literature, as the stereotype has to be pertinent to the targeted person's social identity. As Steele noted, research has indicated "but one prerequisite" to stereotype pressure, "the person has to care about the performance in question," as this makes the possibility of confirming the negative stereotype distressing enough to hinder performance (Steele, 2010, p. 98). In fact, if the stereotype threat is not pertinent to the person's social identity, "stereotype lift" or the enhancement of performance in a particular domain can occur. Stereotype lift happens when an outgroup is negatively stereotyped. For example, men primed with female stereotypes show this stereotype lift in their performance in math (Spencer et al., 2016). In contrast, "stereotype boost" happens when there is the mobilization of a positive ingroup stereotype. That is, stereotype performance boosts result from exposure to positive stereotypes. For example, Asians primed with a stereotype that they are intellectually and academically superior can attain better test scores and grades.

In summary, Steele and other stereotype threat researchers have provided experimental verification for the common experience that when one belongs to a devalued or stigmatized group, at least in particular contexts and settings, one is likely to feel negatively impacted, for example intellectually compromised, psychophysically "stressed out" and uncomfortable in interactions with others who are from different groups. All that is required is that one know about the stereotype (not necessarily believing it is true), though the more stigma aware one is, and the more one cares about one's performance (and thus the more identity threatening in terms of self-conception and status), the greater the negative effect tends to be. As Schmader and Forbes noted in their review chapter, "priming negatively stereotyped individuals with their group membership in an evaluative setting ha[s] led to effects on performance or other outcomes consistent" with stereotype threat theory (2017, p. 250).[12] Moreover, the contingencies that are associated with social identity, whether racial, sexual or political, are "often subtle enough to be beneath our awareness," yet have deleterious impact on our functioning (Steele, 2010, p. 61).[13] Indeed, who cannot empathize with Simone Young, the fifty-seven-year-old world-class white Australian music conductor, and one of the first women to conduct a classical orchestra worldwide, when she painfully observed, "Somehow, if a man gets in front of an orchestra and does a bad job, people say, 'Well, we won't have him back again.' But if a woman fails, they say, 'See what happens when you have a woman conductor'" (Smith et al., 2015, p. 213).

Some psychoanalytic reflections on the heavy cross to bear of stereotype threat

Now that we have a sense for how and why stigma threat can cut so deeply into our narrative of self-identity, including our self-concept and self-worth, the question is what can we do to protect ourselves from this sense of being a devalued if not despised other, the reflected "un-glory" of the social group to which we belong. Perhaps it is worth remembering the counter-intuitive research finding "that individual members of many stigmatized groups, including Blacks, people with developmental disabilities, and people who are facially disfigured, have self-esteem that is just as high as that of individuals who are not members of these groups" (ibid., p. 215). How some people personally shield themselves from much of the deleterious impact of stereotype threat is the subject to which we now turn.

Freud was no stranger to stereotype threat. It was a phenomenon that he had to contend with as he developed and disseminated psychoanalysis. For example, Freud felt that the biggest impediment confronting what he called "the Cause" (i.e., the expansion of psychoanalysis) was anti-Semitism. Freud himself was a "godless" Jew (though he had a strong Jewish identity), and the analysts who came together in his living room in 1902 to create the Wednesday Psychological Society (the world's first psychoanalytic association) were secular Jews. Freud was afraid that psychoanalysis would become so linked with Judaism that it would never have traction in mainstream science. "Our Aryan comrades are," he wrote to a friend, "quite indispensable to us; otherwise, psychoanalysis would fall victim to anti-Semitism" (Freud & Abraham, 2002, p. 72). Thus, Carl Jung was everything Freud could have wished for: gifted, public-minded, a respected member of the scientific establishment—and, most of all, born without a drop of Jewish blood in his Swiss Protestant veins. "Only his appearance," Freud disclosed, "has saved psychoanalysis from the danger of being a Jewish national concern."[14]

This being said, by about 1909, the first cracks in what was later to be a full-blown split between Freud and Jung occurred. Freud ended their relationship in a famous letter dated 1913, based on what can be described as irreconcilable differences, including those related to the future of psychoanalysis. Jung, some believe, showed his "true colors" on the Jewish science issue and the "Jewish problem" in general when he became a Nazi sympathizer and actor, including writing in 1934, "The Aryan unconscious has a greater potential than the Jewish unconscious."[15]

Freud's way of responding to stereotype threat was to deny that psychoanalysis was a "Jewish science," a stigmatizing affliction at the time, even though the great majority of the early devotees to psychoanalysis were Jewish, and some of his elemental discoveries were likely lodged in the Jewish mystical tradition (Bakan, 2004). In addition to his denial of the "Jewishness" of psychoanalysis, Freud used Jung as his real and symbolic medium for "passing" psychoanalysis off as an objective science that had universal application to the non-Jewish majority culture he lived and worked in.

"Passing" is the term used when a person tries to be viewed as a member of an identity group or category other than their own, such as race, ethnicity, caste, social class, sexuality, gender, religion, age or disability status. Passing serves as a way to gain increased social acceptance as well as other material and psychological benefits that may result. Most importantly perhaps, from a psychoanalytic point of view, passing is a way to manage social anxiety of being different, often a despised other, and in this sense, it can be self-sustaining and self-shielding. Jews, blacks and many other minorities have historically attempted to change their accents, word selections, ways of dressing, grooming behavior, names and physicality (e.g., "nose jobs," lip-reduction and hair straightening) in an effort to pass in the eyes of members of the majority and/or privileged group. While passing may achieve acceptance into a perceived higher-status community, it also can propel a person to temporarily or permanently abandon his community of origin. While passing can foster financial security, physical safety and evasion of stigma pressure, it can have negative emotional consequences as a function of the denial/avoidance of one's background, and a feeling of being untrue to oneself, and/or anxiety about being "outed." As one of my financially successful, highly educated black patients once told me, he spent most of his young adulthood feeling he was disapprovingly and offensively viewed as an "Oreo" (a brand of cookie composed of two chocolate wafers with a sweet crème filling). By this he meant he was seen as "black on the outside and white on the inside," that he had embraced the attitudes, values and behavior judged as typical of middle-class white society while repudiating his own ethnic heritage. Conscious and unconscious self-hatred and depression are sometimes the result of this relationship to oneself when passing is the overriding goal. This kind of self-hatred was described by Freud in *Mourning and Melancholia* and in a letter to the Jewish gay essayist Kurt Hiller in which Freud commented on an anti-Semitic letter he received from Theodor Lessing, asking Hiller, "Do you not think that self-hatred like Lessing's is an exquisite Jewish phenomenon"(Marcus & Rosenberg, 1989, p. 46).[16] It also appears in an essay, "Self-Hatred Among Jews" (1941), by Kurt Lewing, the father of social psychology.

It was Anna Freud, Freud's daughter and a brilliantly innovative child psychoanalyst, who dramatically redefined psychoanalytic group membership in a favorable manner, a form of "social creativity" that counters stereotype threat. Social creativity involves strategically introducing and stressing new aspects of social comparison on which a negatively judged group can view itself as superior (Smith et al., 2015, p. 221). In 1977, Anna Freud via a proxy who gave her lecture in honor of the first Freud Professorship at Hebrew University, an International Psychoanalytic Congress held in Israel, noted that

> During the era of its existence, psychoanalysis has entered into connexion [*sic*] with various academic institutions, not always with satisfactory results … It has also, repeatedly, experienced rejection by them, being criticized for its methods being imprecise, its findings not being open to proof by experiment, for being unscientific, even for being a Jewish science. However the other derogatory comments

may be evaluated, it is, I believe, the last-mentioned connotation, which under present circumstances, can serve as a title of honor.

(Stewart-Steinberg, 2011, p. 104)

Anna Freud's referencing of psychoanalysis as a "title of honor" rather than one of shame was a way of reinforcing group self-esteem and distinctiveness, a creative strategy that is sometimes used when group boundaries are perceived as fairly fixed. When group boundaries are more permeable, individuals implement strategies of "individual mobility," fleeing a perceived physical or psychological threat from being a member of a stigmatized group. This sometimes involves group membership suppression, a form of passing, or disidentification or dissociation (Smith et al., 2015, p. 219).

Disidentification in psychoanalysis refers to the casting off of the personal impact of a former identification. It is not simply the opposite of behavioral imitation, the way it is typically understood in social psychology. Generally speaking, in psychoanalysis, identification is said to occur when an individual "extends his identity *into* someone else … borrows an identity *from* someone else …, or fuses his identity *with* someone else" (Rycroft, 1995, p. 76). Disidentification suggest a significant modification of subjective experience and explicit behavior that matches a particular object (i.e., a psychologically significant person). For example, a teenage boy might emotionally and practically distance himself from his mother in order to strengthen his masculine identity. In social-psychological language, disidentification has been defined as an individual's gross reduction of their personal association with a perceived stigmatized group and is regarded as a phenomenon that only "takes place in the mind" (Smith et al., 2015, p. 220). Examples of disidentification are evading cues of membership in such a devalued group, publicly disapproving or discrediting an ingroup member's behavior, and judging oneself to be an exception in word and deed compared to other group members (ibid.).

Dissociation, a vague if not disputed notion in psychoanalysis, has been defined as "the state of affairs in which two or more mental processes co-exist without becoming connected or integrated" (Rycroft, 1995, p. 39). It was called "splitting" by the famous psychoanalyst Donald Winnicott as early as 1960, which contributed to the two terms having roughly the same meaning in the eyes of most analysts. Splitting is a defense mechanism "by which a mental structure loses its integrity and becomes replaced by two or more part structures" (ibid., p. 173). This process can be of the ego and/or the object. In social psychology, unlike disidentification which is described as occurring only in the mind, dissociation pertains to "actual," overt behavioral "escape" from a socially disadvantaged group or the hiding of group affiliation (Smith et al., 2015, p. 120), such as American and English Jews anglicizing their surnames or gay people who remain "in the closet." Goffman describes these attempts to hide or obliterate signs that have become "stigma symbols," such as a person with deteriorating eyesight not wearing bifocals because to do so might indicate old age (1963, p. 92).

What needs to be emphasized is that disidentification and dissociation are only viewed as either in the mind or overt behavior if one regards human existence as lodged in a mind/body duality or split. Social psychologists make this distinction, as discussed earlier in the chapter, and psychoanalysts tend to focus mainly on the mind and not overt behavior in the "real world." Following Heidegger and existential phenomenology, human existence is best conceived as an integrated whole in which the mind and overt behaviors are not discrete domains, but only being-in-the-world. That is, in this view, there is no isolated psyche with its intra-psychic parts or dynamics; existence is not experienced "in the head," nor is it experienced as overt behavior implemented "out there;" rather, being-in-the-world always involves cognitive, affective/kinesthetic and behavioral processes that reflect lived in-the-world experiences. "Existence is *dasein* [being], fundamentally in the world" (Cooper, 2017, p. 46). For example, an African American residing in the totality of circumstances called stereotype threat engages in both disidentification (allegedly in the mind) and dissociation (allegedly enacted in overt behavior) in one form or another. Moreover, he has conscious and unconscious thoughts, feelings and bodily sensations as he enacts his avenue of flight. Thoughts, feelings/kinesthetics and actions are always holistically interrelated, interdependent and interactive, and such a theoretical perspective is perhaps the most illuminating angle of vision when trying to understand stereotype threat as a way of being-in-the-world. This being said, in the clinical context, helping an analysand become aware of his stereotype threat experience as an assemblage of distinct components rather than as a single "thing" with an amorphous shape can be the onset of a critically reflective process of deconstruction. Such a process can potentiate in the analysand a way to respond more skillfully rather than to respond habitually (Segal et al., 2013, p. 166).

It should also be mentioned that when stereotype threat is conceived as a way of being-in-the-world by an observer, it tends to put into sharp focus the intensity of this psychological experience to the target. In particular, most targets of stereotype threat feel like nothing short of a "hunted animal," as the term target implies. I am, for example, thinking of some of my former patients: the light-skinned African man who attempted to conceal his blackness and ancestry and fashioned a white identity; the Jewish woman who not only changed her Jewish-sounding name but got a cosmetic rhinoplasty to make her prominent "Jewish nose" less visible; and most recently, the Hispanic man who felt that he had to go out of his way to demonstrate to non-Hispanics that he was neither a gang member, drug dealer nor illegal immigrant. In all of these cases of stereotype threat, the person's way of being-in-the-world was characterized by feeling "under siege." They all had a perceived sense of privation, blocking and constriction of what was possible in their work, love and everyday lives (Cooper, 2017, p. 47).

Implications for treatment

While stereotype threat has been addressed by social psychologists in ways that have reportedly diminished its detrimental impact, mainly by diminishing the threat such as in identity-safe contexts which led to enhanced performance, for most people going about their everyday lives, the concern is how to best insulate themselves from the toxicity of stigma pressure, or as Goffman calls those visible stigmas that are impossible to camouflage, "stigmatizing affliction[s]" (1963, p. 73). Put simply, how does one protect oneself from a perceived stigma, a "situation of the individual who is disqualified from full social acceptance" (ibid., preface, np), who has, "an attribute that is deeply discrediting" by virtue of his group affiliation (ibid., p. 3)? Given that any stigma involves a "special kind of relationship between an attribute and a stereotype" (ibid., p. 4), say being African American and viewed as inherently "stupid," or Jewish and viewed as inherently "cheap," how can a person develop a way of being-in-the-world that maintains his self-respect and fosters an effective, if not flourishing, existence? Steele describes this overarching goal and opportunity that he suggests all stigmatized people desire, "the good life" (2010, p. 3).

Narcissistic vulnerability

For Freud, and most modern psychoanalysts, it is assumed that man is fundamentally egotistical. That is, he takes his own needs and desires as most important and in most instances he thinks about the other second. In many cultures, human beings seem to be mainly for themselves. Altruistic behavior, even everyday kindness like someone holding the door open for you, is so striking because it is rare. Thus, in modern psychoanalysis, narcissism as a "bedrock" or limit condition of human existence has been defined as a person's "love, regard, and valuation of his or her own self" (Person et al., 2005, p. 555). So-called "normal narcissism," admittedly a clinical value judgment, is manifested in reasonable self-care, self-confidence and pride, while "heightened narcissism" is manifest in vanity, insistence on privilege, overstated claims of superiority over others, or in its extreme, out-and-out grandiosity (ibid.). Finally, and most importantly to understand stereotype threat, "the more a person's narcissism, the more aggressively he or she may react to real or imagined insults, and the greater his or her vulnerability to humiliation and shame" (ibid.).

It is the last aforementioned sentence that I want to focus on, for I believe that to the extent that one's narrative of self-identity (e.g., one's self-concept and self-esteem) is vulnerable to insult, humiliation, shame, and, I would add, guilt, which is often clinically coupled with shame, the more likely he will be susceptible to stereotype threat. While shame and guilt both reflect "moral angst," they have been conceptualized differently. As experimental personality researchers have noted, shame centers on the self while guilt centers on behavior. Shame emerges when people negatively appraise the global self ("I am bad"), while guilt emerges when people negatively appraise a specific behavior ("I did something bad"). Moreover, shame has been found to be a more painful and distressing feeling because, in light of failure and transgression (including the stigmatized person being "authentic" or "inauthentic" in his mode of being),[17] the whole self is judged as deficient and imperfect, leading to feelings of worthlessness, powerlessness and the wish to vanish (e.g., passing). Shamed people often ruminate on how defectively they are viewed by others (Tangney & Dearing, 2002; Tangney & Mahek, 2004), as in people who feel serious stereotype pressure. As Goffman notes about the stigmatized, "shame becomes a central possibility, arising from the individual's perception of one of his own attributes as being a defiling thing to possess, and one he can readily see himself not possessing" (1963, p. 7). Psychoanalytically speaking, shame is lodged in the painful feeling of failure for not behaving in a manner that is in accordance with one's expectations of one's ego-ideal (roughly the ideal conception of oneself rooted in childhood experience), while guilt emerges when a person feels he has violated a prohibition of, say, a moral system emanating from outside the self (e.g., I should be loyal to my ancestry or childhood religion), though embedded in the superego (roughly the conscience). While the shame-filled person withdraws into a system of hideouts because of his "sins" (e.g., disidentification and dissociation), the guilty person typically feels compelled to "confess" his "sins" (e.g., he accuses himself of having a spoiled identity) (Akhtar, 2009, p. 264). Of course, both shame and guilt are operative in most people who perceive themselves to be seriously stigmatized as, to some extent, they are depressed about their fate; shame and guilt co-produce each other in certain contexts, or shame is assimilated into guilt, et cetera.[18] However, here I want to briefly focus on the shame element because it is underappreciated in terms of what may be most morally tragic about the depressive aspect of stereotype threat, but also suggestive of how to surmount its most painful aspects.

"Shame is a soul eating emotion," said Jung (Sanderson, 2015, p. 11), and Kilborne noted that unresolved shame conflicts are especially tragic because the person is ensnared in a paradox "between the longing to be recognized and the terror of being seen" (2004, p. 472). Such a paradox resonates with the person experiencing stereotyped threat who wants to excel in his performance based on his socially unobstructed ability but who dreads being seen as a failure due to his group membership. It is ironic that what makes a person vulnerable to stereotype threat is less academic limitations than academic strengths; in fact, frequently it is the best students who are most prone to stereotype threat effects (Steele, 2010 pp. 54, 94). In light of this painful paradox of wanting to be seen and not seen, there can be an "inability to make a vital connection to anyone" (hence the often depressive "closedness,"[19] avoidant attachment patterns and social isolation of the seriously stigmatized), "together with shame also over omnipotent wishes organized in response to a fear of never being seen or found," hence the defensive narcissistic self-absorption, reversing self-shame into shaming others, self-serving, playing "fast and loose" with the "facts" of reality, and other deceptions (ibid., p. 479; Akhtar, 2009, p. 264). As Goffman notes, the individual attached to his stigmatized category is ambivalent about his condition. He can be both avoidant and hostile depending on the social context, or even enact the stereotype when he witnesses his own kind behaving in a stereotyped manner (1963, p. 107). Indeed, the lives of those stigmatized persons who managed to succeed in their lives, like Anatole Broyard, a light-skinned black American writer, literary critic and editor, who "passed" as a white man (even to his children) until just prior to his death, exemplify many of these aforementioned dynamics (Steele, 2010, p. 65). From my clinical experience working with the seriously stigmatized, they are infused with thoughts, feelings and behaviors that reflect conflicts about acceptance, disclosure and impression management (e.g., they are always "on," "covering" as they handle "normals," or alternating between cowering and showing hostile bravado/triumph over "normals"), aspects that suggest pronounced self-estrangement. Such people appear to be in a "dance of death" with themselves, "they can neither embrace [their] group nor let it go," in part animated by metastasizing lies (Goffman, 1963, pp. 108, 102, 112).

Philosopher Richard Rorty captures the psychologically wounding effect such humiliation has on people's internal conversations when they have the aforementioned warped relationship between an attribute and a stereotype:

> Now that I have believed or desired this [read: I possess a stigmatized affliction and wish to dissociate from my group affiliation] I can never be what I hoped to be, what I thought I was [read: fully human, without a spoiled identity]. The story I have been telling myself about myself—my picture of myself as honest, loyal, or devout [read: accepted for who I "really" am] no longer makes sense [read: I will always be stigmatized]. I no longer have a self to make sense of [read: a self-respecting narrative of self-identity]. There is no world in which I can picture myself living, because there is no vocabulary with which I can tell a coherent story of myself [read: I feel profound self-alienation].
>
> *(1989, p. 179)*

In other words, in the mind of the depressive/stigmatized person, humiliation prevents the integration of events that occurred—acts of omission and commission associated with his spoiled identity and its management—and the ability to sort them into the ongoing, let alone acceptable, story about the self that affirms his self-respect and dignity. Thus, the depressive/stigmatized person lives with a soul-destroying feeling of shame and guilt that ultimately undermines his autonomy, integration and humanity. As such, he often withdraws into his solipsistic, protective cocoon in his work and love life. To make matters worse, he longs to resurrect himself in his own eyes and the eyes of others. He craves feeling self-worthy and lovable to others, a vital validation from a world that he protractedly doubts will ever be forthcoming as he desperately needs and wants. As Erik H. Erikson noted, "doubt is the brother of shame."[20] It is precisely this anxiety-ridden doubt that makes the future appear so dark, gloomy and impossible to bear to the depressive/stigmatized person, especially within the context of serious stereotype threat associated with an identity affliction.

If narcissistic vulnerability makes one susceptible to feeling debilitating humiliation, shame and guilt, and being stigma-afflicted radically disrupts self-esteem and identity, then one way to protect oneself from stereotype threat is to have access to strongly felt, flexibly and creatively applied, transcendent-pointing moral beliefs and values that decisively transform the meaning of the totality of circumstances that constitute the context for experiencing stereotype threat. Strong religious (with or without God) or political beliefs and values function like emotional muscles that act as emotional "shock absorbers." For example, Steele says the single precondition to stereotype threat is that the person has to care about his performance, as this makes the likelihood of confirming the negative stereotype troubling enough to undermine performance (2010, p. 98). Suppose the stigmatized person did not care about his performance the way a victim to stereotype threat typically does. A person with transcendent moral beliefs and values has an "inner center of gravity," as Christian Buchenwald Holocaust survivor Eugen Kogon noted, that is not easily susceptible to humiliation and degradation. This is inclusive of democratic Western society, the normative context for most of the research done on stereotype threat (2006, p. 276). The basic point here is this: when the *raison d'être* of one's whole existence is rooted in a heroic refusal to embrace the standards and values of the hostile majority culture one has been hurled into, it is possible to reside in a dimension of being that is not vulnerable to those hostile demands or subjugating judgments of external reality. In a certain sense, one has proudly and creatively embraced one's stigmatized connection as his limit condition. There is a well-known Talmudic principle that the severity of an insult, like being stigmatized via a stereotype, "is relative to the human dignity of the one who administers it and to that of the one at whom it is directed" (Berkovits, 1979, p. 59). Indeed, Sartre made a similar point when he affirmed the importance of being an autonomous and reflexive subject: "I don't align myself with anybody else's descriptions of me. People can think of me as a genius, a pornographer, Communist, a bourgeois, however they like. Myself, I think of other things" (Kappler, 1964, p. 88). While it is beyond the scope of this chapter to detail how having strongly felt, flexibly and creatively applied, transcendent-pointing moral beliefs and values protectively operates in both everyday life and the extreme situation (Marcus, 1999), when it comes to dealing with actual stigma and stereotyping, one can never be insulted when the hostile, judgmental majority is regarded as having nothing in common with oneself. In short, "A pest does not insult you" (Berkovits, 1979, p. 59), and to again use an animal metaphor, while a biting dog can hurt you, he can never humiliate you.

The last point for consideration is how one can metabolize stirred-up rage associated with stigma and stereotyping. For along with feeling insulted, humiliation, shame and guilt, it is rage that can subvert not only one's performance on important tasks, but it can pollute one's entire self-identity. Rage is best conceptualized as "love outraged," that is, when one anticipates being cherished but is instead violated (Krystal, 1988, p. 82). Such rage responses are typically connected to feelings of having been humiliated, real and/or imagined, though they can be linked to other asymmetrical emotions such as envy (e.g., feeling inferior to the stereotyping majority), unrequited affection (e.g., feeling a possible paramour does not desire you as much as you desire her because of your group affiliation) and hypocrisy (e.g., when the stereotyped stereotypes the majority culture). There are of course a wide range of social contexts connected to stigma and stereotype threat in which a person can feel narcissistic rage, roughly a severe wounding to self-esteem and self-worth. This is especially the case for those at the lower registers of personality and relational functioning who are less likely to have easy access to strongly felt, flexibly and creatively applied, transcendent-pointing moral beliefs and values that are meaning-giving, affect-integrating and action guiding, and allow one to carry on less encumbered by toxic social dynamics.

Indeed, one of the best ways of shielding oneself from being overwhelmed by intense anger or rage in the context of stigma and stereotype threat is to engage in a way of being-in-the-world that can be characterized as engaged disengagement. The great Taoist philosopher Chuang Tzu captures how emptiness, meaning the emptying of the self (i.e., a kind of "unselving or transelving"),[21] that has been inundated by the Tao (roughly the unique source of the universe that determines all things) has a relational thrust that can be applied in the context of stigmatizing and stereotype threat. That is, bracketing the Taoist language for a moment, it is a skillful psychological way of protecting oneself from injury from others, as it promotes detachment and flexible accommodation to the external world. As Beckett famously said, "nothing is more real than nothing" (1956, p. 16). Such a mode of being-in-the-world tends to generate a greater calmness of the mind, as this well-known example from Chuang Tzu suggests:

> If a man, having lashed two hulls together, is crossing a river, and an empty boat happens along and bumps into him, no matter how hot-tempered the man may be, he will not get angry. But if there should be someone in the other boat, then he will shout out to haul this way or veer that. If his first shout is unheeded, he will shout again, and if that is not heard, he will shout a third time, this time with a torrent of curses following. In the first instance, he wasn't angry; now in the second he is. Earlier he faced emptiness, now he faces occupancy. If a man can succeed in making himself empty, and in that way wander through the world, then who could harm him?
>
> *(Watson, 1968, p. 212)*

While the aforementioned Taoist insight may seem unrealistic, as it relates to diminishing the negative impact of stereotype threat, it has been experimentally shown that a related technology of the self, mindfulness training, can alleviate working memory load, a key resource that is connected to stereotype threat effects in performance. For example, it has been reported that a mere five-minute mindfulness exercise eradicated traditional stereotype threat effects. Exactly why this is the case, and for how long the positive effect lasts, requires further research. Stereotype threat has been demonstrated to undermine emotional regulation, such as by diminishing executive resources, and mindfulness has been shown to enhance regulation and relaxation. Mindfulness also dissociates the social cues connected to social comparison from their threatening meaning, permitting the individual to reframe these cues in light of what is factually stated, that he is in a diagnostic condition. In other words, through this reframing a person is less likely to be anxiously concerned about self-definition and identity and can instead focus on achieving performance excellence (Spencer et al., 2016, p. 428; Weger et al., 2012).

Final comment

While Steele and his social-psychological entourage tend to underplay the dispositional side of social identities, that is, a person's "perspectives, emotional tendencies, values, ambitions, and habits" (Steele, 2010, p. 84) and instead emphasize the significance of the "contingencies to which all of that internal stuff is an adaptation," (ibid., p. 151) psychoanalysts tend to view identity and stereotype threat as mainly emanating from an internal psychological condition, such as a narcissistic vulnerability. Of course, external and internal processes related to both theoretical perspectives are at play, processes that co-potentiate and co-produce the stereotype threat effect for a particular person in a particular context. Indeed, Steele is right to say that it is easier to modify the external conditions, the contingencies of social identity, than the internal beliefs and values that are coupled with these contingencies. Hence, from a pragmatic point of view, for policymakers and educators, social psychologists have a lot of good suggestions to reduce stereotype threat effects in stereotyped groups (Spencer et al., 2016; Steele, 2010).

This being said, from the personal psychological perspective, while the importance of strongly felt, flexibly and creatively applied, transcendent-pointing moral beliefs and values in fending off stigmatizing affliction and stereotype threat may seem implausible, or at least overstated to some, the fact is that the findings of experimental social psychology tend to confirm the main thrust of this claim. For example, in two randomized, double-blind field experiments with a control group of European Americans over a two-year period, social psychologists (Cohen et al., 2006) had a group of African American seventh-grade students who were susceptible to stereotype threat regarding intelligence and academic performance engage in a brief in-class writing assignment in which they reinforced their sense of personal worth, or what they called "self-integrity" (ibid., p. 1307). Students affirmed such values as relationships with friends or family or being good at art. Results showed that the racial achievement gap was significantly improved by this targeted social-psychological intervention. As Cohen et al. noted, self-affirmations that encourage self-worth can reduce the stress stirred up in threatening performance situations related to one's group affiliation and stereotypes (ibid.). As Steele (2010) suggested about this and similar studies (see, e.g., Sherman et al., 2013), with one's larger sense of competence and worth put into focus by the writing exercise, poorer early performance in the school semester and additional identity-threatening cues in the classroom were less relevant. This factor inclined the students to be less hypervigilant, loosening up mental capacities and enhancing performance. Moreover, with improved performance came a notable disruption of the usual negative recursive process that was amplified among blacks in the control condition. In other words, says Steele, "without affirmation, early frustrations and threatening environmental cues worried them more, which worsened their performance, which worried them still more, until a full scale down progression was underway" (2010, p. 176). It was through the affirmation of self-defining beliefs and values that one's narrative of self-identity was enhanced and better school performance was potentiated.

However, there is one caveat to the encouraging aforementioned findings. While self-affirmation has been reported to diminish stereotype decrements in many studies, it is not effective at reinstating self-integrity among people who expect it to have this kind of impact (Sherman et al., 2013; Spencer et al., 2016). This implies that strongly felt, flexibly and creatively applied, transcendent-pointing moral beliefs and values need to be more than a one-off assertion or a brief writing exercise. They must sustain the self over time when faced with stigmatizing, stereotype threat or worse. Such beliefs and values have to be both deeply anchored in lived experience and reflection and pragmatically expressed with the fullness of one's whole being.

Notes

1 www.igi-global.com/dictionary/positive-stigma/54128, retrieved 2/12/19.
2 Goffman does not actually use the words "positive stigma" in his book, but he appears to be pointing to this phenomenon when he discusses deviancy in the context of person in a "high-position in some small close-knit groups." See Shih (2004) for a discussion of positive stigma.
3 Following Heidegger, the term being-in-the-world is one I often use. It refers to the fact that we are fundamentally always involved in a context, that is, we have a place in a meaningful totality where we reckon with other things and people. Our relation to the world is always one of active engagement, as we are never radically detached (Polt, 1999, p. 46).
4 It is worth noting that gender stigma has been shown to operate in women's reduced performance in advanced math; however, such stereotype threat effects are not usually seen in advanced English classes where women are seen to excel. Moreover, when math stereotype threat in women is removed, their performance dramatically improves. For example, when women took a tough math test but were reminded beforehand of strong female role models, it eradicated underperformance on the test compared to equally capable men (Steele, 2010, pp. 32, 40, 215).
5 Robert Merton's "self-fulfilling prophecy" may be operative here, which is when an originally false claim or assumption becomes true merely because it was predicted.
6 In G.W. Allport's *The Nature of Prejudice* (1979), first written in 1954, Allport brilliantly describes "Traits due to Victimization" that are still pertinent today.
7 In today's world, it would be judged as ill-conceived if not politically incorrect to ask a subject to mark his race.
8 In their book, drawing from large amounts of diverse data, Herrnstein and Murray (1994) claimed that the distribution of intelligence in the overall population is roughly a normal distribution (the bell curve). Moreover, they alleged that there is one fundamental form of intelligence, rather than a number of independent forms, that predict how well a person will perform academically and when employed, and therefore, how fruitful they will be in society. Racial group differences were also discussed with African Americans not faring well compared to the overall population. The book was criticized because it appropriated a unidimensional theory of intelligence rather than a multidimensional one in which intelligence is viewed as a multifaceted notion, not easily assessed by one variable, and most likely formed as much by environmental influences as by genetic ones. In his discussion of the truth of stereotypes, Helmreich, who reviewed the evidence on the stereotype that African Americans are "stupid," summarized, "there is no clear-cut evidence—either culturally, environmentally, genetically, or anatomically—to support the argument that Blacks are not as smart as whites" (2009, pp. 73, 81).
9 While Steele claims that he "doesn't ignore the internal" (2010, p. 214) to understanding group differences in say academic performance, golf putting and women's performance in math and conversational proximity of chairs (a test of the role of identity threat in interracial interactions), his explanations, at least at times, come perilously close to social-psychological reductionism.
10 https://plato.stanford.edu/entries/integrity/, retrieved 2/20/19.
11 www.social-engineer.org/newsletter/Social-Engineer.Org%20Newsletter%20Vol.%2003%20Iss.%2037.htm, retrieved 2/20/19.
12 Schmader and his colleagues have suggested that stereotype threat is catalyzed when a situation concurrently "primes three incongruent conditions: *I am a member of Group X, Group X is thought to do poor[ly] in this domain, I care about doing well in this domain.*" In other words, stereotype threat happens whenever these three uncalibrated components of self, group and domain are triggered (Schmader & Forbes, 2017, p. 250; Schmader et al., 2008).
13 Steele notes that we "have less direct access to" "moderate" emotions such as "lingering anxiety," and that humans have "limited access to their feelings and to the cause of their feelings," a "limitation of human functioning," a part of "human nature" and "human character" (2010, pp. 116, 115, 215). Steele is clearly not a postmodernist in that he

seems to have a notion of identity and the self that is not culturally, geographically and linguistically situated, but is prewired or hardwired: "Identity threat is a constant presence" (ibid., p.120). He has a similar view of stereotype threat: "a general phenomenon that, in some form or another, in some situations or another, can affect anyone" (ibid., p. 88). I don't subscribe to this foundationalist point of view.

14 https://theweek.com/articles/809415/freud-jung-beginnings-psychoanalysis, retrieved 2/20/19.

15 www.jta.org/jewniverse/2016/was-famous-psychoanalyst-carl-jung-an-anti-semite, retrieved 2/26/19.

16 Freud viewed the origin of Jewish self-hatred in terms of a conflicted relation with one's father. Identification with the aggressor is another psychoanalytic notion that has been applied to help explain this neurotic behavior, as analysts usually view it.

17 Authentic and inauthentic are evocative terms that have a long and complex philosophical and psychological history. I use them here to suggest a person's felt sense of being "real" or "false," and the analyst's ability, admittedly a value judgment, to designate certain behavior as authentic or inauthentic (Marcus, 2017, pp. 92–93).

18 The existential claim that "guilt is our own sense of falling short, while shame is to fall short in another's eyes" (Van Deurzen, 2012, p. 189) is true in certain contexts, but from a psychoanalytic point of view it oversimplifies how the psyche works.

19 "Closedness" versus openness are ways of relating to the world that existentialist Medard Boss (1979) has aptly described. Where focusing on the patient's "closedness" is geared toward helping him see how he restricts his way of being-in-the-world and thus his possibilities for living better, Freud's unconscious is more focused on the camouflaged motives for the "closedness" (Cooper, 2017, p. 49).

20 www.freud.org.uk/education/topic/10575/subtopic/40015/, retrieved 2/27/17.

21 The notion of emptiness has received considerable attention in most forms of ancient religious wisdom and spirituality, including its modern expressions (Marcus, 2003). For example, the great sixteenth-century Jewish mystic, R. Isaac Luria, was preoccupied with the question of how the universe can exist if God exists. His answer was a concept of "*tzimtsum*," translated as "self-effacement" or "self-limitation." The idea was that in order for the universe to exist, God had to limit his being, or conceal himself. Therefore, just as God made room for the universe, the believer should make room in his mind, heart and, most importantly, behavior for God's radiant presence. Self-effacement and self-limitation, that is, emptying oneself of one's inordinate narcissism and selfishness, and being other-directed, other-regarding and other-serving, is what God wants most from the spiritual aspirant (Sacks, 2019, p. 2).

References

Akhtar, S. (2009). *Comprehensive dictionary of psychoanalysis*. London: Karnac.

Allport, G.W. (1979). *The nature of prejudice* (25th anniversary ed.). Reading: Addison-Wesley.

Aronson, J., Quinn, D.M. & Spencer, S.J. (1998). Stereotype threat and the academic underperformance of minorities and women. In J.K. Swim & C. Stangor (Eds.), *Prejudice: The target's perspective* (pp. 83–103). New York: Academic Press.

Bakan, D. (2004). *Sigmund Freud and the Jewish mystical tradition*. Mineola, NY: Dover.

Beckett, S. (1956). *Malone dies*. New York: Grove.

Beilock, S.L., Jellison, W.A. & McConnell, A.R. (2007). Stereotype threat and working memory: Mechanisms, alleviation and spillover. *Journal of Experimental Psychology: General*, 136(2), 256–276.

Berkovits, E. (1979). *With God in hell: Judaism in the ghettos and death camps*. New York: Sanhedrin Press.

Boss, M. (1979). *Existential foundations of medicine and psychology*. S. Conway & A. Cleaves (Trans.). London: Jason Aronson.
Cohen, G.L., Garcia, J., Apfel, N. & Master, A. (2006). Reducing the racial achievement gap: A Social-psychological intervention, *Science*, 313, 1307–1310.
Cooper, M. (2017). *Existential therapies* (2nd ed.). Los Angeles: Sage.
Erçetin, Ş., Gungor, H. & Ackahn, S.N. (2016). Different sides of reality: "Positive stigma." In Ş. Erçetin & H. Bağcı (Eds.), *Handbook of research on chaos and complexity theory in the social sciences (Advances in religious and cultural studies)* (pp. 125–132). Hershey, PA: IGI Global.
Freud, S. & Abraham, K. (2002). Letter of 26 December 1908. In E. Falzeder (Ed.) and C. Schwarzacher (Trans.), *The complete correspondence of Sigmund Freud and Karl Abraham 1907–1925* (pp. 71–73). London and New York: Karnac.
Goffman, E. (1963). *Stigma: Notes on the management of spoiled identity*. New York: Simon and Schuster.
Heatherton, T.F., Kleck, R.E., Hebl, M.R. & Hull, J.G. (2000). *The social psychology of stigma*. New York: Guilford.
Helmreich, W.B. (2009). *The things they say behind your back. Stereotypes and the myths behind them* (4th ed.). New Brunswick, NJ: Transaction Publishers.
Herrnstein, R.J. & Murray, C. (1994). *The bell curve: Intelligence and class structure in American life*. New York: The Free Press.
Kappler, F. (1964). Sartre and existentialism: A spurned Nobel Prize calls the world's attention. Existentialism. *Life Magazine*, 11/6/64, 86–112.
Kilborne, B. (2004). Shame conflicts and tragedy in the The Scarlet Letter. *Journal of the American Psychoanalytic Association*, 53(2), 465–483.
Kogon, E. (2006). *The theory and practice of hell: The German concentration camps and the system behind them* (reprint ed.). New York: Farrar, Straus and Giroux (Original work published 1950).
Krystal, H. (1988). *Integration and self-healing: Affect, healing and alexithymia*. London: Routledge
Lewin, K. (1941). Self-hatred among Jews. *Contemporary Jewish Record*, 4(3), 219–232.
Marcus, P. (1999). *Autonomy in the extreme situation: Bruno Bettelheim, the Nazi concentration camps and the mass society*. Westport, CT: Praeger.
Marcus, P. (2003). *Ancient religious wisdom and spirituality and psychoanalysis*. Westport, CT: Praeger.
Marcus, P. (2017). *The psychoanalysis of career choice, job performance, and satisfaction: How to flourish in the workplace*. London: Routledge.
Marcus, P. & Rosenberg, A. (1989). Another look at Jewish self-hatred. *Journal of Reform Judaism*, Summer, 37–59.
Person, E.S., Cooper, A.M. & Gabbard, G.O. (Eds.) (2005). *Textbook of psychoanalysis*. Washington, DC: American Psychiatric Publishing.
Polt, R. (1999). *Heidegger: An introduction*. Ithaca, NY: Cornell University Press.
Rorty, R. (1989). *Contingency, irony, and solidarity*. Cambridge, UK: Cambridge University Press.
Rycroft, C. (1995). *A critical dictionary of psychoanalysis*. London: Penguin.
Sacks, J. (2019). Parshat Pekudei. *Shabbat Announcements*. Great Neck Synagogue, 3/9/19, 1–2.
Sanderson, C. (2015). *Counseling skills for working with shame*. London: Jessica Kingsley.
Schmader, T. & Forbes, C. (2017). Stereotypes and performance: Revisiting Steele and Aronson's threat experiments. In J.R. Smith & S.A. Haslam (Eds.), *Social psychology: Revisiting the classic studies* (2nd ed., pp. 245–268). Thousand Oaks, CA: Sage.
Schmader, E., Johns, M. & Forbes, C. (2008). An integrated process model of stereotype threat effects on performance. *Psychological Review*, 115, 336–356.

Segal, Z., Williams, M. & Teasdale, J. (2013). *Mindfulness-based cognitive therapy for depression*. New York: Guilford.

Shapiro, J.R. & Neuberg, S.L. (2007). From stereotype threat to stereotype threats: Implications of a multi-threat framework for causes, moderators, mediators, consequences, and interventions. *Journal of Personality and Social Psychology*, 11, 107–130.

Sherman, D.K., Hartson, K.A., Binning, K.R., Purdie-Vaughns, V. & Garcia, J. (2013). Deflecting the trajectory and changing the narrative: How self-affirmation affects academic performance and motivation under identity threat. *Journal of Personality and Social Psychology*, 104(4), 591–618.

Shih, M. (2004). Positive stigma: Examining resilience and empowerment in overcoming stigma. *The Annals of the American Academy of Political and Social Science*, 591(1), 175–185.

Smith, R., Mackie, D.M. & Claypool, H.M. (Eds.) (2015). *Social psychology* (4th ed.). New York: Psychology Press.

Spencer, S.J., Logel, C. & Davies, P.G. (2016). Stereotype threat. *Annual Review of Psychology*, 67, 415–437.

Steele, C.M. (2010). *Whistling Vivaldi: How stereotypes affect us and what we can do*. New York: W.W. Norton & Company.

Steele, C.M. & Aronson, J. (1995). Stereotype threat and the intellectual test performance of African Americans. *Journal of Personality and Social Psychology*, 69, 797–811.

Steele, C.M., Spencer, S.J. & Aronson, J. (2002). Contending with group image: The psychology of stereotype and social identity threat. *Advanced Experimental Social Psychology*, 34, 379–440.

Stewart-Steinberg, S. (2011). *Impious Fidelity: Anna Freud, psychoanalysis, politics*. Ithaca, NY: Cornell University Press.

Stone, J. (2002). Battling doubts by avoiding practice: The effects of stereotype threat on self-handicapping in white athletes. *Personality and Social Psychology Bulletin*, 28(12), 1667–1678.

Tangney, J.P. & Dearing, R.L. (2002). *Shame and guilt*. New York: Guilford.

Tangney, J.P. & Mahek, D.J. (2004). In search of the moral person: Do you have to feel really bad to be good? In J. Greenberg, S.L. Koole & T. Pyszczynski (Eds.), *Handbook of experimental existential psychology* (pp. 158–186). New York: Guilford.

Van Deurzen, E. (2012). *Existential counseling and psychotherapy practice* (3rd ed.). Los Angeles: Sage.

Watson, B. (1968). *The complete works of Chuang Tzu*. New York: Columbia University Press.

Weger, U.W., Hooper, N., Meier, B.P. & Hopthrow, T. (2012). Mindful maths: Reducing the impact of stereotype threat through a mindfulness exercise. *Conscious Cognition*, 21(1), 471–475.

Internet sources

www.igi-global.com/dictionary/positive-stigma/54128, retrieved 2/12/19.

www.social-engineer.org/newsletter/Social-Engineer.Org%20Newsletter%20Vol.%2003%20Iss.%2037.htm, retrieved 2/20/19.

https://theweek.com/articles/809415/freud-jung-beginnings-psychoanalysis, retrieved 2/20/19.

www.jta.org/jewniverse/2016/was-famous-psychoanalyst-carl-jung-an-anti-semite, retrieved 2/26/19.

www.freud.org.uk/education/topic/10575/subtopic/40015/, retrieved 2/27/17.

https://plato.stanford.edu/entries/integrity/, retrieved 2/20/19.

10

SANE VERSUS INSANE

The Rosenhan or Thud experiment (1973)

"Every normal person, in fact, is only normal on the average," said Freud in *Analysis Terminable and Interminable*. "His ego approximates to that of the psychotic in some part or other and to a greater or lesser extent; and the degree of remoteness from one end of the series and of its proximity to the other will furnish us with a provisional measure of what we have so indefinitely termed an 'alteration of the ego'" (1964, p. 235). In psychoanalytic theory, alteration of the ego (roughly, the "I" or personality) denotes modifications the ego suffers as a consequence of age or neurotic or psychotic injuries that it must metabolize and manage. As psychoanalyst Ernst Federn notes, "Alterations of the ego … are an aspect of the normal psychology, as well as of the pathology, of the ego".[1] Thus, Freud was well aware that what constitutes "normal" and "psychotic" is a "provisional measure," a judgment that boils down to an educated guess, made by the diagnostician in a particular set of circumstances: "A normal ego … like normality in general," is "an ideal fiction" (1964, p. 235), and therefore, what constitutes "abnormal" may be viewed similarly. The highly respected psychoanalyst Wilfred Bion aptly noted twenty years later that in the seriously neurotic person, "there is a psychotic personality concealed by neurosis as the neurotic personality is screened by psychosis in the psychotic," and thus, distinguishing these aspects of the personality and discerning how they interact is no small accomplishment (1957, p. 275).[2] There is a "documented unreliability of 'clinical predictions on interview information'" (Tavris & Aronson, 2015, pp. 135–136). Likewise, clinical researchers have noted that "clinical samples of patients with personality disorders are not qualitatively distinct from the personalities of normal functioning individuals in community settings" (Barlow & Durand, 2015, p. 96). In other words, as David Rosenhan suggested in his groundbreaking study (1973, 1975), to judge someone as "sane" (normal) or "insane" (abnormal) is radically perspectival and historically contingent. Depending on one's perspective, the "nature of mental illness" can be judged as "reality, convention or illusion" (Porter, 2002, p. 4).

For example, the psychiatrist/psychoanalyst Thomas Szasz (1961, 1989) famously argued that mental illness—neurosis or psychosis—is neither mental nor an illness. It is merely a set of problems in living that reflect ill-conceived and ill-fated behavior and inadequate coping skills that were learned in childhood and later social experiences. Psychiatry, according to Szasz, has engaged in the medicalization of deviance, a symptom of an underlying illness that needs to be treated by a doctor. While Szasz acknowledged that there are people who have so-called mental illnesses that have organic origins or chemical imbalances in brain chemistry that can be verified by laboratory tests and treated with medications, these treatments are based on physical illnesses and observable behavior, such as the crying, long-standing sadness and anhedonia present in certain depressive conditions. However, when a person becomes deviant in ways that bother others (e.g., they are viewed as nuisances, peculiar or challenging), and these others cannot find adequate accounts for why the person behaves "like that," they infer that he has a "sickness in the head," an illness in the mind, that generated the inappropriate, unacceptable behavior. Mental illness, says Szasz, is a myth that the naïve public has had imposed on it by a psychiatric profession that uses pseudo-scientific jargon to control those people who do not conform to its conception of "normal" and "abnormal" (Henslin, 1995, p. 217). The contributions of R.D. Laing (1967) and Michel Foucault (1967), one an existentially influenced psychiatrist/psychoanalyst and the other a transdisciplinary philosopher, have made arguments that somewhat resonate with Szasz's views of mental illness, especially of madness and its treatment.

Indeed, in the troubled and troubling landscape of modern-day psychiatry (what has been called the "psy" professions, which includes psychologists and social workers), diagnostic labeling and categorization has been used by mental health professionals who have been societally legitimated as "experts," and sometimes (some claim frequently, and others inevitably) this process has deleterious consequences to the individual who has been pathologically labeled, categorized and treated (Rose, 1996, 2019). I present cautionary tales, admittedly extreme, of some abuses of psychiatry. Between January 1940 and September 1942, in what might be seen as a rehearsal for the "Final Solution to the Jewish Question," as the Nazis called it, 70,723 mental patients were gassed, chosen from lists of those whose "lives were not worth living," as judged by nine prominent professors of psychiatry and thirty-nine top physicians. Between 1932 and 1972, under the auspices of the U.S. Public Health Service, hundreds of black mental patients at the Tuskegee Asylum in Alabama were guinea pigs without their knowledge or consent in a notorious experiment to evaluate long-term responses to syphilis (Porter, 2002). Also, worth mentioning was the role of psychiatrists in their support of lobotomy and leucotomy which were enthusiastically performed in the United States such that in 1951 over 18,000 patients had undergone these procedures before it was challenged and overtaken by the psychopharmacological revolution (ibid.). Likewise, more recently, prominent psychiatrists like Bessel van der Kolk (the "PTSD" researcher) have had a major role in "recovered memory therapy" in which adults engaged in therapy without any memory of childhood trauma and emerged believing that they had been sexually abused by their parents or tortured in satanic cults, sometimes for numerous years, without being aware of it when it occurred, and without any corroboration by siblings, friends or doctors. These persons claimed that their therapists facilitated them to remember, while under hypnosis, the dreadful experiences they had suffered as toddlers, as infants, in the crib and sometimes even in former lives. As a result of this self-justifying "closed loop" pseudoscience that ignored the fallibility of memory and the numerous confabulations of recovered-memory cases, many individual's lives were destroyed and many families have never been reunited (Tavris & Aronson, 2015).[3]

In this chapter I describe Rosenhan's brilliantly controversial study that tested the validity of diagnosis in psychiatric hospitals, including its implications for how we understand what constitutes sane and insane, and psychopathology in general, along with some of the negative effects of diagnostic labeling and categorization when it is routinely implemented in both inpatient and outpatient settings. I draw from findings of experimental social psychology (e.g., impression formation, decision-making) that puts into sharp focus the dangers associated with making life-defining and life-altering judgments about the "mental health" and "illness" of patients, including directing them to ingest powerful medications, sometimes for a lifetime. I also discuss the effects of diagnostic labeling and categorization on how an individual understands oneself, one's narrative of self-identity and its influence on one's efforts to maintain a modicum of autonomy, integration and humanity in what Foucault has called a "disciplinary society" (1979). Briefly, discipline is a mechanism of power that controls and standardizes the behavior of individuals in the social body. This is accomplished by regulating how space, time (timetables) and people's everyday activities and behaviors (e.g., drills, posture, movement) are organized. Discipline is imposed with the help of complicated systems of surveillance, including by the psy professions that put forth a reified and substantivized notion of normality.

I should mention from the onset that I am not denying that there are people who have serious psychological problems in living and display severe mental distress, including what phenomenologically can be called psychosis or schizophrenia, but that current psychiatric diagnosis by members of the psy professions in many settings has a dangerous side to it.

This becomes clear when one considers the findings of social psychologist Milton Rokeach. In his wonderful book *The Three Christs of Ypsilanti* (1964), Rokeach described his two-year clinical experience at a state psychiatric hospital where he brought together three paranoid schizophrenics who believed they were Jesus Christ. The patients worked at the same laundry room, ate at the same dining room and slept on three adjacent cots, totally enmeshed in each other's environment. The purpose of the confrontation was to generate the maximum human dissonance Rokeach could contrive; each Christ had to live with two other people day in and day out who believed they were he. Rokeach says he was motivated by his longstanding interest in the structure of belief systems, and he was attempting to clarify what happens when the most basic of all beliefs, i.e., "who I am," was constantly being challenged in a way that it could not possibly be challenged in our daily lives (Evans, 1980, p. 118). As Rick Moody said in his 2011 introduction to Rokeach's book, "Rokeach wanted to see if this procedure would free them from a shared but perhaps incompatible illusion," a new type of confrontational therapy (1964, p. viii). After confronting these three men with contradictions about self-identity, in his afterword written seventeen years later, Rokeach realized that his study "was really a story about a confrontation among four people rather than three … I had overlooked the effects of such a confrontation on my as well as their delusional beliefs and behavior" (ibid., p. 335). Rokeach was referring to his

> God-like delusion that I could change them by omnipotently and omnisciently arranging and rearranging their daily lives within the framework of a 'total institution' … That I really had no right, even in the name of science, to play God and interfere around the clock with their daily lives … I became increasingly uncomfortable about the ethics of such a confrontation. I was cured when I was able to leave them in peace …
>
> *(ibid., p. 336)*

Finally, Rokeach noted that the primary distinction between him and the three Christs was analogous to the size of an eye of a needle: "The main difference between the three of them and the rest of us who are also trying to be God-like is that whereas the rest of us can bring ourselves to admit the impossibility of ever becoming absolute or infinitely moral and competent the three Christs found it difficult to admit such an impossibility" (ibid., p. 338). As Rokeach implied in his afterword, such are the dangers of empowering well-intentioned but arrogant, ignorant and ethically questionable clinicians as they engage the alterity of their suffering patients.

The Rosenhan experiment

During a three-year period, Rosenhan (1973) deployed eight sane men and women (including himself) to be admitted to twelve psychiatric hospitals on the East and West Coasts. Great care was taken to guarantee that none of the pseudo-patients had any psychiatric history or serious problems. Each of the pseudo-patients made a complaint at the admissions desk that they were hearing voices, that uttered the words, "empty," "hallow" and "thud." Rosenhan chose this feigned presenting symptom, an auditory hallucination, because it was not reported in the clinical literature to be determinative of a clinical diagnosis of schizophrenia. Nowhere in the psychiatric literature were there reports of any patients complaining of such an obviously "silly" and "cartoon angst" (Slater, 2004, pp. 71, 65). In the psychiatry of the day, such a diagnosis should have been made based on serious disturbances in thinking, emotion, as well as withdrawnness, and/or bizarre behavior, but not solely based on an auditory hallucination. Also worth noting is that the pseudo-patients accurately provided their actual family history and the circumstances of their current well-functioning life. The exception was for the psychologist in the group, the famous positive psychologist Martin Seligman ("learned helplessness"), who withheld that fact so as not to bias the psychiatric staff (i.e., a professional colleague might be treated differently than a regular inpatient).

The results of the study were stunningly disruptive to the psychiatric establishment: All the pseudo-patients were diagnosed as having psychosis; on eleven occasions the diagnosis was paranoid schizophrenia, and on one occasion manic-depressive psychosis. Moreover, all of the pseudo-patients were admitted to the hospital, where they remained for an average of nineteen days (the longest stay was fifty-two days). All pseudo-patients were given powerful antipsychotic medications, which they feigned taking. As Seligman recalled, "it took me awhile to get the pill thing right, and I was so nervous. I was nervous I'd accidentally swallow a pill if they forced one on me, but I was more nervous about homosexual rape" (ibid., p. 65).[4] In no instance did any of the staff detect that the pseudo-patient was actually sane, even though the pseudo-patient stopped talking about hallucinations immediately after admission was secured and behaved in a "normal" manner. While the pseudo-patients initially had "nervousness" (Rosenhan, 1973, p. 251) at admission to the hospital, it rapidly diminished to nothing, and for the most part they were bored and wanted to get out as soon as they could without revealing their identity and purpose. Only the actual hospitalized patients ever detected that the pseudo-patients were in fact confederates. "You're not crazy. You're a journalist or a professor [referring to the continual note-taking]. You're checking up on the hospital" (ibid.).

Rosenhan notes that sometimes when the pseudo-patients accurately described their past history, at least as they viewed it, the psychiatrists appeared to unconsciously distort or reconfigure information—that is, they gave the pseudo-patient's narrative an unintended meaning that was geared to "explain" the disordered behavior presented on admission. For example, one of the pseudo-patients described a rather close relationship with his mother and a distant one with his father, what is a fairly standard account of both so-called normal and neurotic people. As the pseudo-patient grew up, he became closer to his father and somewhat estranged from his mother, also a fairly common familial scenario. However, the discharge summary put a pejorative "spin" on the pseudo-patient's rendering of the "facts" of his own life, one that was meant to support, if not confirm, his diagnosis of psychosis:

> This white thirty-nine year old male … manifests a long history of considerable ambivalence [a common human experience, according to Freud, and what does "considerable" mean anyway?] in close relationships, which begins in early childhood … Affective stability is absent [absent? No emotional stability ever?]. His attempts to control emotionality [what kind of emotionality? And what does "control" mean?] with his wife and children are punctuated by angry outbursts [verbal and/or physical? What is an outburst?] and, in the case of the children, spankings [spankings were a common forms of discipline at the time—was it harsh or reasonable?] And while he says that he has several good friends, one senses [senses?] considerable ambivalence embedded in those relationships also [What does that mean? All relationships have ambivalence from time to time.].
>
> *(ibid., p. 273)*

Anyone who has worked in the clinical context of a psychiatric setting, inpatient or outpatient, or has heard a case presentation at a clinical conference has chanced upon the kind of narrative "smoothing" that was done by the psychiatrist/staff who wrote the discharge summary. Put simply, members of the psy professions routinely fashion case reports, vignettes and discharge summaries to support their rhetorical strategy that advances their intellectual agenda, sometimes consciously, more often unconsciously. The aforementioned discharge summary is a form of narrative construction, a kind of "storytelling" that is designed to persuade the reader by deploying data analysis and interpretation in a rhetorically magnified and self-serving manner meant to affirm the author's truth-claims about the patient. As Rosenhan notes, the proclivity of the psychiatrists in his study to conceptualize pseudo-patients using a medical model led them to interpret just about any behavior as an expression of their supposed illness. However, since the behavior of the pseudo-patients was totally unremarkable and uneventful, that is, "normal," the only grounds for interpreting their behavior as abnormal or pathological was the fact that they were being evaluated on a psychiatric ward and were affixed with the diagnostic label characterizing them as psychotic. Thus, as Rosenhan noted, "the issue is the diagnostic leap that was made between a single presenting symptom, hallucination, and the diagnosis, schizophrenia (or in one case, manic-depressive psychosis)" (1975, p. 466). Moreover, "clearly the meaning ascribed" to the pseudo-patient's "verbalizations (ambivalence, affective instability) was determined by the diagnosis: schizophrenia. An entirely different meaning would have been ascribed if it were known that the man was 'normal'" (Rosenhan, 1973, p. 253). In Rosenhan's view, the psychiatric diagnosis had little or no pertinence to the pseudo-patient's actual behavior, putting into question the credibility and usefulness of the entire diagnostic process.

To further emphasize the truth of Rosenhan's argument, in response to an affronted hospital administration that challenged Rosenhan to send pseudo-patients to its research and teaching hospital, whom the staff should then detect, Rosenhan consented that in a three-month period he would attempt to send in pseudo-patients. The results were that of 250 new patients, the staff identified forty-one potential pseudo-patients with "high confidence" (ibid., p. 252), with two of these receiving suspicion from at least one psychiatrist and the other staff members. However, in a clever deception, Rosenhan had sent no pseudo-patients to the hospital, again emphasizing that it was the context and setting, including the bias and expectations[5] of those empowered to make clinical diagnoses, and not the actual behavior of the patients, that mattered most in terms of diagnosis/treatment. Over-diagnosis of sanity had replaced over-diagnosis of insanity, at least in terms of the base rate of the research and teaching hospital.[6]

Criticisms of Rosenhan's study

All of the pseudo-patients were diagnosed on two occasions—when they were admitted (based on the aforementioned auditory hallucination) and discharged. Rosenhan correctly notes that it was not proper clinical procedure to diagnose a patient on one symptom, let alone on an auditory hallucination. For example, in many traditional cultures, auditory hallucinations, "hearing voices," are indicative of divine favor and bestow special status on those who experience them (Schaefer, 2003, p. 490).[7] Moreover, it is difficult to discern symptoms of alleged "severe mental disorder" like hearing voices, seeing visions, and exhibiting ecstatic states and trances from life-affirming spiritual experiences (Mohr, 2013, p. 259). To be fair to the well-intentioned hospital psychiatrists, the fact that the pseudo-patients were complaining of hearing voices and were self-hospitalized, presumably because they experienced considerable distress about the voices, one can argue that it was reasonable to view the presenting symptom as more or less in harmony with a diagnosis of psychosis [though why not due to alcohol, drug abuse, organic causes or toxic psychosis, asks Rosenhan (1975, p. 466)]. In other words, Rosenhan may have somewhat overstated his claim that the diagnosis did not have any relation to the pseudo-patient's behavior, though it clearly was lodged in insufficient information and inadequate evidence. What should have occurred is that rather than make a diagnosis, let alone the serious and far-reaching one of psychosis, the diagnosis should have been deferred pending additional data collection [or described as "hallucinations of unknown origin" (ibid.)].

From Rosenhan's perspective, the diagnosis in the discharge summary, "schizophrenia, in remission," rather than diagnosis deferred, reflected the "stickiness" of the psychiatric label. That is, the label became the frame and filter that was used to judge all of the behavior of the pseudo-patients, even if their behavior, the auditory hallucinations, didn't exist anymore. In short, the labels assumed an independent life of their own. Given the fact that the pseudo-patients allegedly acted normally after they were admitted, how can it be claimed that they were schizophrenics, even with the diagnostic qualification "in remission" when they were discharged? Rosenhan is highlighting the disconnect between the diagnosis of "schizophrenia, in remission," and the actual unremarkable, uneventful, normal behavior observed during the pseudo-patients' hospitalization. Thus, as psychologist Lauren Slater noted, Rosenhan's experiment demonstrated that the way the world is perceived is warped by the lens we are looking through, implying that we are "inextricably immanent, suffused with subjectivity" (2004, p. 63).

Robert Spitzer, a psychiatrist, psychoanalyst and the late chairman of the committee that developed the DSM-III (American Psychiatric Association, 1980), wrote two articles (1975, 1976) vigorously criticizing Rosenhan's study. Spitzer was thoroughly, if not arrogantly, lodged in the medicalized view of deviance, telling Slater in a phone call, "I believe in the medical model of psychiatry … Did you read my responses to Rosenhan … They're pretty brilliant, aren't they?" (Slater, 2004, p. 73).[8] The gist of Spitzer's argument was that the use of the term "in remission" was not a typical one used by psychiatrists in most hospitals at the time. In most instances, a discharge summary would characterize a schizophrenic as either somewhat improved or much improved. Thus, says Spitzer, the psychiatrists in the study did indeed identify that the pseudo-patients were normal on discharge and used the term "in remission" to emphasize this conclusion. While Spitzer's argument has some plausibility, the fact is that at the time the DSM-II (American Psychiatric Association, 1968) had the category of "no mental disorder" that could have been applied by the psychiatrists making the diagnosis (the DSM-III had not been published when Rosenhan's study came out). As Davison and Neale noted, quoting from the DSM-II, the "no mental disorder" diagnosis "is used when, following psychiatric examination, none of the previous disorders [the whole range of psychiatric diagnosis] is found. It is not to be used for patients whose disorders are in remission" (1982, p. 77). Thus, if the treating psychiatrists had been attuned to the behavior of the pseudo-patients, they should have used the diagnosis of "no mental disorder" and not "in remission," but this is not what occurred, again reflecting the stickiness of the label of schizophrenia given at admission (ibid.).

Social psychology and diagnosis

To my knowledge, experimental social psychologists have not systematically commented on Rosenhan's study, but there are some important concepts from this perspective that can help illuminate some of the limitations and strengths of Rosenhan's observations.

One methodological criticism of Rosenhan's study raises a serious challenge to his main conclusion. There is no way of knowing whether the pseudo-patients actually acted normally after they were admitted. For example, the pseudo-patients did not request to be released once they were on the hospital ward. Wouldn't a normal person who believed he was improperly and unfairly hospitalized want to be released as soon as possible? In this sense, didn't the pseudo-patients behave abnormally? Of course, what is normal and abnormal in a psychiatric hospital is a judgment call (as it is in ordinary life), and Rosenhan's pseudo-patients had agreed to get hospitalized, and remain there for a while, as part of the research methodology. In contrast, many patients who are psychiatrically hospitalized ask to be released early on, as some feel they have been wrongfully hospitalized. The evaluating staff may judge such requests as indicative of their disease or condition that got them there in the first place (Davison & Neale, 1982, p. 77). As I have said, and what the history of madness demonstrates, is that what constitutes being "crazy," is context-dependent and setting-specific, a judgment made by those who are empowered to do so. This judgment can be very complicated; for example, there are patients who feign the feigning of symptoms so as to convincingly pretend to themselves and others that they are saner and more in control of their lives than they really are (Sass, 1992). In this case, madness is the inability to fake sanity! Moreover, while Rosenhan might claim that, based on self-report (obtained from pseudo-patients and their visitors' notes) and the hospital documentation they reviewed, the pseudo-patients behaved normally, social-psychological studies (including those discussed in this book) have demonstrated that particular situations can sharply alter behavior and be more useful in predicting behavior than knowledge of personality characteristics, which is what mainstream analysts usually prioritize and possibly what the pseudo-patients believed they enacted and experienced while hospitalized [e.g., boredom, "dull and difficult" (Rosenhan, 1975, p. 470)]. In other words, if behavior is context-dependent and setting-specific, including the psychiatrist's diagnosis as Rosenhan claims, then is it not possible that over time, pseudo-patients began to behave similarly to the real patients who may have been properly diagnosed? Or maybe their own personal "craziness" was expressed and they did not realize it since they were in a psychiatric hospital in an extremely stressful environment; they could have begun to unravel without realizing it. As Rosenhan did not provide his "raw" data in a detailed and systematic manner, including the clinical documentation from the hospital ward and the pseudo-patients' notes, et cetera, there is some credibility to this criticism, though Rosenhan has strongly argued otherwise (1975, p. 470).

A social psychologist might say that Rosenhan indicated an important, documented research finding that our motivations and expectations can seriously influence our judgments. Once the pseudo-patients were diagnosed at admission, the "group mind," as it were, had "made up its mind," and the psychiatric staff found it impossible to see, let alone metabolize and embrace, evidence such as the pseudo-patients' normal, unremarkable and uneventful behavior that challenged, if not contradicted, their prior characterization of the pseudo-patients as psychotic.

This research finding calls to mind the work of Irving Janis (1972, 1982), the brilliant originator of the social-psychological phenomenon known as "groupthink." Janis defined groupthink as "A mode of thinking that people engage in when they are deeply involved in a cohesive in-group, when the members' strivings for unanimity override their motivation to realistically appraise alternative courses of action" (1972, pp. 8–9). Groupthink thus involves "a deterioration of mental efficiency, reality testing, and moral judgment." It is rooted in group pressures for conformity, compliance and the avoidance of anxiety and conflict. Groupthink shuns the articulation and critical assessment of opposing perspectives and rejects non-traditional or innovative ideas. As a result of groupthink, premature, ill-conceived and ill-fated decisions are made. For example, Janis describes how groupthink led to disastrous foreign policy decisions such as the failure to expect and foresee the Japanese attack on Pearl Harbor, Hitler's decision to invade the Soviet Union, The Bay of Pigs Invasion debacle and President Lyndon B. Johnson's ruinous prosecution of the Vietnam War. It is possible that Rosenhan's greatly disturbing findings should be included in this list.

Another social-psychological construct, group polarization, may be pertinent to understanding Rosenhan's study. Group polarization refers to the fact that within decision-making groups there is a tendency, after interaction and discussion, for the group and individuals to take more extreme positions, both in terms of risk-taking and cautiousness. Moreover, research has shown that after discussion, group members who at first opposed a subject become more radically against it, and members who were in support of the subject become more aggressively supportive. What this means for group decision-making is that groups who at the onset have a point of view that veers in a particular direction are more likely to embrace a more extreme perspective after interaction with each other. In the context of war and other comparably dangerous decision-making contexts, this can be catastrophic. If group members are inclined to make riskier decisions in a dangerous context, they are more likely to be supportive of doing so after interacting with other group members (Nelson & Quick, 2008, p. 239). When, for example, soldiers with the same opinion about an enemy spend most of their time interacting with each other, their opinions tend to become considerably stronger and more extreme. Such a polarization effect can have obvious detrimental effects on collective decision-making, including in Rosenhan's study where the tight-knit treatment staff regularly convened and the psychiatrists had hardly any contact time with the pseudo-patients ["psychiatrists ... were rarely seen on the wards" (Rosenhan, 1973, p. 253)], which is still the case in many psychiatric hospitals where nurses and other support staff do most of the hands-on clinical care.

A psychiatric diagnosis is made in a relatively brief time (in the inpatient and out-patient settings I have worked in it usually took about a half-hour, though it can take as long as an hour-and-a-half) and has a stickiness and stigmatizing effect, as Rosenhan and Erving Goffman (1961) have noted, which underscores how a person, including a psychiatrist, forms first impressions. These cues, interpretations and inferences that are made can have deleterious effects on the hospital ward patients. Aspects of first impressions that are salient, the cues that attract attention in a specific context, are likely to provide the basis for first impressions, which can be way off the mark, especially in the long-term to understand a person and predict behavior. For example, a psychiatrist might have information about a person's physical appearance (e.g., more attractive patients unconsciously stir up positive expectations, such as what is beautiful is good), their nonverbal communication (e.g., interpretations of emotional expressions vary from culture to culture, especially sadness, disgust and surprise), their chosen environments (e.g., impressions of others can be differently deduced based on how the pseudo-patients used the space they occupied, like their rooms) and some of their behavior (e.g., people draw different inferences from how a person behaves). In the context of an intake diagnostic interview done by the psychiatrist in a busy inpatient setting, these aforementioned factors can negatively influence the type and magnitude of the diagnosis made, though they are hardly ever considered, let alone in a critically reflective and context-sensitive manner (Smith et al., 2015, p. 63).[9]

Social psychologists have pointed out that behavior (thoughts, feelings, actions) is ambiguous and as such can generate a wide range of inferences, depending on what the diagnosing psychiatrist has accessible in consciousness at the time of diagnosis. In many instances and without deliberate intent, what is accessible is automatic, if not unconscious. Expectations, motives and moods are some of the many elements that can influence accessibility. For example, an important source of expectations about people emanates from their group memberships, like age, gender, ethnicity and occupation, and there is a huge literature that has demonstrated how expectations influence social perception (ibid., p. 57). In Rosenhan's study, the psychiatric staff expected their patients to display disturbed behavior, and they were not able to detect the pseudo-patients who were allegedly acting normally.

Likewise, motivation matters in the diagnostic context. For example, a mental representation that has recently been brought to mind also remains accessible for a time, therefore anything that brings the idea to mind—even accidental, immaterial events—can make it accessible and influence interpretations of behavior. The activation of a thought to increase its accessibility and make it more likely to be used is called "priming." Concepts that have been primed can remain accessible and influence later interpretations for as long as twenty-four hours and do not necessarily depend on people's awareness of activation—they can be subliminally influenced. If a diagnosing psychiatrist had simply glimpsed a real patient screaming and/or throwing something without consciously registering it, it would likely make him interpret the behavior of the patient he is engaging in a diagnostic interview with as aggressive.

Other experimentally demonstrated biases may be operative during the diagnostic process: The "primacy effect," when early-encountered information has a greater influence than successive information on decision-making, this being an example of cognitive conservatism (people are slow to change their worldviews and strive to propagate them); the "Golem Effect," when expectations function as self-fulfilling prophecies with negative consequences; and finally, "confirmation bias," when one favors evidence that confirms one's personal beliefs. The point is that there are many kinds of cognitive biases that can be operative during the diagnostic process and, after thirty-five years of reading hospital, clinic and school psychiatric and psychological diagnostic evaluations, I have never once seen any of these aforementioned considerations mentioned, let alone seriously discussed, as having bearing on the diagnosis.

Lastly, moods also matter in the diagnostic context. Emotions can affect not just the nature of the decision but the speed at which it is made. Anger, for example, can lead to impatience and rash decision-making. If the psychiatrist is time pressured and angry (even unconsciously) about something unrelated and personal, the intense thinking that is necessary to provide a credible, if not compelling, diagnosis might not occur. Likewise, if fearful of a patient—and I have treated some violent teenagers and adult gangsters in my day—one has to be mindful that decisions may be clouded by uncertainty and caution, which might make a description and diagnosis of the patient take longer, not necessarily for the better.

Also worth mentioning is that psychiatrists, like all of us, have the tendency to assume that others have internal qualities that correspond to their observable behaviors. Such an assumption is often made even when external factors could have influenced behavior. Characterizing someone as having a personality trait, like schizophrenia, that corresponds to his or her observed behavior (e.g., auditory hallucination) is called "correspondent inference." The idea is that when a correspondent inference follows the initial interpretation of a behavior, it completes a first impression—an initial mental representation (the knowledge-fund an individual has stored in memory) of what the other person is like. This can occur automatically and unconsciously. "Correspondence bias," the belief that people's acts reflect their inner qualities rather than situational pressures, have accounted for the unanticipated findings of many of the classic social psychology experiments, like Milgram's paradoxical finding that ordinary people often obey orders that injure innocent victims. Or in the case of Rosenhan's study, perfectly normal people were diagnosed and treated as psychotic in a state hospital for an average of nineteen days and were misdiagnosed as "schizophrenic, in remission" when released. The diagnosing psychiatrist and treatment staff assumed that one behavior they observed at admission, the pseudo-patient's auditory hallucination, must reflect the person's inner characteristics (i.e., schizophrenia) even though other causative alternatives of the situation might explain the behavior (e.g., the auditory hallucination was a harmless, transient phenomenon; a self-serving fabrication relating to family dynamics; a result of alcohol or drug abuse; organically caused; or from toxic psychosis, which vanished as quickly as it came and was not evident during weeks of hospitalization).

I have only skimmed the surface of the social psychology research on impression formation and decision-making, but it should be apparent that making a conventional psychiatric diagnosis in an inpatient setting, as in Rosenhan's study, or in other clinical settings, let alone a credible one, is a very dicey enterprise. There are many criticisms of actual diagnostic practice, specifically of psychiatric classification, the main ones being that diagnostic classes are heterogeneous and they are neither reliable nor valid. In fact, as Barlow and Durand noted in their discussion of the DSM-5 (American Psychiatric Association, 2013), "it has been clear to most professionals involved in this process that an exclusive reliance on discrete diagnostic categories [like in the Rosenhan study] has not achieved its objective in achieving a satisfactory system of nosology" (Barlow & Durand, 2015, p. 95). Moreover, in addition to the problems of comorbidity (the concurrent existence of two chronic diseases or conditions in a patient) and the uncertain boundary between diagnostic categories, "little evidence has emerged validating these categories such as discovering specific underlying causes associated with each category. In fact, not one biological marker, such as a laboratory test, that would clearly distinguish one disorder from another has been discovered" (ibid.).[10] Finally, "It is also clear that the current categories lack treatment specificity," for example, cognitive therapy, psychoanalysis and antidepressant drugs are effective for many diagnostic categories that are conceptualized as dissimilar (ibid.). For all of these reasons, "it may be time for a new approach" to diagnosis (ibid., p. 96). Before tentatively addressing what a new approach to diagnosis might look like, one that has been called "biopsychosocialcultural" in character (Rose, 2019, p. 177), a word about the social construction of psychopathological categories is necessary.

A Foucauldian gloss on the social construction of psychopathology[11]

As Foucault has noted, historically speaking but also at present, the invention and elaboration of "psychopathologies" by the psy sciences is a manifestation of bio-power (i.e., biopolitics) in that it creates a population of people labeled as "sick" or "mentally ill." They have specific behavioral manifestations or symptoms of this alleged sickness that are designated as calcified entities called psychopathologies. Indeed, as Foucault has shown, the fertile breeding ground for the birth of the psy sciences was the "dividing" practices or ordering procedures and the grid of calculability and interpretability with which they are associated. This included the instantiation of psychoanalysis as an authoritative, norm-generating, governing discourse and treatment for these alleged psychopathologies. Foucault's genealogical studies that included psychiatry further amplified this subtle individualizing and totalizing of social dynamics through use of a concept he termed the "surfaces of emergence." This term was meant to indicate the emergence of psychopathology as a sedimented, observable thing that came into existence.

Foucault used this concept of surfaces of emergence to examine the amorphous, power-generating collection of institutional, physical and administrative mechanisms and knowledge structures "within which the troubles or problem spaces condensed that were later to be rationalized, codified, and theorized in terms such as diseases, alienation, dementia, neurosis" (Rose, 1996, p. 61). Such mechanisms and structures like the family, the workplace, the faith community and medicopsychiatric sites (e.g., the clinic and psychoanalysis), within which the amorphous difficulties and problematic "spaces" solidified (such as the upsurge/creation of so-called "conversion hysteria" in Freud's era and "disorders of the self" in ours), later became rationalized, codified and theorized in notions such as disease and neurosis (ibid.). Surfaces of emergence can be conceptualized in terms of a "dis-ease" appearing within society. Today, people feel uncertain, stressed out and worried; this "dis-ease" is problematized by authoritative spokespeople and given a name like the Age of Anxiety, the Age of Violence or the Age of Virtuality. A solution to the problem is developed by experts, like therapies of adjustment and adaptation. Finally, an institution, such as the psy experts, implements and enforces the solutions.

In other words, the notion of surfaces of emergence helps explain how psychiatry came to define its own discourse, and thus created what became definite objects of discourse. The point is that these amorphous difficulties and problematic "spaces" took form within societal contexts, and psychoanalysis and related disciplines developed systems of visibility, labeling diagnostic vocabularies (e.g., "normal" and "pathological") and cure (e.g., "healthy"/"adaptive" and "unhealthy"/"maladaptive")[12] that gave these difficult people/"spaces" and their alleged medicopsychiatric conditions and resultant ways of being socially and self-governed (ibid., pp. 61, 70). These dualistic, binary terms that are generated by dividing practices reflect a power/knowledge moral discourse about what people prefer others to desire and what they determine others should be capable of being and doing (Phillips, 2005, pp. 33, 126). In other words, analysands and analysts appropriated a way of thinking/feeling and acting in terms of what their alleged medicopsychiatric problem was, how it got there and how to "fix" it (not realizing that "it" refers to what we would call a social construction rather than a substantivized entity). In fact, by the time the analysand reaches the analyst's office he has almost always made efforts to diminish the negative impact of the alleged "problem" in his life and interpersonal relationships. In other words, he has been normalized into a strategy of power that he does not recognize is operative. This strategy is for the analysand to passively fashion himself as a "subject," a process that becomes active "subjection," that is, a form of domination.

In our time in the United States, "managed care," the system of health care in which patients, including those with "mental health illness," agree to visit only certain doctors and hospitals, and in which the cost of treatment is monitored by a managing company, personifies such government of the person as it inscribes the patient's identity/subjectivity and dictates the patient's behavior. Moreover, there are competing sites of power/knowledge trying to dominate how the person is governed and self-governs within the medicopsychiatric community. Examples include different psychiatric groupings [e.g., psychoanalytically oriented psychiatrists took the lead in writing the first *Diagnostic and Statistical Manual* (DSM-I, American Psychiatric Association) in 1952, and medical and cognitive behavioral psychiatrists the current one in 2013 (DSM-5,

American Psychiatric Association), both of which are expressions of bio-power],[13] and pharmaceutical, bio-medical and insurance companies (mainly for financial self-interest). By the time the average suffering patient, client or analysand turns up at the psychiatrist, psychologist, social worker or psychoanalyst's door, she has been inundated with different versions of her so-called "mental health illness" or distressing condition and has usually unknowingly embraced a way of thinking about this problem and "managing" it. The vocabularies of the medicopsychiatric apparatuses have been internalized such that a person's life is narrated using those unexamined, expert-driven categories of thought, feeling and action. In other words, individualized identity, with its multiplicity of "voices" and idiosyncrasies and "worries and troubles," has been disciplined. This includes the analysand taking on the "practical cognitive skill" (Lear, 2015, p. 55) that constitutes the psychoanalytic system. Such a system uses normalized values and criteria like "unhealthy," "irrational," "unreasonable," "immature," "infantile," "neurotic" and "maladaptive" to describe ambiguous, ambivalent and ever-shifting distress, the idiosyncratic trajectory of the analysand's "worries and troubles." By uncritically embracing this "practical cognitive skill," the analysand's otherness and right to be different (e.g., productively original and eccentric) is forfeited as he attempts to shape himself using these normative values. In this way, the analysand becomes visible to the analyst, the purveyor of the authoritative science of psychoanalysis, while the analysand is willingly disciplined to understand, speak, enact and judge himself through a decidedly normalized and normalizing psychoanalytic perceptual grid. Such a subjectified person fits in nicely with the political goals of advanced capitalist, liberal democratic forms of governance (Rose, 1996, pp. 172, 195).

A good example of the way that the psy sciences create the "sick" object and discipline is child psychiatrists and child psychoanalysts who have played a significant part in taking behavior which is perfectly acceptable and desirable in one social context and re-describing it in another context as pathology and mental illness that requires therapeutic "correction." The prevalence of the diagnosis of Attention Deficit/Hyperactivity Disorder (ADHD) reflects how behavior that was once viewed as an endearing sign of American childhood is now seen as pathology. Such behavior does not fit into today's management-oriented, norm-governed conception of the person that permeates our society and largely determines our judgments about what behavior is regarded as "appropriate" or "inappropriate." Rather than ask ourselves the tougher questions about the social and discursive conditions that tend to generate these "disruptive" children, or analyze the assumptions underlying the institutions that are empowered to engage in such labeling and dividing practices, we isolate those children who do not conform to these management-driven behavioral norms.

I am not denying that there are children who can be diagnosed with ADHD due to their serious problems with sustaining attention, as well as hyperactivity and impulsive behavior, but I am troubled by the way the term ADHD is a manifestation of a rhetoric of rejection via the implementation of an unchallengeable, taken-for-granted norm. The point is that such norm-based classifications should be made with "fear and trembling," and not as a routine matter that de-individualizes the child and does not adequately consider its potentially dangerous ramifications for the child and family.

Today, Tom Sawyer and Huckleberry Finn would probably both be diagnosed with ADHD and a conduct disorder. While "Tom Sawyer may have been a slob, a truant and a hedonist; he may have picked fights with strangers for no apparent reason," like so many children with so-called ADHD, "he was also resourceful, spirited and deliciously clever. Huckleberry Finn was an illiterate outcast, but as a long-term rafting companion he had no peer" (Angier, 1994, n.p.). In our current context, Tom and Huck would most likely be segregated from those children who could "produce," compete and keep up with the tremendous cognitive and technical demands that characterize the "successful" child. Tom and Huck would almost definitely end up in a special education class with the other "disruptive" children—frequently, this includes a disproportionate number of minority students and the poor, where they are under continual observation, assessment and management by teachers, psychologists and parents. These "special ed" students are stigmatized for the rest of their educational careers. In some cases, it is a psychoanalytically based or informed diagnostic/treatment regimen combined with a neuropsychologically-based child psychiatric one that supports this.

A similar kind of normalizing dynamic has recently taken place when the prestigious World Health Organization's 2018 diagnostic manual judged that too much video gaming was a mental health condition. "Gaming Disorder" is categorized as another form of addictive behavior. The way that ADHD and Gaming Disorder have been diagnosed calls to mind Rosenhan's experiment. The point is that it is necessary to problematize the way that mental health professionals and others reflexively and unwittingly diagnose/treat/normalize people, for this has potentially dangerous de-individualizing, dehumanizing and de-personalizing effects on people's lives.

Thus, following Foucault, my approach is to problematize the notion of psychopathology typical in mainstream psychoanalysis and the psy professions. To achieve this requires using this term cautiously and critically in a way that calls to mind some of the insightful criticisms of mainstream psychiatric and psychoanalytic labeling and diagnosis emanating from "anti-psychiatry" authors. Indeed, skepticism toward all inherited notions, especially those that are taken for granted as "true," appears to be called for (Sass, 1992, p. 141). While detailing all of this is beyond the scope of this chapter, my suggested alternative (not replacement) term for psychopathology (i.e., problems in living and mental distress) is best viewed as a "floating undefined signifier." That is, this term is meant to be phenomenologically suggestive rather than used as a substantivized and reified term, always mindful that its meaning is context-dependent, setting-specific and bound by the present regime of truth in which it is historically situated.

In summary, the problem with the mainstream notion of psychopathology is that it is used by psychoanalysts and other psy experts to engage in diagnostic/therapeutic practices that use norm-generated binaries that become the criteria for judging others, with negative consequences for the individual. As Foucault noted about the "carceral network," as he called it,

> The judges of normality are present everywhere. We are in the society of the teacher-judge, the doctor-judge, the educator-judge, the 'social worker'-judge; it is on them that the universal reign of the normative is based; and each individual, wherever he may find himself, subjects to it his body, his gestures, his behaviour, his aptitudes, his achievements.
>
> *(1979, p. 304)*

A society that is defined by the medicopsychiatric norm involves a system of surveillance and control, a continuous visibility, a permanent classification of individuals, the generation of a hierarchy qualifying, instituting limits and imparting diagnostics. The norm becomes the standard for evaluating individuals, with potentially dangerous consequences in terms of truncating individual autonomy and expression. The analysand becomes a "diminished self," one who cannot speak his own truth in his own words, who cannot be a "witness" to his own life and sufferings. Without being willing and able to claim his own voice as he tells his pained story, he has, in effect, been psychiatrically and psychologically colonized (Frank, 1995, pp. xvi xxi, 10).

I want to again emphasize that I am not denying there is something that is phenomenologically present when the suffering analysand turns up to the analyst's office that can be reasonably called psychopathology. However, the term must be used with the understanding that it has only functional, discourse-specific usefulness and does not encompass the analysand's unique way of being-in-the-world. As Foucault noted, under sovereign power, deviant behavior was seen as a moral lapse or sin that didn't define the person's whole identity; however, with the medicalization of deviant behavior (i.e., a manifestation of bio-power), deviant behavior such as homosexuality defined the identity of the person in toto, and therefore whatever the person did was to be understood as being generated from that designation. One of Foucault's most famous phrases in this regard was, "[t]he sodomite had been a temporary aberration; the homosexual was now a species" (1990, p. 43). This being said, it is entirely compatible with Foucault's and Rosenhan's theses that homosexuality was removed from the DSM in 1975 after a vote from American Psychiatric Association psychiatrists, emphasizing the context/setting-susceptibility to what is considered a diagnosable psychiatric/mental disorder (Slater, 2004, p. 79). Rather than be a "natural fact," homosexuality, and for that matter other forms of so-called mental illness, is a consensual "cultural construct" (Porter, 2002, p. 3) that is impacted by politico-cultural and socio-intellectual factors (ibid., p. 214).

Toward a solution to the diagnosis problem: A biopsychosocialcultural model

Rosenhan's brilliant study, one that has been replicated to some extent by other pseudo-patient studies (Loring & Powell, 1988; Slater, 2004; Temerlin, 1968)[14], emphasized that the perceptions and behavior of the diagnosing psychiatrists and treatment staff were largely controlled by the situation, rather than being motivated by malevolent disposition. As Rosenhan noted, "in a more benign environment, one that was less attached to global diagnosis, their behaviors and judgments might have been more benign and effective" (1973, p. 257). Indeed, as psychiatrist Pat Bracken has said, "In reality, most psychiatric diagnoses are nothing more than a particular way of formulating and naming a person's problems" (2002, p. 4). The main disadvantage to diagnosis and the medical framing/filtering of diagnosis is that it can conceal the reasons for our pain and suffering: "It is often presented to patients as 'the truth' of their condition and serves to silence other possibilities. Psychiatric diagnosis is often little more than a simplification of a complex reality and by formulating an individual's experiences in terms of pathology it can be profoundly disempowering and stigmatizing" (ibid., p. 4). However, diagnosis can in some instances be helpful. It can be

> a means whereby a person in chaos is given a framework that can assist in reordering his or her world. It can also allow an individual to shed some responsibility for his/her suffering and behavior [e.g., reduce self-blame and judgment]. It gets health professionals and others involved and offers a set of therapeutic options
>
> *(ibid.)*

and it can be a useful shorthand with which members of the psy professions communicate.

While "dimensional" or "spectrum" approaches, those that describe clusters of disorders that allegedly share specific fundamental biological or psychological features, have been considered an improvement to conventional diagnosis in the DSM-5 (e.g., "Asperger's syndrome" is now incorporated into "Autistic spectrum disorder"), "it is clear at this point that research is not sufficiently advanced to attempt a wholesale switch to a dimensional or spectrum approach, so the categories in DSM-5 for the most part look very much like the categories in DSM-IV with some updated language and increased precision and clarity" (Barlow & Durand, 2015, p. 96).

Perhaps a somewhat different diagnostic practice can make things better. "Formulation," says Foucauldian-inspired sociologist Nikolas Rose (who has been caring for a seriously psychiatrically impaired wife for over forty years), rejects trying to categorically assign individuals to a specific diagnostic category based on their symptoms, bio-markers or brain structures. Rather, formulation "seeks to make sense of a person's current difficulties in terms of aspects of their current situation, for example, their relationships, their experiences at work or in unemployment, their housing and financial situation, and indeed their own ways of making sense of their situation, and accounting for their distress" (Rose, 2019, p. 187). Such an approach includes elements of a person's life history that they consider pertinent, or that might seem pertinent to the professional making the formulation. Moreover, it would lead to an agreed upon treatment strategy that requires a good therapeutic alliance between patient and doctor/therapist to address each of the distressing current conditions. The focus would be on patterns of capability, impairment and resilience that would help clarify the types of support that might be necessary to give (ibid., p. 93), especially since most forms of mental distress are intimately tied to realistic problems of poverty, precarity, violence, exclusion and other forms of hardship in people's personal and social lives (ibid., p. 148). Also, says Rose, formulation, where feasible, would utilize a wide range of local and community-based resources, such as drop-in centers, self-help groups and community organizations (e.g., religious institutions) that bring together likeminded people in mental distress. Formulation might also include time-limited, palliative use of psychiatric medications for specific conditions, as such drugs are not an effective solution to the experience of most forms of mental distress, regardless of the country's income level (ibid., p. 148). Thus, one of the important assumptions of this formulation-based approach is "difference is not pathology, and we have more to learn from recognizing such diversity than we gain from insistence on an ideal of normality" (ibid., p. 188). Indeed, as the authors of the WPA-Lancet Psychiatry Commission on the Future of Psychiatry noted (Bhugra et al., 2017), "formulation" that specifically "takes into account the social context, contributory risk and protective factors, and developmental change" on the way to developing a treatment strategy, "is unlikely to be replaced by a purely biological or investigative approach and in its ideal form should continue to be based on an integrative biopsychosocialcultural formulation" (quoted in Rose, 2019, p. 177).

Where a DSM-5-based diagnosis is a label, a formulation is more like a narrative construction that strives to take into consideration the totality of circumstances of a person's life, focusing on their problems in living and mental distress. Instead of considering "What is wrong with you?," like in the Rosenhan study and conventional psychiatric diagnostic labeling, the formulation asks, "What happened to you?" and therefore, the best way of answering this question is to tell a compelling story about the person's way of being-in-the-world as in the biopsychosocialcultural approach (Pryor, 2019).

Final word

Undoubtedly, Rosenhan's path-breaking experiment that asked the question, "If sanity and insanity exist, how shall we know them?" (1973, p. 50) was a critical catalyst for asking the even more important question in our era, "If mental disorder exists, how shall we know it?" (Rose, 2019, p. 22). That is, Rosenhan put into radically sharp focus the fact that mental disorders are socially and contextually governed and are mainly social phenomena in which the diagnostician's mind-set and setting animate their perceptions of what they claim they see and know, as well as how they act. This is especially true when the stimulus is ambiguous, as is human behavior (Rosenhan, 1975). Reality, in other words, comprises our efforts to see it (Sass, 1992).[15] Thus, when a person's problems in living and mental distress lead them to a psychoanalyst or psychotherapist's office, or even worse, to a psychiatric hospital, those caregivers who are responsible to help these suffering souls must never forget, as Freud noted, that the difference between them and us turns on incredibly small hinges. Indeed, any diagnostic process demands that the evaluator's way of being is animated by humility, a moral sensibility that embraces, nurtures and affirms, "there but for the grace of God go I;" by skepticism, the mark and pose of the educated mind faced with the infinite mystery of the other's otherness; and by compassion, the passion of passions, the non-indifference to the suffering of the other. For as all of the great Eastern and Western ancient religious and spirituality traditions have emphasized (Marcus, 2003), great compassion necessitates great wisdom so as to bear fruit, and great wisdom necessitates deep and abiding compassion as the inspiration and drive for effective action in the service of the other's freedom, well-being and happiness (Goldstein & Kornfield, 2001, p. 107).

Notes

1 www.encyclopedia.com/psychology/dictionaries-thesauruses-pictures-and-press-releases/ego-alteration, retrieved 4/3/19.
2 As Sass notes in his important study of madness (1992), "Schizophrenia involves exaggerations or diminutions of normal processes rather than anything so radically distinct" (p. 384). He further notes that the "central feature of the schizophrenic mind" is "disconnectedness, an unmooring from practical concerns and accepted practices that allows consciousness to drift in unexpected and unintended directions, and to come to rest in strange orientations" (ibid., p. 127). Needless to say, such a characterization of schizophrenia involves the clinician's decision-making processes that are not only heavily value-laden, but involve making subtle and highly contestable judgments that are context-dependent and setting-specific, as Rosenhan's study demonstrates. Sass appears to be somewhat allied with a medical model, as he describes schizophrenia as a "disease" (ibid., p. 27), the "most severe of mental illnesses" (ibid., p. 399). Rather troubling to me is that in Sass's 595-page study of madness and modernism, Rosenhan is never mentioned.
3 According to Tavris and Aronson (2015), the therapist's claims were lodged in lingering Freudian and pseudo-Freudian notions "about repression, memory, sexual trauma, and the meaning of dreams and on their confidence in their clinical powers of insight and diagnosis. All of the claims these therapists made have since been scientifically studied. All of them are wrong" (p. 127).
4 In Rosenhan's study (1973), he described the physical and verbal abuse of hospitalized patients in which their powerlessness and depersonalization was evident.
5 Rosenhan was aware of the remarkable study done by Rosenthal and Jacobson (1966) on the impact of teachers' expectations on student performance. The Pygmalion or Rosenthal Effect occurs when others' expectations of a target person positively impacts the target's performance, which is a form of self-fulfilling prophecy.
6 It should be noted that Rosenhan's study was published in *Science*, the premiere journal of the American Association for the Advancement of Science, hence its scientific challenge to the validity of psychiatric diagnosis and the medical model, was that much more incendiary.
7 One cannot help but recall Mother Teresa's train ride from Calcutta to Darjeeling for her annual retreat on September 10, 1946. According to a Vatican source, it was then that she received her "inspiration," her "call within a call." On that day and over the course of the next weeks and months, by means of interior locutions and visions, Jesus revealed to her the desire of His heart for "victims of love" who would "radiate" His love on souls. "Come be My light," He begged her, "I cannot go alone" (Marcus, 2017, p. 51). Likewise, Socrates frequently referred to his *daimon*, roughly, the voice of his guardian angel, that did not tell him what to do, only what not to do. "Hearing voices" need not be negative, it can be uplifting and instructive.
8 According to psychologist Gary Greenberg, Spitzer, the editor of the DSM-III, was drenched in "cynicism." He "acknowledged to me that he was responding to the fact that 'psychiatry was regarded as bogus,' and who told me that the book [the DSM-III] was a success because it 'looks very scientific. If you open it up, it looks like they must know something'" (Greenberg, 2019, n.p.).
9 I have liberally relied on Smith et al. (2015, pp. 55–94) in reporting the research findings on perceiving individuals.

10 Barlow and Durand (2015) have noted that, "Given the attention" schizophrenia has received in terms of the extensive research on "its causes and treatment … you would think the question 'What is schizophrenia?' would by now be answered easily. It is not" (p. 477). That is, "it is not easy to point to one thing that makes a person 'schizophrenic'" (ibid., p. 478), rather it "is a number of behaviors or symptoms that aren't necessarily shared by all people who are given the diagnosis" (ibid., pp. 478–479). Finally, they note, "Individuals who have schizophrenia have varying symptoms, and we find their causes vary as well" (ibid., p. 479). Put simply, what constitutes so-called schizophrenia (let alone schizophreniform and schizoaffective disorders) appears to be radically contested, reflecting a nosology that is in near conceptual disarray.

11 This section is based on my work with philosopher Alan Rosenberg, to be detailed in our forthcoming book, *Psychoanalysis as a Philosophical Way of Life* (in preparation). When I use the pronoun "I" here, I mean "we."

12 I am not against the notion of adaptation per se, for as Darwin noted, the animals that are most likely to survive are not the smartest or strongest, but the ones that can adapt. What I *am* against is how experts use the socially constructed notions of adaptation to normalize people.

13 The "depsychoanalization" of the diagnostic criteria used in the DSM-III occurred by 1980 when all references to psychodynamic processes had been removed from the description of dependent personality and other disorders (Bornstein, 2000, p. 334).

14 Slater (2004) claims she replicated Rosenhan's study almost exactly, but she never produced evidence of this claim.

15 As Foucault argued, madness, including all psychopathologies, are not reducible to psychology, that is, to ontological entities. Rather, he says, we need to comprehend madness in terms of how a specific social order problematizes particular forms of experience, of how madness emerges as an object of deliberation and concern (Rosenberg, personal communication, 5/2/19).

References

American Psychiatric Association. (1952). *Diagnostic and statistical manual of mental disorders*. Washington, DC: Author.

American Psychiatric Association. (1968). *Diagnostic and statistical manual of mental disorders* (2nd ed.). Washington, DC: Author.

American Psychiatric Association. (1980). *Diagnostic and statistical manual of mental disorders* (3rd ed., text rev.). Washington, DC: Author.

American Psychiatric Association. (2013). *Diagnostic and statistical manual of mental disorders* (5th ed.). Arlington, VA: Author.

Angier, N. (1994). The nation; The debilitating malady called boyhood. *The New York Times*, 7/24/94. Retrieved from www.nytimes.com/1994/07/24/weekinreview/the-nation-the-debilitating-malady-called-boyhood.html.

Barlow, D.H. & Durand, V.M. (2015). *Abnormal psychology: An integrative approach* (7th ed.). Stamford: Cengage Learning.

Bhugra, M.D., Tasman, A., Pathare, S., Prieve, S., Smith, S., Torous, J. 7 Chiu, H.F.K. (2017). The WPA-Lancet psychiatry commission on the future of psychiatry. *The Lancet Psychiatry*, 4(10), 775–818.

Bion, W. (1957). Differentiation of the psychotic from the non-psychotic personalities. *International Journal of Psychoanalysis*, 38, 266–275.

Bornstein, R.F. (2000). Dependent personality disorder. In P. Brooks & A. Woloch (Eds.), *Whose Freud? The place of psychoanalysis in contemporary culture* (pp. 334–352). New Haven, CT: Yale University Press.

Bracken, P. (2002). *Trauma: Culture, meaning and philosophy*. Hoboken, NJ: Wiley.

Davison, G.C. & Neale, J.M. (1982). *Abnormal psychology: An experimental clinical approach* (3rd ed.). Hoboken, NJ: Wiley.
Evans, R. (1980). *The making of social psychology: Discussion with creative contributors*. New York: Gardner Press.
Foucault, M. (1967). *Madness and civilization: A history of insanity in the age of reason*. London: Tavistock.
Foucault, M. (1979). *Discipline and punish: The birth of the prison*. New York: Anchor.
Foucault, M. (1990). *The history of sexuality, Vol. 1: An introduction*. R. Hurley (Trans.). New York: Vintage.
Frank, A.W. (1995). *The wounded storyteller: Body, illness & ethics* (2nd ed.). Chicago: University of Chicago Press.
Freud, S. (1964). Analysis terminable and interminable. In J. Strachey (Ed. &Trans.), *The standard edition of the complete psychological works of Sigmund Freud* (Vol. 23, pp. 211–253). London: Hogarth Press. (Original work published 1937).
Goffman, E. (1961). *Asylums: Essays on the social situation of mental patients and other inmates*. Garden City, NY: Anchor.
Goldstein, J. & Kornfield, J. (2001). *Seeking the heart of wisdom: The path of insight meditation*. Boston: Shambhala.
Greenberg, G. (2019). Psychiatry's incurable hubris. Book review. *The Atlantic*. April 2019 issue. Retrieved from www.theatlantic.com/magazine/archive/2019/04/mind-fixers-anne-harrington/583228/.
Henslin, J. M. (1995). *Sociology: A down-to-earth approach* (2nd ed.). Boston: Allyn and Bacon.
Janis, I. (1972). *Victims of groupthink: Psychological studies of policy decisions and fiascoes*. Boston: Houghton Mifflin.
Janis, I. (1982). *Groupthink: Psychological studies of policy decisions and fiascoes* (2nd ed.). New York: Houghton Mifflin.
Laing, R. D. (1967). *The politics of experience*. New York: Pantheon.
Lear, J. (2015). *Freud* (2nd ed.). New York: Routledge.
Loring, M. & Powell, B. (1988). Gender, race, and DSM-III: A study of the objectivity of psychiatric diagnostic behavior. *Journal of Health and Social Behavior,* 29(1), 1–22. doi:10.2307/2137177.
Marcus, P. (2003). *Ancient religious wisdom, spirituality, and psychoanalysis*. Westport, CT: Praeger.
Marcus, P. (2017). *The psychoanalysis of career choice, job performance, and satisfaction: How to flourish in the workplace*. London: Routledge.
Mohr, S. (2013). Religion, spirituality, and severe mental disorder: From research to clinical practice. In K. Pergament (Ed.), *APA handbook of psychology, religion, and spirituality, Vol. 2, An applied psychology of religion and spirituality* (pp. 257–273). Washington, DC: American Psychological Association.
Moody, R. (2011). Introduction. In M. Rokeach, *The three Christs of Ypsilanti*. New York: New York Review of Books.
Nelson, D.L. & Quick, J.C. (2008). *Understanding organizational behavior* (3rd ed.). Mason, OH: South Western Cengage Learning.
Phillips, A. (2005). *Going sane: Maps of happiness*. New York: HarperCollins.
Porter, R. (2002). *Madness: A brief history*. Oxford: Oxford University Press.
Pryor, L. (2019). Mental illness isn't all in your head. *The New York Times*, 3/12/19. Retrieved from www.nytimes.com/2019/03/15/opinion/preventing-mental-illness.html.
Rokeach, M. (1964). *The three Christs of Ypsilanti*. New York: New York Review of Books.
Rose, N. (1996). *Inventing our selves*. Cambridge, UK: Cambridge University Press.
Rose, N. (2019). *Our psychiatric future: The politics of mental health*. Cambridge: Polity.
Rosenhan, D. (1973). On being sane in insane places. *Science*, 179, 250–258.

Rosenhan, D. (1975). The contextual nature of psychiatric diagnosis. *Journal of Abnormal Psychology*, 84, 462–474.

Rosenthal, R. & Jacobson, L. (1966). Teachers' expectancies: Determinates of pupils' IQ gains. *Psychological Reports*, 19, 115–118.

Sass, L.A. (1992). *Madness and modernism: Insanity in the light of modern art, literature and thought.* Cambridge: Harvard University Press.

Schaefer, R.T. (2003). *Sociology* (8th ed.). Boston: McGraw Hill.

Slater, L. (2004). *Opening Skinner's Box: Great psychological experiments of the twentieth century.* New York: W.W. Norton and Company.

Smith, R., Mackie, D.M. & Claypool, H.M. (Eds.) (2015). *Social psychology* (4th ed.). New York: Psychology Press.

Spitzer, R. (1975). On pseudoscience in science, logic in remission and psychiatric diagnosis: A critique of Rosenhan's "On being sane in insane places." *Journal of Abnormal Psychology*, 84(5), 442–452.

Spitzer, R. (1976). More on pseudoscience in science and the case for psychiatric diagnosis. *Archives of General Psychiatry*, 33, 459–470.

Szasz, T. (1961). *The myth of mental illness: Foundations of a theory of personal conduct.* New York: Hoeber-Harper.

Szasz, T. (1989). *The myth of the rights of mental patients.* New York: Liberty.

Tavris, C. & Aronson, E. (2015). *Mistakes were made (but not by me): Why we justify foolish beliefs, bad decisions, and hurtful acts.* Boston: Mariner Books.

Temerlin, M. (1968). Suggestion effects in psychiatric diagnosis. *The Journal of Nervous and Mental Disease*, 147(4), 349–353.

World Health Organization. (2018). *International statistical classification of diseases and related health problems* (11th Revision). Retrieved from https://icd.who.int/browse11/l-m/en.

Internet sources

www.encyclopedia.com/psychology/dictionaries-thesauruses-pictures-and-press-releases/ego-alteration, retrieved 4/3/19.

INDEX

Page numbers followed by "n" refer to notes.

For Product Safety Concerns and Information please contact our EU representative GPSR@taylorandfrancis.com
Taylor & Francis Verlag GmbH, Kaufingerstraße 24, 80331 München, Germany

www.ingramcontent.com/pod-product-compliance
Ingram Content Group UK Ltd.
Pitfield, Milton Keynes, MK11 3LW, UK
UKHW020159200926
475702UK00004B/526
9780367415594